Ship of Death

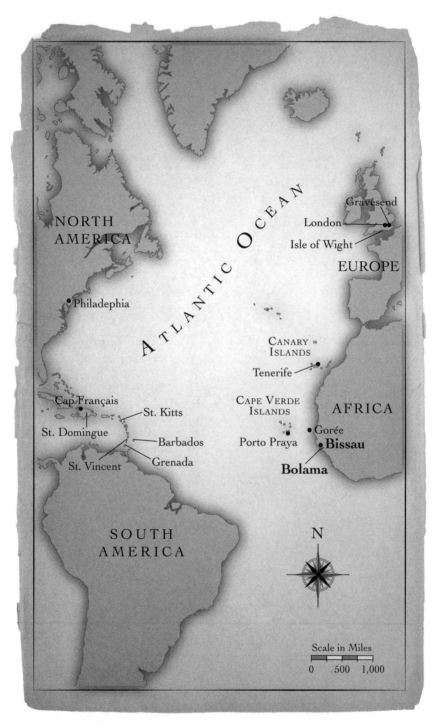

The *Hankey*'s ports of call, 1792–93. Map drawn by Michele Angel.

Ship of Death

A Voyage That Changed the Atlantic World

ɷ

BILLY G. SMITH

Yale UNIVERSITY PRESS

New Haven & London

Published with assistance from the Annie Burr Lewis Fund.

Yale University Press books may be purchased in quantity for educational, business,
or promotional use. For information, please e-mail sales.press@yale.edu (U.S. office)
or sales@yaleup.co.uk (U.K. office).

Designed by James J. Johnson.

Set in Bembo type by Westchester Book Group.

Printed in the United States of America.

Library of Congress Cataloging-in-Publication Data

Smith, Billy G. (Billy Gordon)

Ship of death : a voyage that changed the Atlantic world / Billy G. Smith.

page cm

Includes bibliographical references and index.

ISBN 978-0-300-19452-4 (hardback)

1. Hankey (Ship : 1784)   2. Yellow fever—Guinea-Bissau—Bolama Island—History—
18th century.   3. Bolama Association.   4. Epidemics—History—18th century.   5. Yellow
fever—Caribbean Area—History—18th century.   6. Yellow fever—United States—
History—18th century.   7. Bolama Island (Guinea-Bissau)—Colonization.   8. Antislavery
movements—Great Britain—History—18th century.   9. Abolitionists—Great Britain—
Biography.   10. Bolama Island (Guinea-Bissau)—History—18th century.   I. Title.

RA644.Y4S58 2013

614.5'41096657—dc23

2013018243

A catalogue record for this book is available from the British Library.

This paper meets the requirements of ANSI/NISO Z39.48–1992 (Permanence of Paper).

10 9 8 7 6 5 4 3 2 1

To Michelle

ဘာ

Contents

ια

Preface

This is an adventure story about the late-eighteenth-century voyage of a single ship, with the unassuming name of the *Hankey,* that changed world history. It is a tale that sprawls back and forth across the Atlantic Ocean, as the antislavery ship and its passengers sailed from Britain to West Africa to the Caribbean to North America and then returned to London. But it is considerably more than that. It's an account of idealistic early abolitionists in Britain and their failed attempt to establish a free colony in Africa, the West African peoples who encountered and interacted with the settlers, a successful slave revolution in Haiti that the colonists inadvertently assisted, a series of international yellow fever epidemics that incubated on the *Hankey* and bloomed in Philadelphia and many other parts of the Atlantic world, and the geopolitical transformation the abolitionists sparked that greatly expanded the territory of the new United States. Spreading yellow fever wherever it sailed, the ship and its passengers played a significant role in causing or at least shaping each of these events.

This is also a forgotten story. Rarely do historians uncover events that not only changed history but also are virtually unknown to all but the most specialized scholars, yet the chronicle of the *Hankey,* though infamous during the decades following its voyages in 1792 and 1793—doctors debated it in newspapers and magazines, officials from Spain to New Orleans argued about whether to quarantine

arriving vessels, inhabitants of the lands along the Atlantic rim lived in
fear of another devastating epidemic—gradually fell into obscurity. By
the mid-nineteenth century, it had all but disappeared from the public
memory. I pieced together the journey of the *Hankey* and its aftermath
primarily from records deposited in specialized archives and libraries.
Following one clue after another, I visited institutions in Scotland and
England, took a detour to France, and scoured half a dozen archives
on the east and west coasts of the United States, traveling from Boston
to Worcester to Princeton to Philadelphia to Annapolis to Washington, D.C., and then on to San Francisco and Los Angeles. (The Inter-
net also proved invaluable as an additional research tool.)

I first came across a reference to the *Hankey* more than a decade
ago at the American Philosophical Society in Philadelphia in an ob-
scure, unpublished medical manuscript written during the city's 1793
epidemic. The author, Dr. Jean Devèze, mentioned that a British ship
filled with antislavery colonists had moored for six months off the
coast of West Africa, and then sailed on to the West Indies, where it
spread yellow fever. I was intrigued, but suspicious of the account's
validity. Why would Britons migrate to West Africa to form a colony
at the end of the eighteenth century? I knew about the outpost of
Sierra Leone settled primarily by free black people from London and
Nova Scotia about this time, but I had never heard of an effort to
form another settlement several hundred miles to the north. British
ships sailed to West Africa in the eighteenth century for a single purpose: to buy slaves. Never, I thought, did they drop off pioneers. It
did not make sense. Moreover, why would these colonists then sail
to the West Indies? And could the *Hankey* really have set off a severe
outbreak of yellow fever in those islands during the era of the revolution in Saint-Domingue (now Haiti)? It took several years for
me to follow up on these questions, in part because I live in Montana,
a considerable distance from the relevant archives, and in part because
I was engaged in other writing projects. However, my curiosity remained.

Uncovering the story turned into an adventure in historical de-
tection that sent me on a journey covering thousands of miles across

several continents. Individual pieces of the tale began to emerge out
of manuscripts and old books in a host of institutions. I visited the
Library of Congress in Washington, D.C., for three days to finish
research for another book, and I saved the final day to scan the library
holdings about the *Hankey.* I had just begun reading an account written by William Pym, a physician in the West Indies in 1793, who
claimed that the ship carrying antislavery white colonists from Africa
had introduced an entirely new disease, a mysterious "Bulam fever,"
to the Caribbean. At mid-morning, however, an alarm went off and
everyone had to evacuate the library because of a bomb scare. Authorities did not allow us to return to the reading room that day and,
frustrated, I had to catch an airplane home that evening. I remained
dubious about the tale.

A few months later, while participating in a conference in Philadelphia, I dropped by the library of the College of Physicians. They
had dozens of books from the 1790s and early nineteenth century
wherein doctors debated one another, often in the most rancorous
terms, about the numerous contemporary outbreaks of yellow fever
in the United States, Europe, and the West Indies. Was the disease
contagious (it's not), should ships be quarantined because they carried
polluted cargoes, what treatments should be used, and, most important, what had caused this pandemic? The *Hankey's* name kept
reappearing in the accounts, with the authors accusing one another of
lying about it, especially with regard to the date it arrived in Grenada.
All seemed to agree that it carried a disease, but if it docked after the
epidemic on that island began, then it could not be the cause of the
affliction. The story was still a mystery to me, but it was becoming a
bit more intriguing.

To get to the roots of the voyage, I flew to London, where I spent
ten days. I had gone hoping to find some hard evidence, but if none
appeared, I figured that I would at least enjoy the charms of one of
the liveliest cities in the world—no small attraction to a Montanan.
The sources were so rich that I spent all ten days and most evenings
in libraries and archives. The murky two-hundred-year-old story was
beginning to take shape. At the Library of the National Maritime

Museum in Greenwich, I found documents from Lloyd's of London recording voyages taken by the *Hankey,* including a journey to Africa in 1792, but, strangely, no trips after that. The British Library in London yielded a brief firsthand account of the ocean voyage to "Bulam" (currently called Bolama), which I could now identify as an island off the coast of Guinea-Bissau. The Public Records Office at Kew was a treasury of information. The "Committee Minutes of the Black Poor in London" described the only black people who ended up at the colony of Bolama. The planning documents of the expedition, along with the organizers' radically democratic constitution, were there as well. The contemporary correspondence with His Majesty's secretary of state for the Home Department revealed a great deal about the origins and early problems of the *Hankey.* It also contained an enigmatic 1793 order to sink the ship, with all of its cargo and even its crew, if necessary! The long-lost log of the *Hankey* likewise turned up in Kew, confirming that the ship had arrived in Grenada immediately before an epidemic of yellow fever broke out—a crucial point in the medical debates I had discovered earlier at the College of Physicians. The tale was turning out to be a true one.

I returned to Montana with the basis for a new book, but I still required more evidence. At about this time, serendipitously, the library at my institution, Montana State University, was offered a free, one-week trial of the computerized version of the London *Times.* Access to this site was beyond the budget of my institution, but I took advantage of the offer, spending late nights during the next week searching the newspaper online. The *Hankey* appeared in many articles. A few authors identified the ship as having sailed from the West Indies to Philadelphia, at that time the capital of the new United States, just before the outbreak of a horrendous epidemic there in 1793. From the City of Brotherly Love the disease radiated outward during the next dozen years, spreading to every major urban port in the United States and to a good number of municipalities in Europe. It was the first pandemic of yellow fever in the Atlantic world. The story had just become not only bigger but also more significant in its implications.

However, my research was far from complete. I spent a week at the American Antiquarian Society in Worcester, using their marvelous collection of eighteenth-century sources, most of which can be searched by computer. I flew to the Huntington Library in a suburb of Los Angeles (not an unattractive escape for someone in the midst of a Rocky Mountain winter) to read the papers of one of the organizers of the antislavery expeditions to Africa. I bought a ticket to Paris, searching the Archives Nationales for traces of Philip Beaver, a leader of the colonists who had spent time in France in the 1780s and was influenced by Enlightenment philosophers. My quest proved bootless; this was the only archive that held nothing for me (though the French food was fantastic). I considered traveling to Bolama, but discovered that Guinea-Bissau is today a narco-state and a bit too dangerous even for an intrepid Montanan.

I tracked down several firsthand accounts of the colonists and of the organizers of the Bolama expedition at the Library Company of Philadelphia. It was the place worth spending some time. I applied, successfully, for a sabbatical and for a fellowship from the National Endowment for the Humanities, which allowed me to spend half of a year at the Library Company, where I read every available source and began drafting book chapters.

Returning to Montana, I completed the manuscript over the next few years. Ironically, during that time, Google Books scanned many of the books and pamphlets I read previously in a host of archives and libraries. I can now find facts and check my footnotes from the comfort of my home. It is certainly more efficient and surely the way in which scholars will mostly work in the future. But I shall miss the adventure of journeying around the world to solve a historical mystery.

This book focuses on ordinary people—working men and women, servants, slaves, soldiers, Britons, Africans, and Philadelphians—documenting and analyzing how they constructed and maintained their own lives, confronted the international forces that affected them, and, in the process, helped form the larger Atlantic world. Most of them toiled in obscurity, but they nonetheless deserve considerable credit for their contributions, both good and bad, to setting the foundation for our modern world. Seventy-five years ago, the playwright Bertolt Brecht wrote a poem about reading history. Brecht posed the questions "Who built Thebes of the seven gates?" and "In what houses of gold-glittering Lima did its builders live?" This book addresses analogous queries: Who built the Atlantic world? How did they do it? By following the *Hankey* as it crisscrossed the ocean, I address these and related questions, seeking a better understanding of seemingly anonymous humans doomed to silence unless historians dig deeply in the records for evidence that will give them voices.

Slavery and the slave trade were at the center of the Atlantic world, and they are at the heart of the story in this book. In Albert Camus's great novel *The Plague,* the disease symbolizes the evils of fascism, which can be eradicated only when ordinary people fight against it. In a somewhat similar fashion, the struggles to eradicate the yellow fever epidemics also entailed a clash by ordinary people against the evils of slavery and naked exploitation.

The voyage of the *Hankey* linked many of the communities and international forces that rotated around slavery, like planets circling a sun. Without the slave trade to protest, the British adventurers probably would not have set their sights on the island of Bolama, in West Africa, nor would a handful have stayed on after the *Hankey* left. Without the international commerce in humans that began on their shores, the Bijago and *grumettas* (hired workers) of the region would not have faced the severe struggle simply to maintain their freedom. In the absence of racial bondage, the oppressed people of Saint-Domingue would not have been compelled to wage a bloody revolution, nor would European troops have been required to fight them. Had he not lost Saint-Domingue, Napoleon might have held on to the Louisiana Territory, changing the course of U.S. westward expansion. Without slavery, Philadelphia and other Atlantic port cities would not have suffered some of the worst epidemics in modern times. If slavery had not existed, the *Hankey* would not have sailed on a route that connected communities in West Africa, the West Indies,

North America, and Europe. And yellow fever would not have gained such a large foothold in the Atlantic world. History would have taken a different course.

In many ways, then, this is a story that resonates in our own era of intensified globalization and capitalism, the growth of both wealth and inequality, the transference of industries from affluent to poorer countries, the increasing threat of disease on a worldwide scale, and the degradation of the environment—issues which cross national borders so easily today. People living in rural communities, villages, towns, and cities are all affected by what happens in other parts of the earth. In other words, the voyage of the *Hankey* is a human story with relevance for our own times.

ᘎᘏ

Acknowledgments

I have been fortunate for all the help I have received during the years
I was researching and writing this book. Friends, family, colleagues,
students, research assistants, librarians, archivists, and other profes-
sionals generously provided assistance. Various institutions gave additional support. I sincerely thank them all.

I would like to express my gratitude to all the archivists and
librarians, especially those at the Library Company in Philadelphia,
for their invaluable assistance. For their financial support, I thank the
National Endowment for the Humanities as well as the following at
Montana State University: the Scholarship/Creativity and Sabbatical
programs, INBRE, and the Office of the Vice President for Research
(Tom McCoy). Donovan Webster played a huge role in helping to
craft significant parts of the chapter drafts when I was struggling. I
much appreciate the dedication of John Paine, Jane Sunderland, and
Lisa Thomas, all of whom were invaluable in shaping the story and
crafting the language. At Yale University Press I likewise thank Christopher Rogers for believing in this book and Susan Laity for performing
a spectacular editing job. My agents, Sandy Dijkstra and Elise Capron,
and their staff were extremely adept at guiding the manuscript to the
right press. They were also very patient. I much appreciate Michele
Angel's work in drawing excellent maps for this book.

For their help at Montana State University, I extend my deep appreciation to Anita DeClue, a graduate student who researched and wrote an outstanding M.A. thesis about the yellow fever epidemics in Philadelphia; Paul Sivitz, my co-director of the Philadelphia Mapping History project; and Stuart Challender, Tara Chesley-Preston, Alice Hecht, and Alex Schwab. Mike Zuckerman generously invited me to present my early work on this book at his salon in Philadelphia, where he acclaimed me one of the two best standup comedians among early American historians; faint praise indeed. In addition, I thank David Large, Dale Martin, Adrienne Mayor, Mary Murphy, Simon Newman, Josh Ober, Michael Reidy, and Bill Wyckoff for their friendship and for conversations about history.

I have purposely saved the most important acknowledgments for last. My daughter, Sage Smith, a talented artist, has provided support throughout the long process of putting this book together. Michelle Maskiell, my wife and a professor and scholar in her own right, was not only a continual inspiration for the book but also the major reason it was eventually completed. Her research, writing, editing, and engagement with all matters intellectual shaped the book into what it is, providing what is most good and valuable in it, especially in the sections about West Africa and about women. Her life partnership has shaped my own life in similar but even more powerful, wonderful ways.

Ship of Death

CHAPTER I

The *Hankey*

రిలు

The *Hankey,* like all wooden vessels of its time, whispered to its inhabitants. In the early morning dawn, its anchor and rigging lines tugged and groaned in the breeze. The timbers of its hull made lulling sounds in the estuary's sometimes slapping roll. The vessel was a fully rigged ship: it contained a foremast in front, the tallest mast, the mainmast, in the center, and a shorter mizzenmast at the back; square sails hung on all three. The *Hankey* was a relatively large oceangoing vessel for its time, designed to sail across the Atlantic with a 260-ton cargo or the equivalent weight in passengers. When constructed in northern England in 1784, it had been remarkably fine and stout. Now its timbers creaked when they moved, beginning to show their age.[1]

Waiting to depart on the *Hankey* this morning in March 1792 were 120 British residents of varying social stations, their ages ranging from infancy to late middle age. With its bottom sheathed with copper to protect it against the boring worms common in the tropics (the ship's regular destination), the *Hankey* stood ready to transport these pioneers to an unknown land on the West African coast. A grand experiment was about to begin. The same spirit that animated abolitionists from Manchester to Massachusetts and would lead to the ending of the Atlantic slave trade in 1807 by Britain and in 1808 by the United States moved these future colonists.

Two other ships awaited the expedition's departure in Gravesend, where the river Thames flows into the sea. The *Calypso* was a slightly larger, 290-ton vessel, and the *Beggar's Benison* was a small, slow, 34-ton cutter, designed merely to ferry people and goods from the London docks down the river to the port of Gravesend. As its name suggested, after leaving Gravesend anyone who died aboard would be committed to the ocean rather than given a grave on land. That would become the final destination for all too many of the 275 colonists spread among the three ships.

All three ships were laden with the possessions of the colonists, along with "British merchandise, to a very considerable amount," meant to pay native Africans for their land and labor. Each vessel—in the description of papers presented that day to Henry Dundas, His Majesty's secretary of state for the Home Department—also carried British subjects who expected to travel to the island of Bolama, on the western coast of Africa, to "lay the foundation of a permanent settlement on the said coast, there to cultivate sugar, cotton, indigo, and other productions of the torrid zone."[2]

According to their group's charter, the colonists were determined to accomplish this goal by *hiring* rather than *enslaving* Africans—a rare concept at the time. This was a central thrust of the expedition. By demonstrating that Africans could work more effectively as free people than as bound laborers, the colonists expected to show their home nation that Africans could be "civilized" in the manner of Europeans. "Civilizing Africa," one colonial supporter claimed, was "the most effectual means for abolishing the slave trade." The colony would thus illustrate that the buying and selling of human beings was unnecessary to the success of colonial ventures—a model that might overturn the overseas slave trade. Halting the raging tide of slaves across the Atlantic Ocean, the colonists hoped, would abolish slavery itself.[3]

Even though they possessed scant resources, at least half a dozen women contributed a portion of the capital needed for this expedition, reflecting the enthusiasm displayed by late-eighteenth-century British women in the opposition to the slave trade and slavery.

Mrs. Sarah Duppa donated fifteen pounds, as did Charlotte Walker, an unmarried woman in Manchester. In 1787 abolitionists had targeted women's support in that city, appealing in the *Manchester Mercury* for "female aid" based on the "Humanity, Benevolence, and Compassion" that were "expected in and particularly possessed by that most amiable Part of the Creation." C. B. Wadstrom, one of the Bolama expedition's organizers, admired the women for their fiscal donations, which were all "the more remarkable as, in general, their property is not so much at their own immediate disposal as that of the Gentlemen." The Swedish abolitionist declared, "This is one instance among many to show how warmly the Ladies interest themselves in liberal and humane enterprises. To what sublime degrees of humane feeling and heroic virtue might not mankind arrive if, in union with the sex, they would always set before them the amiable pattern of female goodness?"[4]

Many Manchester female and male workers were already dissatisfied with the region's nascent factory system, and while they did not have money to contribute to the subscription for founding the colony, they could apply to join as workers. Other than the "dark Satanic Mills" memorialized by William Blake, they had few options available to them.[5] The venture also drew interest in London's Old Bailey courthouse. In this era criminals might be sentenced to transportation out of England for committing major or even minor crimes, including the theft of a loaf of bread. So many men and women applied from Manchester and London to join the expedition that the organizers cut off applications and hired an additional ship.

Some of the middle- and upper-class supporters left records of their ideas about the venture and its potential role in abolishing the slave trade. To Philip Beaver, a leader of the new colony, the trip was "an experiment to ascertain whether those Africans, already free, are capable or not of being drawn by industry, cultivation, and commerce from their present debased situation to hold a responsible rank among the nations of the earth. If we fail, they will be just where they were." However, the optimistic Beaver noted, "If we succeed, it promises happiness to myriads of living and millions of unborn people."

Like Christopher Columbus, these adventurers hoped to change the world. The voyage of the *Hankey* did change the world, but not in the way Beaver imagined.[6]

The leaders of this British humanitarian experiment had met regularly in London's coffeehouses and pubs since the previous November. They hired the two larger ships and purchased the *Beggar's Benison* outright. They made the other arrangements with great haste, leading to oversights they would subsequently regret. Excited by the possibilities of their adventure, they felt that they were now ready to sail. The old hands among the sailors were more cautious, since they knew about the dangers that lay ahead, if only through rumors circulating among seamen. As a ditty common among British mariners who sailed to Africa held:

> Beware and take care
> Of the Bight of Benin.
> For the one that comes out,
> There are forty go in.[7]

The rhyme was sadly predictive: few sailors on the expedition to Bolama ever returned home.

The would-be colonists had written a democratic constitution, radical for its time, as well as agreements setting out regulations for behavior. They likewise had divided up the land they planned to purchase and had engaged the services of people with necessary skills, including a doctor, a surveyor, and a tailor, to see to their needs. On its voyage from the London docks, the *Hankey* paused briefly at Greenwich so the ship's clocks could be set to the exact time, which would enable the sailors to calculate the ship's longitude during the voyage. Yet when they arrived at Gravesend, they received disappointing news. Home Secretary Henry Dundas had not approved the colony's constitution, ostensibly because the enterprise did not have sufficient funding. Dundas sympathized with the proslavery lobby, and he proposed to phase out the slave trade so gradually that it would never actually end. Against the background of the ongoing French

Revolution, protests in Britain, and the objections of proslavery West Indian planters in England, the government did not want to encourage a wild-eyed group of radicals to plant a colony in Africa.[8]

The government's disapproval, Philip Beaver noted, cast "a considerable gloom over all our minds." Britain's endorsement would legitimate land claims and contracts in the colony as well as the authority of Bolama's leaders over the settlers. In addition, the powerful British navy might provide occasional assistance. The expedition's organizers appealed the decision, presenting petitions to the home secretary describing their personnel, their honorable intentions, and a final argument about how the venture would benefit their homeland. They also asked their prominent supporters, including the future mayor of London, to pull strings with the Privy Council. As they waited for a response, they decided to move all three ships to the Isle of Wight, on the southern coast, to "wait the issue of our Memorial."[9]

In the late eighteenth century, an era of fervent British colonial optimism had dawned, despite the recent loss of most of England's American colonies. The British people, especially merchants and officials, determined to explore far-flung locales and exert their command over the peoples there. Britons increasingly turned a covetous eye from west to east, especially toward India and China, to increase their wealth.

They likewise cast their gaze south, toward Africa, which was considerably closer and seemingly ripe for exploitation. Since the middle of the eighteenth century, prominent Britons had advocated the extension of trade through the settlement of Africa. During the Seven Years' War, in 1758 British troops took Saint-Louis, an island off Senegal, from the French. Britain subsequently claimed a wide swath of African hinterland, called it Senegambia, and created the first crown colony on the continent. The British went on to establish a colony in Sierra Leone in the late 1780s, and in 1795 they seized South Africa from the Dutch. A new era of empire was unfolding, one that would become known as Britain's imperial century. Before

World War II and the resistance movements by indigenous peoples finally eroded the British Empire, the Union Jack flew above the heads (whether they liked it or not) of one in four people around the world.[10]

The British built their empire in the eighteenth and nineteenth centuries, following the examples of Portugal and Spain, which in the previous centuries had built powerful overseas holdings. They made commercial and political inroads in South Asia with the East India Company. In East Africa, they established colonies that would eventually stretch the length of the continent, from South Africa all the way to Cairo. In the Pacific, the crown sent Captain James Cook to stake claims on the Australian continent and New Zealand, while also establishing footholds in Indonesia, Malaysia, Melanesia, and Micronesia. Singapore and Hong Kong fell to British control, while Japan's leaders decided to accept British trade rather than submit to the likelihood of colonial occupation. Across the vast, sparsely populated plains of Central Asia, British imperial agents and operatives of the Russian tsars played the imperial Great Game for local tribal loyalties. The British feared that Russia was looking for a land route to invade India, the jewel in Britain's imperial crown.[11]

Colonization, many Britons reasoned, led to both a more robust national economy and increased personal wealth. In private meetings and public forums across Great Britain, speculators weighed the commercial possibilities of colonizing different areas of the globe. Numerous groups lobbied government officials to establish colonies and extend the empire.[12]

In this acquisitive environment, a group of six former British naval and military men—friends who had mustered against the Dutch in 1787, the Spanish in 1790, and the Russians in 1791—first met at Old Slaughter's Coffeehouse just off High Holborn in central London. The coffeehouse had long been a hangout for radicals, from William Hogarth, the engraver of lower-class life, to Benjamin Franklin and his deist club. Currently, Thomas Paine and Mary Wollstonecraft often worked there, writing their tracts on the rights of men and women.[13]

On November 2, 1791, the half dozen former officers formed a society to establish themselves as colonists of a potential location on the western coast of Africa. Before long, the group—comprising Henry Hew Dalrymple, John Young, Sir William Halton, John King, Robert Dobbin, and Philip Beaver—had identified the island of Bolama off what today is the nation of Guinea-Bissau, "in the 11th degree of north latitude" as "the spot . . . the best adapted to the commencement of our undertaking." They quickly outlined their goals, which included a proposal to hire rather than enslave the native peoples in Africa and to "publish to the world" their plan.[14]

Enthusiasm ran high at the initial meeting. The men decided to hire rooms to meet on subsequent occasions, and to convene again on November 9, when they would draw up their proposals. At that meeting they determined to make their colonizing aspirations known to the prime minister and issue a call for subscriptions from people in London and Manchester to support their adventure. (Appealing for subscriptions was a popular eighteenth-century strategy to raise money for public or private enterprises, such as building hospitals or libraries or even selling books.) They would "sail the moment our subscriptions would enable us, and take possession of the island."[15]

The plan sounded so easy. The noble idea of non-enslavement as the foundation for colonization in West Africa spread like a fire driven on the wind. The British movement to end the slave trade was still young, but it had attracted a great deal of attention. Ordinary people and public officials alike soon were offering broad support. On November 19, the group of six met again and appointed a secretary.

The group had already endorsed universal adult male suffrage, even for men without property—a radical position at the time. At a meeting three days later, however, came the first proof that their commitment to equality had limits. Philip Beaver noted in his diary of this meeting: "It was resolved that no female should be admitted as a settler on her own account."[16] Even had they read them, Wollstonecraft's feminist arguments would have carried little weight for this group of antislavery males.

By November 28, the group had taken on more subscribers, disbanding and reconstituting itself as nine principal colonists instead of six. At the meeting on January 13, 1792, the number of subscribers to the colony rose to thirteen. Three weeks later, it was twenty. Acting almost purely on faith, each man put up money in return for a promise of real estate in a faraway place. As one critic at the time observed caustically, the Bolama organization was peddling land in a colony whose whereabouts was uncertain and whose ownership was unclear. The total funds collected from subscribers ideally would be sufficient "to charter one ship, and purchase a sloop together with the necessary provisions, ammunition, etc. for the maintenance of forty families."[17]

The planners calculated that establishing the colony would require forty paying subscribers in addition to a host of servants and laborers who pledged their work in return for transportation and the promise of land. Speculative fever for the settlement of Bolama rose quickly, faster than the organization could make the necessary arrangements for a colony of this magnitude. Money from subscribers and applications to join as servants and laborers poured in from the newly industrializing city of Manchester; nearly half the subscribers came from that city. The Bolama organizers soon had more volunteers and funds than they needed.[18]

With their personnel in place, the nascent colonists fitted out the ships with a new suite of sails. They loaded their provisions aboard, and they set sail. With an amazing lack of foresight, however, they had neglected to bring any carpenters' tools or to include people who knew how to build houses. The leaders had a general idea of where they were going but did not know precisely how to locate Bolama. Once they found it, the plan was to purchase the island rather than seize it. For this they would require a local pilot to steer them to Bolama as well as to help find the current owners. They would also need someone with local knowledge and the linguistic and political skills to negotiate the purchase of the land. Apparently these requirements did not occur to the leaders until after the ships had crossed the ocean.

Their official charter for the colonization continued to languish in the home secretary's office through weeks of bureaucratic delays. As the French Revolution across the channel grew increasingly more radical, the British government became more suspicious of the democratic and antislavery goals of the Bolama enterprise. After the people aboard the three ships had sailed the short distance from Gravesend to the Isle of Wight, their frustration mounted. They feared that the rainy season, a bad time to start a new colony, might soon arrive in western Africa. Morale plummeted in the tight confines of the ships. The free African colony of Bolama waited like a glorious sunrise, and the small-mindedness of government officials posed the only impediment to riches, a new life, and a chance to remake the world.

While it was moored at Mother Bank, a port on the Isle of Wight, smallpox broke out on board the *Hankey.* The outbreak began because two of the colonists, Hannah and Joseph Riches, had concealed their toddler's illness so that they would be allowed on the vessel. Following a screaming fever, the infant developed the characteristic dimpled pustules produced by the virus. Everyone understood the gravity of the threat: smallpox was both deadly and extremely contagious. Yet after some discussion, the leaders decided that the family could stay. Five people jumped ship a day later. Philip Beaver ousted four others for disruptive behavior, part of his attempt at "regulating the internal discipline of the *Hankey.*" Like those travelers who missed the sailing of the *Titanic,* they were the fortunate ones.[19]

Finally, the impatient pioneers received word that the government had once again denied their charter. The good intentions claimed by the Bolama Association could not overcome the radical aspects of their constitution in the eyes of Britain's bureaucrats. Frightened by the threats of domestic unrest, Prime Minister William Pitt was poised to lead Britain's own persecution of political radicals, including antislavery activists. The colonists now faced a stark choice: they could either abandon the project entirely or continue to Africa without official sanction and government support. After painful discussions, they decided to set sail.

The convoy of three ships finally weighed anchor, loosed sheets, and got under way on the morning of April 11, 1792. As the tiny fleet set off, the wind faded, forcing the vessels to retreat to the nearby port of Yarmouth. At noon, as the boats struggled into the harbor, Hannah Riches gave birth to a healthy baby girl. It seemed like a good omen. That was offset, however, as night came on, when a child newly infected with smallpox died. In addition, during the *Hankey*'s first day on the open sea, the young daughter of a wealthy traveler and an older male laborer died of causes not recorded in the ship's documents. Both were committed to watery graves, events that tempered enthusiasm for the trip ahead.[20]

Calm skies without a puff of wind continued for the next two days. Then, on the morning of April 13, a stiff breeze filled the sails, enabling the ships to navigate the spectacular cliff and rock formations known as the Needles on the western end of the Isle of Wight. As they headed out to sea, soon losing sight of the last point of British soil, some passengers compared their forthcoming adventure to the explorations of Christopher Columbus three centuries earlier. Their voyage to West Africa, they believed, would change history in a similarly dramatic fashion. They had no way of knowing how right they were.

Once at sea, the ships separated. The *Hankey* could easily outdistance the little cutter *Beggar's Benison*. The *Calypso,* a flyer, outran them both. All three vessels were soon on their own. The dispersion of the ships did not unduly worry their captains, since they planned to rendezvous in Tenerife, in the Canary Islands southwest of Spain. Unfortunately, they made no backup plan should any of the ships fail to reach anchor. As the winds increased and the height of the waves rose, many of the passengers—nearly all landlubbers—grew seasick. The ships pitched and rolled with some violence, making loud noises as the frames creaked and the cargo shifted. The *Hankey* had an additional disadvantage in that its captain, John Cox, was new to the job and unaccustomed to the vessel. Cox had worked for the British East India Company, shipping to and from India in the late 1780s, although he apparently had never served as a captain before this trip to Africa. It is not clear from the records why he replaced Captain Sundies, who had commanded the *Hankey* for most of the previous decade. Cox would prove to be a less than stellar commander throughout the journey.[21]

In the midst of the widespread seasickness aboard the *Hankey,* Philip Beaver, a Royal Navy lieutenant on half pay, retained the sure footing of an experienced saltwater man. He voluntarily helped the passengers adjust to life on board. As a "democrat" and a "liberty man"—terms used to describe British radicals and reformers at the time—Beaver took pride in performing the menial but necessary chores of caring and cooking for the ill, seeking to translate his abstract political commitment into the realities of everyday life. Beaver's performance of these duties won him admiration among the seasick colonists, while his example of leadership would make the settlers willing to follow him during the trying months to come.

Yet performing menial work did not mean that Beaver considered his shipmates as equals, regardless of his radical politics. The task of cleaning up his shipmates' vomit, for example, he dismissed as women's work. Like many in the middle and upper classes, Beaver privately referred to workers and the poor as "rabble," considering them, as a group, to lack the self-discipline, industry, and frugality associated with the enlarging middle class. Beaver and the other subscribers considered the servants and laborers and their families necessary adjutants of the colonial experiment, but not capable of being equal citizens of the future colony until they internalized these "civilized" values.[22]

Being aboard a ship in the eighteenth century, as the great Samuel Johnson once remarked, was "like being in a jail with the chance of being drowned." Indeed, Johnson continued, "a man in jail has more room, better food, and commonly better company."[23] One hundred and eighteen men, women, and children endured severe trials on the *Hankey*. Few of the people on the voyage had ever sailed on the open seas, and they were struggling to adapt to the closeness of extremely limited shipboard space. The colonists may have dreamed of a more egalitarian society, but their place in the literally upstairs-downstairs living arrangements depended primarily on their social position. Having paid a substantial fee to support the effort, the twenty-four male subscribers, with their seven wives and eight children, enjoyed the relative luxury and comforts available in private or semi-private family staterooms on deck. Subscriber John Paiba, an affluent former ship captain, paid sixty pounds for his subscription to the colonial venture, a sum that netted him a private cabin and a thousand acres of land in Bolama. He brought his wife and his adult son and namesake, who came with his wife and infant child and had himself invested thirty pounds for the promise of five hundred acres on the African island.[24]

Among the passengers lodged in the "between deck" were three dozen indentured servants who couldn't pay the subscription fee. Most had pledged to work for the colony in return for their ocean passage and a promise of land—a method the British had used to attract colonists since the founding of Jamestown. Some of these poorer men brought their families, who were crowded into confined quarters in the hold. Aaron and Ann Baker spent the voyage packed into the second or third level belowdecks. A tailor who earned a modest living in Britain, Aaron hoped to achieve financial success in Bolama. In particular, the Bakers wished to raise funds for dowries for the three unmarried daughters accompanying them on the trip.[25]

A few men and women went out as personal servants. James Watson accompanied Philip Beaver in that capacity. A former slave who had won his freedom by fighting for the British during the American Revolution, Watson was the only black passenger on board. No written record exists that might illuminate Watson's motivations for signing up for the trip, but he would prove to be one of the most valuable, steady pioneers on Bolama.[26]

The poorer passengers stayed topside as long as possible, day and night, since conditions in steerage were cramped and crowded. When the extra people milling about on deck interfered with the work of the mariners, exasperated sailors would chase them below. Those in the hold spent most of their time either crouched in the limited, dark spaces or lying in lattice hammocks, since the four and a half feet between decks scarcely allowed adequate headroom for them to stand. A few family bunks designed to hold three or four people lined the sides of the ship, but lying in them often made the passengers even more seasick, since it amplified the roll of the waves.

Travelers belowdecks ate their meals huddling around tapers or lanterns, amid crates, barrels, and their own personal belongings stacked throughout the hold. The *Hankey* measured 110 feet from bow to stern and about 30 feet at the beam. But the passengers had a few compensations for their discomfort. Even in such cramped circumstances, the poorer migrants on this trip enjoyed considerably more room than the three hundred Irish indentured servants the *Hankey* had carried from Dublin to Philadelphia a decade earlier.[27] In addition, since the *Hankey* had recently carried sugar from the West Indies to Britain, the steerage compartment exuded a sweet smell during the initial days of the cruise.

But the pleasing odor slowly gave way to the stench of people and animals, in particular smells arising from the "necessary tubs," which were filled with a fetid mixture of feces and vomit. The chickens, pigs, sheep, and goats—on board to feed the first-class passengers and to start flocks and herds in the Bolama settlement—occupied the belowdecks area and the small boats strapped to the sides of the ship, further adding to the noxious odors and uncomfortable conditions.

Rats, cats, and cockroaches also scurried about the ship. Like most people of the time, the passengers, especially the farmers, were used to living in close proximity with pests. More upsetting, however, were the lice that annoyed travelers throughout the voyage, a pestilence that would remain during the months the ship anchored offshore at Bolama. As they sailed, the dissonant sounds of people cooking, babies crying, goats bleating, hens clucking, people retching, and the ship's timbers creaking carried on incessantly. In good weather, female passengers hung a network of clotheslines on the deck. The lines sometimes interfered with the work of the mariners, but it allowed the colonists to try to dry garments that always seemed damp.[28]

The laborers all ate ghastly food: salt meat, sea biscuits, dried peas, and a little cheese. The diet concerned Philip Beaver because of its monotony and the threat of scurvy, an often fatal disease that was just becoming known at the time to be the result of poor diet, especially lack of fresh fruit and meat. Beaver planned several stops at ports off the coast of West Africa to obtain fresh provisions, especially limes, which the Royal Navy was beginning to use to stave off the ailment (the origin of the derogatory name "Limey" for British sailors). In the meantime, he issued sauerkraut and mustard to the passengers and crew in hopes of preventing the disease. As for the wealthier travelers, the meat from slaughtered animals aboard and fresh milk from goats made them less susceptible to illness from malnutrition and vitamin deficiency. Yet the longer the passengers traveled under the unsanitary conditions of the ships, the more vulnerable to diseases they all became.[29]

To pass the time, male and female passengers in the *Hankey*'s steerage probably engaged in a good deal of singing—an activity especially popular among sailors, who favored bawdy sea shanties. The wives of servants and laborers spent most of their time caring for children. The poorer passengers drank a great deal of gin, while those in the fancier cabins imbibed claret and port. The crew, commonly called "Jack Tars" because they wore waterproof, tar-impregnated hats, traditionally knocked back an ounce of bumbo or grog (rum and sugar) every four hours, three or four times a day. During periods of long exposure to the sun, the sailors also received extra rations of wine.[30]

The late eighteenth century was a time of hard drinking for both the British and their North American counterparts. People typically started with "small beer" for breakfast, and then sipped more potent beer or rum throughout the day and into the evening. On average, Americans downed five gallons of alcohol each year, more than twice the consumption rate today. Taking breaks from work to drink alcohol was as common as our modern coffee or tea breaks.[31]

One of the activities on board that was probably encouraged by alcohol was gaming. An early form of bridge called whist, which started as a pastime among the lower classes and was subsequently adopted by the affluent, was probably the preferred card game for both passengers and sailors. Another entertainment, faro, had gained popularity among the English poor. It was fast paced with easy-to-learn rules. Some of the passengers wagered either badly or too obsessively, and they lost favorite items of clothing and jewelry during the voyage. A handful of the migrants lost their land claims in the new colony. Embracing emerging middle-class values, the council of the Bolama Association on board the *Hankey* condemned the "pernicious effects" of all this gambling, fearing it would create "the dissolution of all industry, frugality, good order, and good morals." After all, if they were going to teach Africans the virtues of Britain's "superior" civilization, they needed to set a good example. The expedition's leaders decreed that debts incurred through betting would not be payable when they reached their new home. We might confidently wager that the new policy did not delight the gamblers who had won.[32]

The male council members also expected their wives to be models of industry, frugality, good order, and good morals. These women probably did embroidery or other needlework when shipboard conditions permitted. This was a favorite pastime for aspiring middle-class women, who were expected to set an example of industriousness without stooping to the ordinary chores left to servants.

The seafaring colonists sailed for a week along the Atlantic coast of France. Before the revolution, Beaver had spent a year there, in 1783, learning to speak the language fluently. The calls for liberty, equality, and fraternity resonated with him and many of the other colonists, who sympathized with the early, less violent stages of the revolution and wanted to institute some of its ideals in a new democratic society in Africa. Now, three years after the revolution began, as the ships skirted its shores the new leaders in France were starting to execute their enemies on the guillotine—soon to become the symbol of the bloody chaos that would engulf the country. To protect its revolution, France was also declaring war on the politically reactionary countries of Austria, Prussia, and Sardinia, which all opposed the Revolution, thereby initiating the lengthy French Revolutionary Wars. These ideas of freedom and democratic independence would reshape the colonies in the Caribbean and South America over the next few decades, including Saint-Domingue (present-day Haiti), the most valuable French colony at the time. The *Hankey* would inadvertently assist in that reconfiguration.

As the *Hankey* approached the northwest African coast at the end of April, tension among the crew and passengers increased. They stared apprehensively toward the eastern horizon, searching for Barbary pirates from the northern African coast, who would seize non-military vessels and hold well-to-do passengers and sailors for ransom by their relatives and home nations, while enslaving the hapless poorer passengers. As a lightly armed civilian ship, the *Hankey* would have to surrender at the first sight of a craft with cannon and a heavily armed crew of corsairs. Although both Britain and the United States paid tribute to protect their ships from raids, there were no guarantees of safe passage. This time, however, all the expedition's ships, though each was sailing alone, would escape unnoticed.[33]

Turning their gaze westward, the travelers eventually spotted the Canary Islands, which meant the ship was 275 miles east of its rendezvous point in Tenerife. For centuries, the convoluted tides and winds in the region, exacerbated by complex currents flowing between the Atlantic and the Mediterranean, had deceived the dead reckoning of mariners. Many ships had been wrecked on the dangerous African coast, some ending up aground where the barren Sahara met the ocean. Captain Cox could hardly claim this excuse for missing his destination, however. Measuring longitude using precise timepieces had become a standard practice for British captains since the 1760s. The *Hankey*'s being so far off course caused some to question his sailing skills. Indeed, his poor seamanship continued to be an issue throughout the ship's long journey.

The Canary Islands served at the time as a way station for seafaring traders. These islands were among the first to be conquered on fledging voyages from the shores of Europe, although the Portuguese had learned early on that superior weaponry alone did not ensure military victory. The difficulties that Europeans had encountered while trying to conquer the Canaries should have served as a warning

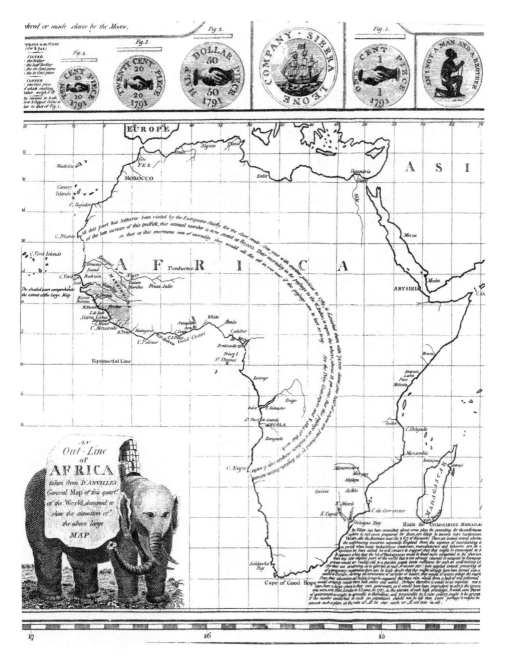

Africa as imagined by the colonists. Detail of the "Nautical Map intended for the Use of Colonial Undertakings" drawn in 1794, based in part on information provided by the Bolama expedition. Note at the upper right the antislavery symbol and slogan: "Am I Not a Man and a Brother." From Philip Beaver, *African Memoranda, Relative to an Attempt to Establish a British Settlement on the Island of Bulama. . . .* (London, 1805), frontispiece. Courtesy the Library Company of Philadelphia.

to the Bolama colonists. They may have envisioned transforming Africans into a civilized, hardworking people, but indigenous groups all along the African coast had long experience in resisting European invasions.

Approximately eighty thousand Vincheai lived in the Canary Islands (inhabiting seven of the thirteen isles) when the Genoese and Portuguese began trading there and raiding the area for slaves in the fourteenth century. Their ancestors had probably floated to the archipelago from southern France, the Iberian Peninsula, and northwest Africa about three thousand years previously. The incomers made contact with the ancient Phoenicians and Carthaginians, and became part of the mythology of the Greeks and Romans. Europeans had imagined the islands as the Garden of Eden, the Elysian Fields, or remnants of the legendary lost continent of Atlantis.[34]

There was good reason for these imaginings. The moderate temperatures caused by Gulf Stream and Mediterranean currents, the splendid beaches, and the ample stores of food encouraged notions of paradise. These "Fortunate Isles," the Roman author Pliny the Elder claimed in the first century C.E., "produce all the goods of the earth [and] all the fruits, without sowing or planting." Yet the fortunate lands allegedly lay at the end of the world, where vessels could find no wind to sail, and the sun set permanently in the ocean.[35]

The Canary Islands were not named for their lovely greenish-yellow-and-brown canaries. Rather, the vicious giant black mastiffs that were also to be found in the area had impressed an early Roman maritime expedition, and the sailors had named the islands after the Latin word for "dog," *canis*. Europeans continued to use this Roman name for the group of islands. While the fourteenth-century invaders called the people living on the islands Guanche, the native inhabitants called themselves Vincheai.

Between the time of the Romans and the appearance of Portuguese explorers looking for wealth and slaves, the Vincheai had developed largely in isolation. This seclusion ensured that, like Native Americans, they possessed no immunity to the diseases common to

Europeans and Africans. (Few events have proved to be as threatening to the survival of an isolated group of people as the arrival of foreigners.) In addition, also like most Native American societies, the Vincheai had, technologically, a Stone Age culture. The consequences, as was so often the case during European conquests, were catastrophic.

Most Vincheai made comfortable homes in the thousands of caves located in the mountainous volcanic terrain of the islands. They improved the spacious caverns, constructing multilevel dwellings with partitioned rooms and wooden floors. Today these caverns are among the most ancient continually occupied residences in the world. The local peoples also transported and stacked enormous rocks to build large, circular houses near the sea, where the elite retreated during the warmer months. Caves were also used as sepulchers: the Vincheai practiced mummification, which they carried out with an expertise equal to that of the ancient Egyptians. The embalmers would use sharp obsidian blades to remove the organs from the bodies, and then wrap the dead in ornately decorated tanned goatskins to dry. Dozens of sepulchral caves existed in Tenerife; one grotto, discovered by the Spanish three decades before the arrival of the *Hankey,* contained a thousand mummies.[36]

The challenges of life on a mountainous set of remote islands fortuitously prepared the Vincheai to resist foreign invaders, making them resourceful and hardy. To care for their sheep and to hunt goats, they had learned to scale the rugged valleys and graveled mountainsides. They created a system of long-distance communication by means of extremely loud whistling in a sort of proto-Morse code. (In the early seventeenth century, one curious if somewhat dull-witted English traveler reportedly lost his hearing for two weeks after asking one of the island inhabitants to whistle in his ear.) In popular games, boys perfected their skills by throwing pointed rocks to kill pigeons, an important food source, and by waging wrestling contests. When the Portuguese came to conquer their islands, the Vincheai began adapting their strengths to defend against these attacks from abroad.

For nearly a century, the Vincheai, using literally sticks and stones, warded off assorted European warriors equipped with metal swords, armor, firearms, and cannon. The conflict began in 1402, when French knights attacked the small eastern Canary Islands, overwhelming their tiny populations within a few years and establishing an outpost there.

The Portuguese, not wanting to miss out on the spoils, attacked the larger and better-defended islands of Gran Canaria and Tenerife beginning in 1415. When thousands of invaders with more than a hundred horses landed on their beaches, the Vincheai were ready, having warned one another via their elaborate system of whistles. They greeted the soldiers hotly with a hail of large sharp obsidian rocks. Following this deadly rain came eight-foot javelins, capable of penetrating the chainmail worn by the Portuguese mounted on horses. Sticks with fire-hardened and sharpened points were hurled next. After their early battles, the Vincheai enhanced their fighting techniques. Imitating their foe, they made shields from the bark of the dragon tree, a substance hard enough to protect against sword blows and even bullets. Gran Canaria had gotten its name not because of its size but because of the bravery and cleverness of its defenders.

Finally, in 1466, the Portuguese abandoned the idea of conquering the Canaries. As they left, however, they captured hundreds of prisoners, claiming them as spoils of war, and shipped them as slaves northwest to the Madeira Islands. There, Portuguese settlers had already cleared the uninhabited archipelago by burning its forests. The Canary Island slaves built canal systems to carry water from the wetter districts in the north to drier ones in the south, where the valuable sugarcane plants consumed a great deal of water. Before long, the Madeira Islands became the most profitable sugar-producing region in the Atlantic. The riches produced by the new colony whetted the appetites of Europeans for further conquests. Meanwhile, the Vincheai had the misfortune of being among the first agricultural slaves transported over the open ocean by Europeans. Forced enslavement subsequently became the basis for the plantations and a mercantile, capitalist system that would come to dominate the Atlantic trade.

It should be noted that racial differences were not the critical factor in the Europeans' decision to enslave the Canary Islanders. They
considered the Vincheai *white* rather than black since most of them
had copper-colored skin and fair hair. Rather, Europeans justified
enslaving the Vincheai because of their supposed cultural inferiority
and their status as spoils of war. From this time forward, however,
racism linked to skin color would increasingly be used as an explanation of Europeans' right to enslave other peoples. Notions of racial
superiority gained in popularity as the African slave trade and con-
comitant growth of the plantation system developed into highly lucrative industries for European empires.

As would often occur during the centuries to come, when one
European power failed in its efforts at conquest, another assumed its
place. Following the Portuguese, the Spanish made their own attempt
to colonize the Canaries. In 1478, Queen Isabella and King Ferdi-
nand ordered the invasion of Gran Canaria. Like the Portuguese, the
Spanish would pay dearly, but so would the Vincheai.

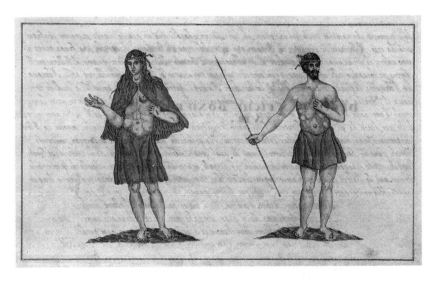

Vincheai men. An image of two light-skinned Vincheai as depicted in the late
sixteenth century by an Italian artist and engineer. Although they fought fiercely for a
hundred years, the Vincheai were eventually enslaved by Europeans. From Leonardo
Torriani, *Alla Maesta del Re Catolico, descrittione et historia del regno de l'isole Canarie. . . .*
(1590).

The Vincheai took refuge in their mountains, conducting a guerrilla campaign. On Gran Canaria they fought a bloody defensive war against Spanish control for the next five years before finally being conquered. Local resistance on Tenerife was even fiercer. The inhabitants repelled an invading force in the 1460s and another in 1490. Two years after Columbus set sail in search of new lands, they killed hundreds of Spanish soldiers at an ambush in the mountains. The relentless conquistadores attacked yet again the following year, eventually exhausting Vincheai resources.

The Spaniards enjoyed the advantage of biological allies. A host of diseases, to which the isolated Vincheai had not been exposed and thus possessed no immunities, burned through the islands. At the height of the epidemic, as many as a hundred inhabitants of Tenerife died each day—a staggering number given their small population. Vincheai corpses grew so abundant that domesticated dogs fed on their former owners.

Those indigenous peoples throughout the Atlantic world who survived the initial wave of devastation created by smallpox and measles were forced into slavery. Many indigenous peoples of the American interior recuperated and reorganized their societies within a few generations. However, when European invaders continually harassed the original inhabitants, they ensured that these societies would fall apart. The Vincheai resisted for a century but ultimately became casualties of European imperialism.

Besides making slaves of many of the local people, the Spanish conquerors disrupted the ecological balance of the islands by introducing several species of flora and fauna from Europe. The colonizers harvested thousands of indigenous goats from the mountains, for example, and imported burros—stronger and more easily domesticated livestock—to fill the niche. The donkey population exploded since it had no natural predators, and the animals grazed many landscapes clean in a few years. To stop the destruction, the Spanish had to slaughter hundreds of burros.

The Vincheai's former home became strategically vital as the staging area for Spanish and Portuguese expeditions to explore beyond the edge of their known world, especially the terra incognita of the Americas. Prevailing winds (eventually named the "trade winds") blew southwest from the Iberian Peninsula, carrying ships directly to the Canary Islands and then on across the Atlantic. In 1492, Columbus charted what became the standard route for such voyages, sailing from Spain to Gran Canaria, where he restocked provisions and made repairs. Before continuing across the ocean, he witnessed the eruption of the great volcanic mountain that gives Tenerife its name. The island later became the first port of call for many of the nineteenth-century scientists who changed European knowledge of the natural world. Both Charles Darwin and Alexander von Humboldt set the foundation for their careers by exploring Tenerife.

B y April 1792, the *Hankey*'s crew and nascent colonists were sailing south along the African coast, although its leaders were probably not focused on the natural history of the Canary Islands. Like so many other vessels, the Bolama expedition ships stopped there for supplies. However, Beaver and his crew found obtaining these much more difficult than they had anticipated.

The *Hankey* tacked westward into a strong breeze for five days before coming close enough to the island of Gran Canaria to anchor. The Jack Tars worked the davits and launched a small jolly boat bearing Beaver and two oarsmen. They hoped to find a ship's pilot to guide them to a safe harbor on the island, where they could procure fresh provisions and water. Beaver expressed a fear that their Spanish hosts might attack any British contingent landing there since tensions ran high between their two countries. Landing on a rocky beach near Las Palmas, Beaver found a French-speaking Catholic priest, to whom he explained the situation. The cleric warned them not to approach the town but offered to carry a message from Beaver and the *Hankey* to the governor. Ever the impatient man of action, Beaver waited only a few hours, and then decided to enter the city gates. The guards promptly arrested him and his two assistants and locked them in a tower on the beach.

Like all ports, Las Palmas feared diseases carried by arriving ships. Europeans living in isolated circumstances were as vulnerable to imported infections as the indigenous peoples were. The island's Spanish governor eventually visited the prison tower but kept his physical distance from Beaver and his men, refusing to approach closer than ten yards for fear of catching smallpox, typhoid, typhus, or a host of other ailments. Shouting over the roar of the surf, the governor's interpreter agreed to send several pilots to the *Hankey* and, if they gave the ship a clean bill of health, to sell them provisions the following day.

Beaver took the pilots back to the *Hankey* for the night, and then returned to the beach the next morning. By that time the local bureaucrats had changed their minds about trading with the British. Perhaps the pilots had given a signal that not all was well aboard the ship. Fearing that the pilots might have contracted communicable diseases, the governor refused to accept them back. He requested a bill of health to certify that the *Hankey* did not carry sickness and had not embarked from an unhealthy port. Beaver claimed that he had forgotten to bring the papers, which were usually required of ship captains. Most likely, he did not want to reveal that smallpox had already claimed the lives of some of the passengers. Beaver instead blustered at the governor and his emissaries, complaining about his detention the previous day and demanding that food and water be supplied to his ship, as it would have been by any other "civilized people." Finally, he appealed to the governor's sense of masculinity by pleading the dire necessity of "refreshments for the women" aboard the *Hankey*.[37]

After lengthy negotiations, local officials grudgingly agreed to sell items at a much higher price, suggesting that their reluctance may in part have been a bargaining strategy. They also took appropriate precautions against the spread of disease, ordering Beaver to drop his coins of payment into a jar filled with vinegar, widely believed to guard against maladies. Meanwhile, laborers brought fresh fruit, vegetables, meat, milk, and chocolate to the shore. They vanished before the foreigners had loaded the new provisions into the jolly boat and returned to the *Hankey,* where the passengers gorged themselves on the fresh food, the first they'd tasted in weeks.

Luck seemed to be turning their way. With newly shifting winds blowing toward their rendezvous point with the *Calypso* in Tenerife, Captain Cox, Beaver, and the other leaders decided to take advantage of the favorable conditions. A day later, they anchored at Tenerife's largest port, Santa Cruz, marveling at the huge volcano that smoldered on the island. Health officials once again questioned the captain and crew about disease, especially smallpox, which fortunately had disappeared on board. The *Calypso,* however, had not been so lucky. Infested with smallpox when it docked four days earlier, it had to flee precipitously rather than have officials quarantine the passengers for the minimum of a fortnight. During its panicked departure, the *Calypso* had sailed without leaving word of a future rendezvous point with the other Bolama colonists. The *Hankey* resupplied with lemons, oranges, bananas, and pomegranates while waiting for the *Beggar's Benison;* the colonists also purchased corn kernels and the seeds of other edible plants to sow in the new colony, and secured barrels of fresh water from a nearby aqueduct.

The stop led to further delays. At a local Tenerife pub, several passengers from the *Hankey* became involved in brawls with the locals, and Beaver had to engage in protracted negotiations to secure their release. When the *Beggar's Benison* appeared, Peter Hayles, a seemingly experienced sailor who was living on the island, expressed a desire to sign on as a crew member. His offer pleased the *Beggar's Benison*'s captain, who needed able hands. Unknown to him, Hayles was a pirate being hunted by authorities, which may have explained his eagerness. Ironically, despite his checkered past, Hayles would prove to be one of the colony's most hard-working and loyal members in the difficult days to come. In perhaps the first written use of the term, Beaver would later describe Hayles as a man "worth his salt."[38]

The problem of finding the *Calypso* remained since the expedition had made no backup provision for a failure to rendezvous in the Canaries. Beaver and the other expedition leaders took a wild guess as to the *Calypso*'s next destination. The *Hankey* and *Beggar's Benison* sailed southwest, reaching Saint Jago (present-day Santiago) in the

Cape Verde islands two weeks later. Disappointment awaited them, however. The *Calypso* was not lying at anchor in the harbor.

The two ships resupplied at Saint Jago, and Beaver purchased livestock for Bolama. Bullocks, cattle, donkeys, and dozens of goats, sheep, and poultry crowded into the above- and belowdecks on the *Hankey,* as well as the jolly boat hanging at the side of the ship. The animals displaced the passengers, driving most of them all the way down into steerage for the remainder of the voyage.

More important than resupplying or even finding the *Calypso* was the expedition leaders' belated realization that they knew neither the exact location of Bolama nor how to get there. They decided to seek out knowledgeable locals, and they caught the favorable winds southeast to Bissau, one of the Portuguese "factories" (as slave-trading posts were called) on the west coast of Africa. At Bissau, merchants purchased slaves and herded them into forts, holding them until slave captains showed up to buy them. Designed to produce a product (in this case, African slaves), these factories actually resembled the early industrial plants beginning to take shape in Britain. The merchandise, a bound labor force millions strong, became the foundation for European mercantile and capitalist expansion in the eighteenth century.

When Beaver and Captain Cox landed at Bissau, they were disappointed not to find the *Calypso*. Frustrated, they set off in search of a pilot who could guide them to Bolama. Portuguese authorities did not react well; they immediately arrested the two men on suspicion of being pirates. Representatives of both Portugal and Spain had now imprisoned him during the voyage, Beaver noted with irritation, while Britain was at war with neither nation. Indignant at having his national dignity insulted, Beaver quarreled with the governor, calling him a "half savage." The governor promptly jailed him for a few days, until Captain Cox, reluctantly, produced official papers explaining the purpose of their voyage. (In fact, the colonists did not have official sanction from the British government, so, technically, they were acting illegally.)[39]

Bissau's governor remained suspicious even after freeing Beaver. He continued to investigate the purpose of their voyage, threatening to transport all the Bolama colonists to Portuguese Brazil as slaves. His hostility can in part be explained by the avowed aims of the colonists: officials at a West African slave-trading post could hardly be expected to react sympathetically to a group of foreigners arriving with plans to destroy their livelihood. But Beaver's belligerence had ratcheted up the inherent tension of the situation.

The *Hankey* and *Beggar's Benison* had now journeyed to within several hundred miles of Bolama. The voyage had been bearable, and "at this time," Beaver commented, "there were not any sick [passengers] on board the *Hankey*."[40] Their dream seemed within reach, even if hostile bureaucrats had stymied them temporarily. Meanwhile, all on board continued to ask the same worrisome question: Where was the third ship of their small armada?

"There are many humorous things in the world," Mark Twain would remark during the height of the imperial century, "among them the white man's notion that he is less savage than the other savages."[41] In our own cynical times, when lofty but sometimes disingenuous rhetoric about the ideals of democracy are often bent to disguise self-interest, dismissing the idealism of past reformers and radicals committed to bettering the world seems too easy. The dedication of these people to the idea of ending one of the world's great evils and improving conditions of life for Africans was wildly optimistic. Building a new colony was a life-stakes gamble for Beaver and his associates, but it was based on their very real belief that they could improve humankind.

CHAPTER 2

The British Colonists

ᔐ

What motivated this group of Britons, mostly middle- and working-class white residents of London and Manchester, to dream of establishing a colony in Africa, a place that many of them feared was both barbaric and dangerous to the health of Europeans? As in all human endeavors, their motivations varied from person to person. But their incentives grew out of the events and circumstances of their everyday existence within the context of the larger Atlantic world. The horrors of the slave trade and the enormous profits realized from that commerce outraged the moral sensibilities of many of the migrants, spurring them to follow their conscience and create an outpost of freedom in Africa. Economic considerations also played a role. While a handful of affluent voyagers envisioned the colony as a way to even greater wealth, many if not most of the immigrants, especially laborers and servants and their families, fled Britain out of economic desperation. The nascent industrial system that would soon sweep through Europe and America was already taking a toll on working people in England. A new start in Bolama offered one of the few viable alternatives to life in a factory, in poverty, in jail—or all three.

Two incidents with which the colonists might have been familiar, a court case in the 1770s and the voyage of a slave ship in the 1780s, helped fuel the antislavery movement that in 1792 stretched across the

Atlantic world, from Britain to America to France. The court case involved a slave, James Somerset, who sought to gain his freedom in England; the slave ship was the *Zong,* whose notorious voyage was one of the most tragic in a long string of heartbreaking catastrophes, outraging even those who had become hardened to stories of cruelty and death aboard the slave ships. What happened on the *Zong,* and what happened after the ship returned to London, inspired Britons to found the first abolition society in their history.[1]

In early September 1781, a ship owned by two former mayors of Liverpool, a city that was deeply involved in financing and managing the slave trade, sailed from West Africa toward the West Indies carrying a cargo of more than four hundred slaves, most of them from São Tomé, an island off the African coast. The commander, Captain Collingwood, embraced the idea of "tight packers": that captains should load as many slaves as possible on board, accepting the probability of a higher mortality rate during the Atlantic crossing than if fewer people were chained in the hold (the "loose packer" scheme). It all came down to profits and free, unfettered markets for captains and merchant ship owners. Whoever transported the most slaves across the ocean earned the most money. There were no other restrictions on the slave traders' decision making.

Badly overloaded with Africans and ineptly commanded by Captain Collingwood, the *Zong* foundered as the commander lost his bearings several times during the voyage. The vessel took twelve weeks to cross the Atlantic, three weeks longer than usual. Supplies, especially water, began to run low. Many Africans locked in the hold died; most of the others grew sick and weak. Realizing that his emaciated cargo would draw very low prices in a Caribbean port, Captain Collingwood decided to throw the slaves overboard so that he could collect money from the company that had insured the human cargo.

Collingwood ordered the crew to toss the bound men, women, and children into the ocean under the pretext of a shortage of water on the ship, which he claimed would eventually kill them all anyway. Shackling the slaves together in long chains, the sailors slid fifty-five

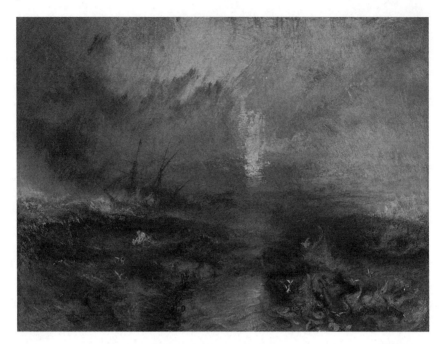

J. M. W. Turner, *The Slave Ship,* 1840, oil on canvas. The story of the *Zong* is believed to have inspired Turner's powerful painting, alternately titled *Slavers Throwing Overboard the Dead and Dying, Typhoon Coming On.* Note the shackles on the drowning people in the foreground. Museum of Fine Arts, Boston, Henry Lillie Pierce Fund/The Bridgeman Art Library.

of them overboard on November 29. They killed forty-two more the next day. Even after a heavy rainfall had refilled the water barrels, Collingwood ordered twenty-six more slaves murdered the following day. Ten jumped overboard of their own accord, asserting at least some control over how and when their lives ended. Although this brutality was but an extreme form of the violence integral to the slave trade, news of the calculated murders drew outrage throughout the Atlantic world. It had a galvanizing impact on both Britons and Americans, inspiring many to question the trade and some to create antislavery societies.

When the *Zong* returned to Britain, its owners duly filed a claim with the insurance company to reimburse them for their lost cargo. The insurers took the case to court in 1783. Olaudah Equiano, who had bought himself out of slavery and now lived in England, brought the case to the attention of Granville Sharp, the lawyer in the 1772 Somerset case. Lord Mansfield, the Lord Chief Justice, who had also served as judge in the Somerset case, came down on the side of the owners, instructing the jury that "the matter left to [them] was whether it was necessary that the slaves were thrown into the sea, for . . . the case of slaves was the same as if horses had been thrown overboard." Following the reasoning that because it was permissible to destroy livestock for the safety of the ship, it was also acceptable to kill people held in chains, the jury ruled in favor of the ship's owners.[2]

The insurance company appealed. Ultimately, three justices, including Mansfield, decided that the slaves on board should be considered human beings rather than livestock. Therefore, the company did not need to pay the *Zong*'s owners for the lost cargo. However, the court refused to prosecute the captain or crew for murder. The logic seemed more than a bit twisted to many observers, who had already begun to question the morality of the slave trade following the celebrated Somerset case. In 1772, it had garnered notice on both sides of the Atlantic, raising public awareness of the injustice of slavery during an era when the rhetoric of liberty and equality was widespread.

James Somerset, born in Africa, had been sold as a slave in 1749 to a merchant from Scotland, one Charles Steuart, who lived in Norfolk, Virginia. Traveling to London on business several decades later, Steuart brought Somerset with him as a personal servant, a position he had held in both Virginia and Massachusetts. In 1771, when it appeared that his master might sell him, Somerset took flight, but was apprehended by a London slave catcher. Steuart immediately had Somerset chained belowdecks on a ship bound for the British plantation colony of Jamaica, where the captain had orders to sell him.[3]

A writ of habeas corpus freed Somerset temporarily, and he sought aid from Granville Sharp. The lawyer had assisted other runaways previously, had spoken out forcefully against racial bondage, and was a leader of the tiny early abolitionist movement. Sharp envisioned this as a test case on the legality of slavery. At stake was not merely the freedom of one person but the very meaning of liberty itself in Britain. He organized a team of sympathetic lawyers for Somerset's defense. Supporters of slavery, especially absentee West Indian planters living in London and Liverpool, perceived clearly the threat to their valuable holdings in human beings, estimated at well over a hundred million dollars in today's terms. Not surprisingly, they rallied around the government prosecution.

The Somerset case became a cause célèbre, covered by newspapers, debated in coffeehouses and taverns, and embraced enthusiastically by the black community in London. A significant number of Britons came together for the first time to crusade against slavery in their homeland. Trying to avoid the wider implications of ending racial bondage in the entire nation, Lord Mansfield, the judge, offered a narrow decision that freed Somerset and decreed that owners of slaves could not forcibly remove them from Britain. However, the press reported and the public widely believed that the assertion by the defense had been confirmed legally: "As soon as any slave sets his foot on English ground, he becomes free."[4]

Britain's small slave population celebrated the victory, even as they realized that neither slave owners nor the state was prepared to free most of the people currently in bondage. The court's decision, however, afforded slaves a powerful new advantage in dealing with their masters. Now that they could not be sold abroad, many slaves found they could bargain more effectively for better living conditions or, occasionally, even for their freedom. Nor was the Somerset case an isolated decision. In Pennsylvania, the legislature passed a law in 1780 forbidding masters to sell their human chattel out of the state. The power of owners declined once they were left with fewer options for disciplining recalcitrant slaves. Owners became more willing to improve conditions to ensure the reliable behavior of their human property. In some instances, masters agreed to free their slaves after a certain number of years of faithful service.

Benjamin Franklin, who was living in London at the time of the Somerset case as the official representative of several American colonies, took note of the ruling, as did many other colonists, especially slave owners. Franklin expressed disgust at the legal decision. He complained to Anthony Benezet, a prominent abolitionist friend in Philadelphia, about British hypocrisy for celebrating their "virtue, love of liberty and equity in setting free a single Negro," while simultaneously disregarding pleas from the Americans for increased freedom to control their own affairs. Franklin's statements surely stemmed in part from the fact that, while in London, one of his own slaves ran away and secured his liberty. Franklin displayed a typical slave owner's repulsion at the Somerset case, shared widely in the American colonies. Although he would become president of the Pennsylvania Abolition Society in the late 1780s, Franklin was not yet a convinced antislavery advocate.

The Atlantic slave trade was a huge industry internationally, comparable to the oil business or high finance in our own times. It involved the movement of enormous numbers of people and products among the West Indies and the four continents that bordered the Atlantic Ocean. It was a business which made both individuals and nations rich. Merchants made a fortune in the enterprise, intermediaries made a handsome profit, and sailors found jobs. Given the stakes, European and American nations struggled and fought wars for centuries over its control. During the years of the slave trade, from 1501 to 1867, the Spanish carried 1.1 million Africans, the French 1.3 million, the Dutch about 550,000, and the United States about 300,000 to the West Indies and the American continents. The Portuguese topped them all, forcibly moving 5.8 million humans, mostly to Brazil. To destroy a business that enriched so many people would require a great deal of moral and economic persuasion.

Traffic in enslaved humans bound for the Americas peaked during the 1780s and 1790s. Hundreds of ships carried more than eight hundred thousand Africans each year. During those decades, the British Empire was the largest slave trader in history, transporting roughly one-quarter of the people removed from Africa. Before the British slave trade ceased in 1807, the nation's ships had relocated more than three million Africans—including untold thousands who perished during the infamous Middle Passage.[5]

In 1789, the politician William Wilberforce organized a parliamentary campaign to halt Britain's participation in the Atlantic slave
trade. Two years earlier, nine Quakers and three Anglicans had met
in a printing shop, inspired by Christian idealism and Enlightenment
humanitarianism to establish the Society for Effecting the Abolition
of the Slave Trade. It was a modest beginning for what would become
one of the most important, successful movements in world history—
the effort to end the slave trade and, eventually, the institution of
slavery itself.[6]

Wilberforce's maneuverings were linked with several attempts by
Parliament to reform the British Empire following its defeat in the
American War of Independence. Wilberforce injected the moral zeal
of the antislavery movement into the political debates. The Protestant
majority of Britons were "all guilty" of profiting from the trade in human beings, he argued. Instead of enslaving Africans, Britain should
focus on converting the "heathens" to Christianity. Wilberforce's
parliamentary leadership complemented the inexhaustible energy of
Thomas Clarkson, a founding member of the Society. Over the next
two years, Clarkson traveled thirty-five thousand miles on horseback
around England, interviewing twenty thousand sailors about conditions on slave ships. He also collected and displayed the tools of the
slave trade—thumbscrews, leg shackles, branding irons—as testimony to the violence inherent in the institution.

Clarkson shared his evidence with Wilberforce's committee, and
its publications created a stir among the British populace. In his travels across England, Clarkson had also inspired and helped organize
dozens of local antislavery societies. Ordinary women and men rallied
to the cause. Most of them could not express their political opinions
at the ballot box: the property qualifications of the time limited the
franchise to the country's wealthier men. But the antislavery advocates circulated petitions, donated money, and organized an effective
boycott of sugar, since so many slaves shed their blood in the course
of its production.[7]

In 1791, Parliament rejected Wilberforce's slave-trade abolition
bill, swayed by the powerful lobby for West Indian planters, whose

slaves produced rum, coffee, tobacco, and sugar for British markets. The following year, the House of Commons voted to phase out the slave trade, but the decision was undermined by both the procedural cleverness of Home Secretary Henry Dundas and a new war with France.

Yet just as the slave trade was international, the movement against it also stretched across the Atlantic. British abolitionists like Thomas Clarkson had long been in touch with their American counterparts, including the Quaker Anthony Benezet. They also contacted the French Société des amis des noirs in the late 1780s. Yet for the majority of Europeans and North Americans in the late eighteenth century, shipping people in chains seemed little different from transporting sugar or flour or cloth or horses, in part because the profits were so great. It took a great deal of time and a tremendous amount of effort and sacrifice for Britain and America to end the slave trade and eventually slavery itself. The United States required a civil war finally to abolish the institution.

The British who sailed on the three ships toward Bolama, whether by individual choice or by the simple fact that they were involved in the enterprise, were part of the international antislavery movement.

The Bolama expedition members consisted largely of pioneers born of the European Enlightenment. They imagined themselves sailing away from a troubled England toward a bright future that would include both prosperous Britons *and* prosperous Africans. They planned to improve the world through their own example, seeking both to do good and to make a better living. Although, as with so many commoners who lived during the eighteenth century, there is little written evidence about their beliefs and motivations, a good deal of circumstantial evidence provides a basis for identifying and interpreting their aims.

Most of them were quite ordinary people. Two-thirds signed on as laborers or personal servants because the only way they could afford to pay for their passage was with their promise of work. These colonists did not leave personal statements or letters for historians to analyze; most left behind only their names and a few scraps of information, often just the date of their deaths.

Scholars, however, have been able to piece together information about the environment in which they lived and died, too often young. Britain underwent profound economic and social transformations in the late eighteenth century, which resulted in rising misery for many of its inhabitants. The effects of trade on a global scale combined with the growth of industrialization remade England and Scotland. Britain began the painful process of transformation from a rural to an urban society. As agricultural workers migrated to metropolitan centers in search of work, living conditions in the overwhelmed cities deteriorated. Life became "nasty, brutish, and short," in the words of the political philosopher Thomas Hobbes. More than half of the inhabitants of London could not earn sufficient wages to put food on the table every day. Many had to take refuge in gloomy institutions like the almshouse or workhouse. Others landed in jail for stealing bread, sticks of firewood, or other necessities of life, and then were sentenced to transportation. One of every five babies in Britain's capital died in infancy, and adults, on average, lived only until their early thirties. It was little wonder that many of the poor found comfort in cheap gin.[8]

Several of the Bolama pioneers were in trouble with the law. John Frasier had served three months in jail for stealing a shirt. Authorities whipped Thomas Blake for pilfering a pair of boots. After falling into debt, others faced jail or transportation. In 1784, Thomas Griffiths suffered banishment from England for seven years for larceny. He returned to his native land in 1791 and the next year was sentenced again. This time, the judge gave him a choice: expulsion or a meeting with Jack Ketch, the popular name for the executioner. "Depend upon it," Samuel Johnson once cynically remarked, "when a man knows he is to be hanged in a fortnight, it concentrates his mind wonderfully." Griffiths, like Frasier and Blake, chose to join the expedition to Bolama.[9]

A few of the other passengers had also been sentenced by the courts to transportation out of Britain. Their choice to join the voyage probably had less to do with the ideals espoused by the Bolama Association than with the orders of the court. During the American Revolution, when offenders could no longer be expelled to the Americas, Britons looked initially to Africa as a possible destination for felons. Ultimately, they settled on Australia, sending the First Fleet, loaded with prisoners, to Botany Bay in 1788.[10]

Many of the workers hailed from Manchester, the home of the earliest factories in England and a city that supported the antislavery movement. Several of the colonizers, like William Bennet, a laborer aboard the *Hankey,* had lost their jobs; they also saw a parallel between their own working lives and the enslavement of African peoples. Many laborers complained about their state of semi-bondage in the early factories. From their perspective, the richest classes imposed similar conditions on workers everywhere, since the control of labor was an important means to wealth. Even within the close confines of the association's three ships, the poorer migrants to Bolama had little interaction with the wealthy philanthropic men who sat on the council.[11]

Thomas Bell, one of the laborers, was a deeply committed democratic man, in the parlance of the time. A staunch antislavery advocate, he was a proponent of a more egalitarian society in Britain and the Atlantic world generally. He was also politically active. Because he owned no property, he could not vote. Instead, he occasionally took to the streets to support a range of political causes, not all of which were focused on democracy in Britain. Authorities arrested him several times, first for participating in the Gordon Riots in 1780 and then for joining the annual rowdy and politicized celebrations named for Guy Fawkes. This infamous rebel had helped devise the Gunpowder Plot of 1605 to overthrow the king, blow up the House of Lords, and restore a Catholic monarch to the English throne, and his effigy was burned every year to drunken outcries of approval. Bell joined the Bolama expedition in part because of his radical political commitment to help end the buying and selling of human beings.[12]

Bell had worked as a weaver for most of his life. In the early 1780s, he and his wife, Ann, opened the Three Jolly Weavers, a gin shop, in

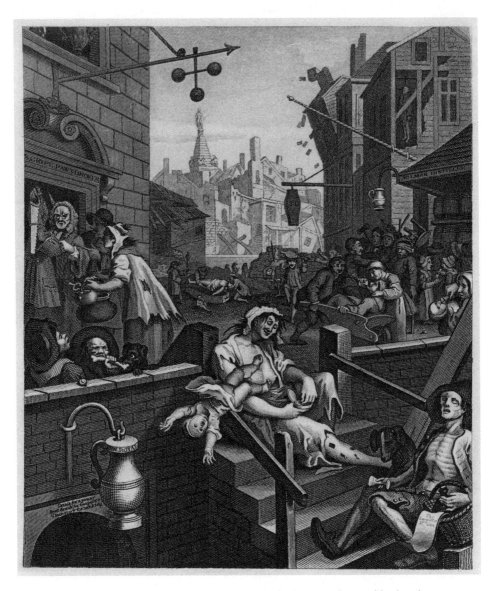

William Hogarth, *Gin Lane,* 1751. The impoverished Saint Giles neighborhood portrayed here was home to many free blacks, who later moved to Sierra Leone, as well as to some of the white men, women, and children who migrated to Bolama. From a re-engraving by Samuel Davenport. Wikimedia Commons, commons. wikimedia.org.

the front parlor of their house, which was located in a back alley accessible only through a narrow, twisting passageway. Thomas was carrying on the tradition of his grandmothers, both of whom had run gin shops in London after the Dutch had introduced the alcohol to Britain. The popularity of gin had exploded in the mid-eighteenth century, akin to the boom in crack cocaine in the United States during the 1980s. The impact of gin was equally deleterious, especially for the British poor. It became such a concern that socially conscious artists like William Hogarth began drawing lurid images of the horrors of gin, which they set against the virtues of English beer.

The Three Jolly Weavers became a gathering place for white political radicals as well as for a few "blackbirds of Saint Giles"—as British officials disdainfully called unemployed black Londoners who lived in the neighborhood. The gin parlor also served as a bawdy house. In a 1785 trial of another man, Thomas Bates, for passing counterfeit money at his establishment, Bell admitted that prostitution sometimes occurred there, though without his consent. "The staircase goes at the back of the street door," Bell explained, "and a man gave a woman a bad half guinea to lie with her all night. The man was taken up for tendering this bad half guinea." Bell noted to the court that he ran a respectable business, "and there never was a man for a felony in any respect, taken out of my house." Regardless of Bell's testimony, the jury found Bates guilty, and the judge sentenced him to transportation to Africa.[13]

Not long afterward, when his wife died, Thomas Bell decided to head for Africa. He was fed up with England and its undemocratic ways and tired of having few financial prospects. He signed on for a berth on the *Hankey* for his young child and himself, hoping to start a new life.

A personal servant to Philip Beaver, James Watson was the only black person on the *Hankey*. Like thousands of others, Watson had emancipated himself during the American Revolution, most likely responding to the promise of freedom offered by British officials: if slaves left their masters and joined Loyalist forces against the revolutionaries, they would be freed. Watson survived both the violence of the war and the diseases that accounted for most of its casualties. He made his way to England, probably leaving with the British armada when it evacuated America in 1783. The paucity of the historical record obscures him from our view today. We know only that he stayed on Bolama until the bitter end, and then moved to Sierra Leone, where other black refugees from the American Revolution had established a colony of free people.[14]

We likewise know little about the fifty-eight adult women, including seventeen personal servants, on the Bolama expedition. Their names appear solely on the passenger lists or in journal entries noting when they gave birth or when they died. The accounts of the expedition written by the four male authors almost totally ignore the women, reflecting the prevailing masculine views of "the sex," as men commonly referred to females at the time. Still, historians' general knowledge about the era can supplement the clues available about a few individuals.

Women in both Britain and North America helped make up the ranks of idealists and radicals; a few even embraced the new feminist ideas expressed by Mary Wollstonecraft. The antislavery movement attracted an especially large number of female adherents. Women were unable to vote or even to address public meetings, but they made their views known in other ways. They enthusiastically boycotted sugar and other items produced by the blood of slaves, and they helped organize petitions against the barbarities of slavery. Unlike leaders of the Bolama expedition, however, abolitionist women could not hold official positions. Long-standing social conventions prevented it, even within radical organizations like the Bolama Association.

Still, the women on the expedition often participated in the decision to join it. Like their husbands, the wives of the Bolama Association members would have been moved by its antislavery ideals as well as by the desire to improve their families' financial position. The late eighteenth century in general was a time of considerable transition in gender and marriage relations. The new Romantic trend advocated a marriage of companions, where both men and women selected their own mates. These new types of union emerged ideally from affection and love rather than the practical property considerations of traditional arranged marriages. In principle, women had more say in making decisions within such marriages, including whether to take such a major step as migrating to Bolama. It should be noted that poorer families already tended to be more egalitarian in their decision making, if only because both marriage partners had to cooperate for the family to survive.[15]

Women like Ann Baker fell into this second category. Ann may well have opposed the slave trade. As the wife of tailor Aaron Baker, she most likely hoped that the new colony would help ensure her family's financial security. Baker helped tend her husband's shop in London; she sewed and took in boarders. She also cared for her aging father and her three unmarried daughters, who needed dowries. Yet as was often true for the lower classes in the preindustrial world, all of Ann and Aaron's hard work was insufficient to earn them a living wage. They continued to fall deeper and deeper into debt. The Bakers struggled simply to make ends meet on a daily basis, much less to provide for the future of their family. They took their three unmarried daughters with them when they moved to Bolama, leaving two married daughters in London.[16]

Elisabeth Curwood, the wife of an affluent subscriber and council member of the Bolama Association, more likely had a traditional eighteenth-century marriage. Her husband may have simply informed her that they were moving, without consulting her views. John Curwood was one of the few survivors who made it back to England, and his opinion of the expedition was frequently sought afterward by medical and government authorities. Elisabeth did board the *Hankey* with John when the ship limped out of Bolama harbor toward home in 1793, but she died two days later. All their children also perished in the colonization attempt.[17]

Only a handful of women traveled to Bolama without a husband, all as personal servants to wealthy subscribers. Most of them were probably young, with few other prospects. Patience Bates was one of these servants. She could not realistically hope to own any land in the colony since she was a woman. Originally from Manchester, Bates may have lost her job when the new mills led to the replacement of unskilled laborers' positions. She fell on hard times after she made her way to London. In early 1792, a judge found her guilty of stealing a book and a few articles of clothing. Sentencing Bates to a year in jail, he offered her the alternative of joining the Bolama expedition as a personal servant. She was one of the few people who survived the entire ordeal, eventually returning home to England on the *Hankey*.[18]

A few particulars about Hannah Riches and her husband, Joseph, can be pieced together from offhand comments contained in Philip Beaver's account of the expedition. Beaver's brief remarks about this couple are colored by his stereotypical thinking about women. At the beginning of the voyage, Hannah and Joseph were packed into the *Hankey*'s tight accommodations belowdecks. Knowing that she would not have been allowed to bring a child with smallpox aboard, Hannah hid her infected child's condition; it was discovered when another young person caught the disease.

Beaver initially damned Hannah Riches's deception about her child as "inconsiderate and almost inhuman conduct," in fact a "crime." After finding out about the subterfuge, the association council decided nonetheless to allow her and her child to remain on board. The child had already been on the ship for nineteen days, and therefore "the seeds of all the danger" of the infection spreading "had already taken root." After more thought, Beaver concluded that Hannah Riches's behavior resulted both from "the feelings of an affectionate wife, about to be separated from a husband whom she fondly loved" and from the anguish she felt about a separation from her child. "It was a crime committed by feeling; it was a crime that might be committed by a virtuous woman, but that could not have been committed by a completely vicious character." Beaver surely never asked Riches what she thought. Instead, he dismissed her offense as the result of the feelings natural to any woman, even a member of the working class.[19]

Once on Bolama, Hannah Riches engaged in customary women's work. She helped cook the meals, a lengthy process given the primitive conditions of the settlement. She engaged in the laborious task of washing clothes. She likewise cared for her children, tended the small farm animals like chickens, and helped plant the vegetable garden. She appeared in Beaver's journal as treating the sick— virtually a full-time task once the majority of settlers grew ill.

Hannah's husband, Joseph, and her very young daughter and namesake died within a week of each other in early December 1792. If she felt grief and despair, Beaver didn't mention it. He wrote cryptically toward the end of his account: "Hannah Riches, discharged to go home." She was the last surviving British woman on Bolama. She had made an arrangement, on her own, with the captain of a slave ship to take her to the West Indies. After that, like so many women and commoners, Hannah Riches disappears from the historical record.[20]

About the leaders and supporters of the colony, modern scholars know a great deal more. Primary among them were an idealist, an adventurer, a "Jew King," a Loyalist, and a future mayor of London.[21] What motivated these Bolama colonists can be uncovered, to a large extent, through their own words.

Short, rotund, and pale, with soft facial features, forty-year-old Henry Hew Dalrymple appeared on the witness stand before the British Parliament in August 1789 and testified before William Wilberforce's committee about the horrors of slavery. He was a man of considerable character, with high ideals and a deep commitment to ending the traffic in human beings. Dalrymple's ethical principles were the primary reason he organized the Bolama Association. For him, racial bondage was morally wrong because, insofar as they were all humans, all people were essentially the same. "In natural capacity," Dalrymple responded under questioning by the parliamentary committee, "the Negroes are equal to any people whatever." He added that in temper and disposition, "they appear to be humane, hospitable, and well disposed." He believed that if they were provided with the opportunity and taught to be consumers and workers, Africans would be "as industrious as Europeans." (Industriousness was a prized Western bourgeois value that he felt would help civilize all of humanity.) These views challenged widely accepted notions about the inferiority of blacks, marking Dalrymple as considerably more radical than American political revolutionaries who owned slaves, or even non-slaveowners like John Adams.[22]

Dalrymple disputed the commonly held idea that Africans did not mind enslavement and probably even benefited from bondage. He drew on his firsthand experience while stationed as a British Army officer at the slave station of Gorée, in West Africa, and as a member of a Caribbean slaveholding family. Dalrymple testified to Parliament that free Africans lived in a "happy state" in their homeland and that slavery dehumanized them. Dalrymple likewise attacked the pervasive European belief that most Africans became slaves as legitimate prisoners of war inside Africa. The arguments Dalrymple used were beginning to undermine the justification of the slave trade; they were small but important steps in the long, uphill struggle.

Born in 1752 to an affluent family on the Caribbean island of Grenada, Henry Dalrymple—like the sons of many other West Indian planters—was sent to England to be educated when a young boy. There Dalrymple pondered deeply about the meaning of British liberty and whether Africans were the equals of Europeans. In 1773 he sailed back across the Atlantic for his first visit in years to his family's 250-acre cocoa plantation. The brutality of slavery that he witnessed in the Caribbean shocked him. In the marketplace of Saint George, the largest town on the island (and coincidentally a port the *Hankey* would eventually use as a refuge), "Negroes were flogged every day by the particular orders of their masters. They were tied down upon the ground," Dalrymple later testified to Parliament, and "every stroke brought blood and very often took out a piece of the flesh."[23]

Slaves endured extremely arduous working conditions on Caribbean plantations, laboring twelve or fifteen hours a day to produce sugarcane, cocoa, and coffee. To save costs, most owners provided them with only minimal food, shelter, and clothing. Some masters literally worked their slaves to death, since it was less expensive to buy new human replacements than to furnish livable conditions day to day. The "general opinion" among planters, Dalrymple noted with outrage, was "that it is more profitable to import slaves and work them out than to breed them."[24] The punishments for slaves were equally horrifying. Branding, whipping, and using thumbscrews and iron muzzles were common techniques for curbing black workers on the plantations; slaves were even hanged as object lessons. A telling statistic of this savage system was that the average life expectancy of a new arrival from Africa was seven years.[25]

Dalrymple's personal views about slavery had evolved over time. Having joined the British navy during the American Revolution, he found himself stationed in 1779 as a lieutenant at Gorée, a European slave-trading post on the west coast of Africa. "Because he held slaves himself in the West Indies," Dalrymple visited the continent frequently, "with a view of knowing the situation" about Africans and their own feelings about human bondage. After interviewing dozens of indigenous people, both Africans and those of French-African ancestry, Dalrymple became convinced that Africans did not want to be slaves—a radical idea about race in both Europe and North America at the time.[26] Dalrymple and other antislavery advocates like him were considered bold to question the slave trade on the grounds of humanity and morality.

As the *Zong* case moved through courts in the 1780s and eventually concluded with the affirmation that slaves were to be legally treated as human beings rather than as analogous to cattle, Dalrymple had become convinced that the practice of slavery was not only morally wrong but also clearly inhuman. After he inherited his father's plantation in 1788, he freed all his slaves. Dalrymple also agreed to testify about the horrors of slavery before the British Parliament. These were actions unheard of among West Indian planters, and a true indication of his dedication to abolishing the slave trade.[27]

Following Dalrymple's testimony, a group of antislavery proponents who were planning a new colony in Africa approached Dalrymple about joining their endeavor. Olaudah Equiano, soon to be a prominent leader in the movement, had joined with white abolitionists to seek a place where a mixture of white and black colonists might retreat and live in freedom. The group agreed to appoint

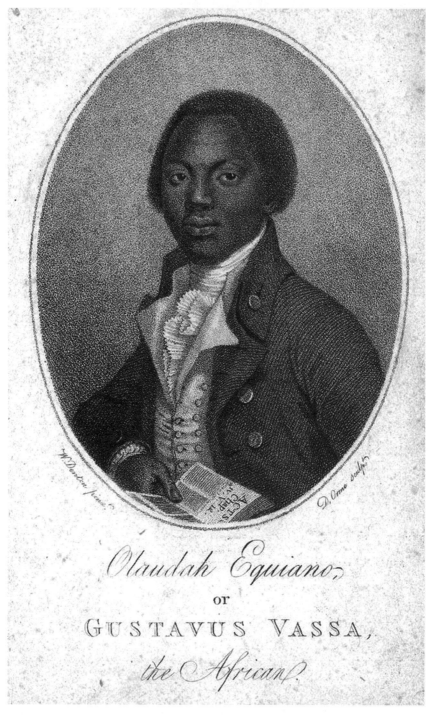

Olaudah Equiano,
or
GUSTAVUS VASSA,
the African

Olaudah Equiano (1745–97) was an important leader of the British antislavery movement and active in organizing the Sierra Leone colonial effort. His autobiography describing his life as a slave and his purchase of his own freedom challenged popular notions in Europe and North America that Africans were inferior beings. From Equiano, *The Interesting Narrative of the Life of Olaudah Equiano, or Gustavus Vassa, the African. . . .* (London, 1789).

Dalrymple as the first governor of Sierra Leone. However, Dalrymple wanted to include a much larger contingent of military men than did the colony's organizer. The white directors, pushed by black potential migrants in London, argued that a relatively small number of pioneers would be helpless against a concerted attack by Africans, so it would be best to create a nonmilitarized colony. After squabbling for a few weeks, the group dismissed Dalrymple before the ships ever launched from England.[28]

Dalrymple very quickly decided to organize his own expedition to Africa. He contacted a few former naval officers he knew, including Philip Beaver. During their twice-weekly meetings in Old Slaughter's Coffeehouse, the newly christened Bolama Association drew up a radical constitution to define the new colony. It emphasized a republican government where "sovereignty resides in the people." It provided for universal adult male suffrage regardless of wealth or race. Most important, the document outlawed slavery in the proposed new colony. To minimize the "undue influence of Property," and to make certain that the outpost would not become dominated by large plantations, as in the West Indies, the constitution specified that settlers could hire only one African laborer for every forty acres of land they owned. In addition, the colonists pledged to settle only where they could purchase land from local people—quite a departure from previous European colonizing efforts.[29]

Far more revolutionary than the U.S. Constitution, the Bolama agreement reflected these Britons' radicalism. The provisions for a new society to be governed with a political order so fundamentally challenging to the contemporary British system alienated British officials, who would later decline to approve the document. The journey proceeded without government sanction, which meant that it was questionable whether the Bolama Council officials possessed the legal power to establish a colony or enforce contracts in Bolama.

Dalrymple's dismissal by the Sierra Leone organizers should have been an early warning that he lacked a number of leadership skills, including the ability to make or enforce timely and difficult decisions. Had he taken decisive action with regard to arranging the purchase of

Bolama Island before the colonists disembarked, following the expedition's principles established in London, he might well have saved lives and slowed the cascade of misfortune that inundated the colonists. Although an admirable idealist, Dalrymple was both a poor planner and a poor organizer of the practical, everyday details that were essential to establishing a successful colony. Dalrymple ultimately did not stay long on Bolama. After returning to England, he died of a mysterious ailment, probably contracted in Africa.

Born in Lewknor, Oxfordshire, in 1766, Philip Beaver was the son of the local parish curate. His father died suddenly when Philip was eleven, leaving Beaver and his mother destitute. Unable financially to care for her son, Beaver's mother accepted an offer from British naval captain Joshua Rowley to take the boy to sea as a midshipman on HMS *Monarch*. After his mother let him go, Beaver's life of adventure began.[30]

Beaver witnessed his first naval action in the English Channel, off Ushant, France, on July 27, 1777. By December, he had proven himself indispensable to Rowley—recently promoted to rear admiral. Rowley asked Beaver to join HMS *Suffolk* for an Atlantic crossing to the West Indies to defeat the Americans in their War of Independence. There, the *Suffolk* joined the British fleet and remained until 1783, by which time Admiral Rowley had promoted Beaver to the rank of commissioned lieutenant. After two years of service in Jamaica, Beaver sailed back to Britain. He remained on naval service afterward, but spent some time living quietly with his mother in Boulogne, a seaport in northwest France just across the English Channel. There he became familiar with the ideas of French Enlightenment thinkers, especially Montesquieu, who was antislavery in principle but not too disturbed if Africans were the ones in bondage. Beaver returned to active service in 1790 and 1791 to assist in British naval mobilizations for possible conflicts with Spain and Russia, then went on half pay when the wars failed to materialize, available for call-up in case of future emergencies.[31]

Beaver, with his prominent aquiline nose, clean-shaven face, and luxuriant nest of brown hair, carried the blue wool and gold braids of his British naval officer's uniform with upright dignity. His experiences had left him serious, fiercely disciplined, idealistic, adventurous, and largely solitary. His service at sea had been marked by a series of successes. There is no record of his tyrannizing over his crew (unusual for the age) or of any jealousy or threat felt by his superior officers. Though self-taught, he was a rapacious and omnivorous reader. A story circulated that during one cruise he brought aboard the entire *Encyclopaedia Britannica.*

Beaver's steady upward climb on his career ladder cemented his position within the middle class. He was deeply committed to its values. Hard work, frugality, delayed gratification, independence—he believed these virtues had saved him from a life of destitution and debasement. They might also save the world if only others learned and practiced them.

Beaver initially heard of the embryonic program to colonize Bolama in 1791, when the twenty-five-year-old was hatching a plan to walk across the African continent on foot. Talk of exploring the "dark continent" was everywhere in Britain, and the Scottish explorer Mungo Park would soon make several expeditions into West Africa, which would earn him enormous popularity in England. When Dalrymple approached Beaver about the Bolama plan, Beaver immediately responded in a positive fashion. "I knew nothing of what would be expected from me, nothing of the plan, except that it was humane," Beaver later wrote. "All that I knew was that a colony was to be established, and among uncivilized tribes, and that was enough for me."[32]

His unique mix of personal characteristics and belief in self-improvement by example fired his interest in civilizing Bolama, while his time in France during the tumultuous rush toward revolution may have helped fuel it. The breadth of his naval voyages had provided him with an appreciation of other cultures, while his egalitarian ideals meshed with the proposals of the Bolama Association. Creating a colony that would treat all human beings with dignity and respect appealed to his sense of mission.

Philip Beaver would prove to be the most important person on the Bolama expedition. One of its few survivors, he wrote a book detailing his adventures in Africa, his understanding of what happened, and, from his perspective, what it all meant.

The inclusion of John King as a Bolama Council member demonstrates how broad the Bolama organization was theologically. Growing up during the Enlightenment, the age of rationalism, many of the colonists were not deeply religious. Their deism and agnosticism differentiated them from other members of the abolitionist movements in both Britain and America, many of whom drew inspiration from Quakerism, Methodism, and other sects of Christianity. Once on Bolama, the colonists engaged only in perfunctory Sunday Bible readings. Their inclusion in the colonial venture of several Jews, including John King and Joseph Montefiore, displayed extraordinary tolerance for the times.

King was born in 1763 in London as Jacob Rey, son of Moses Rey, a Jewish street trader from Gibraltar or North Africa. Jacob received his education in a charity school run by the Spanish and Portuguese in London. In 1771, the school apprenticed him at a business owned by a Jewish merchant. After finishing his tutelage and Anglicizing his name to John King, he worked for an attorney and learned the workings of commerce. Eventually, he became a broker, finding advantageous returns for wealthy clients. King proved good at his work, efficiently and quietly matching needy (and sometimes public) individuals with money loans to tide them over during difficult financial periods. There was nothing untoward or illegal about his practices; Lord Byron (great-uncle of the famous poet) was among the prominent individuals who used King's services. Yet despite the hardship and complexities of his work, the people he helped held him in low regard. Antisemitism ran deep through most of British society in the eighteenth century, and his success inspired a mean-spirited nickname throughout London: the "Jew King."[33]

Given this climate, it is not surprising that King was implicated in several scandals, including allegations of fraud. But public criticism and even disdain did not mar his streak of social generosity. In 1775, he contributed a hundred pounds sterling (a substantial amount) to a charity school in appreciation for his education. He had become an

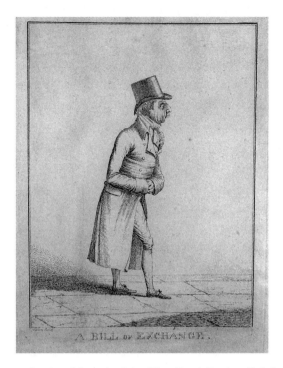

A caricature reputed to be of financier John King (Jacob Rey), called derisively the "Jew King," a member of the Bolama expedition. He returned to Britain on the *Calypso*. Courtesy the Jewish Museum of London.

outspoken critic of the British government by the 1780s and a force for radical social change, claiming to have met Tom Paine as a younger man and been influenced by his thinking. With the prospect of colonization of Bolama, King seemed to believe he could achieve still more prosperity while "doing right" by the people of Africa who were, in the eyes of most Britons, badly in need of European cultural models. As the *Hankey* sailed for Bolama, King was looking forward to an adventure that would lead to fulfilling work gilded by generous remuneration for his efforts. King would stay for only a short time on the island.

Benjamin Marston possessed an idealism equal to Dalrymple's and Beaver's. He was born September 30, 1730, making him sixty-two at the time of the journey to Bolama and the oldest colonist. A socially prominent businessman in the American colonies, he had made the tragic mistake of choosing the wrong side in 1776, a choice that shaped the rest of his life.[34]

Born to a mother from the Winslow family, which traced its American roots back to the *Mayflower,* and a father educated at Harvard College who had become a wealthy, prominent merchant in Salem, Massachusetts, Benjamin Marston grew up in comfortable circumstances. He attended Harvard, graduating in 1749 with a degree in law. After graduation, he sailed to Britain to make the Grand Tour, eventually returning to Boston, where in 1755 he married Sarah Sweet from the nearby town of Marblehead. The couple relocated there soon after their betrothal. Once settled, his wife's family, the Sweets, asked him to participate in a series of lucrative business partnerships jointly with his new brothers-in-law, Jeremiah Lee and Robert Hooper.

Hooper was numbered among the most prosperous businessmen in Massachusetts. By the time Marston joined the partnership, Hooper was deeply entrenched in the Atlantic trade. He purchased virtually all the fish brought into Marblehead, shipped it to ports in northern Spain, receiving gold and silver in payment, and then bought manufactured goods in England that he subsequently sold in Boston. This Boston-Spain-England commercial route is but one example of how the Atlantic Triangular trading networks could enrich merchants buying and selling in each port of call. Such commercial arrangements were crucial, enabling eighteenth-century British merchants to bring, for instance, Indian textiles to African markets and Southeast Asian spices to Europe.[35]

Marston learned his lessons in commerce quickly from his brothers-in-law. By the mid-1770s, he owned a store on Marblehead's King Street, several other shops and warehouse facilities, and three slaves. He had a large, distinguished house in town, plus many real estate holdings in the countryside. Along with his brothers-in-law, Marston's merchant group traded regularly with London, using at least three large ships, which they owned collectively.

He was also an important civic official. Marblehead's voters elected him moderator of town meetings no less than fourteen times between

1765 and 1774. He served on several of the city's management committees, including those for the construction of public buildings, relief to the poor, and public education.

Once fighting broke out at Lexington and Concord, Marston decided to remain loyal to the British crown. Royal Governor Thomas
Hutchinson fled the troubled colony for England in May 1775, having
been driven out by violent crowds. Always despised by the lower
classes—who had once torn down his house during a riot—the ar-
rogant Hutchinson was nonetheless beloved by many well-to-do
merchants. Before he left, Hutchinson received a document signed by
more than two hundred prominent merchants, lawyers, and clergy.
These men asked Hutchinson to carry back to London the message
that they had highly approved of his work as governor, and they desired a restoration of peace and British rule in their colony that would
lead to renewed commercial prosperity. Benjamin Marston numbered among the signatories.

On November 24, 1775, revolutionaries overturned the Marston
family's orderly, gracious life. A group of rioters attacked and ran-
sacked his house that evening, taking his money and ledgers, shatter-
ing his furniture, and carrying off the many books in his beloved
library. Marston fled with his wife, crossing Massachusetts Bay in an
open boat and arriving at the British garrison outside Boston under
cover of darkness. There he found protection from the rebels and
sympathy from other rich Loyalists. But he never saw his home again.
He also lost his wife during this time of bitter transition.

On March 17, 1776, as Marston was busy collecting debts in
Marblehead, Gen. William Howe received orders to evacuate the
British garrison from the city. Howe transported all British troops
and Loyalists by ship to Halifax, Nova Scotia. With a portion of the
250 pounds that he had been able to reacquire, Marston sailed to the
West Indies, bought supplies, and returned to Halifax to sell his wares
to the British Army. During the course of several voyages to the Caribbean, bad luck, robbers, and awful weather dogged him, resulting
in ever-diminishing returns on his investments. During one journey,
when a January gale forced his ship to land in the wilderness 130 miles

south of Halifax, he took refuge among a tribe of Indians for a month
and had to eat his own dog to survive. When he finally made his way
to Halifax in 1782, he was down to his last guinea.

The following year, Marston began anew. He had taken up work
as a surveyor, traveling through the British Maritime Provinces and
along the Miramachi River in New Brunswick. Still, the job proved
to be sporadic in nature. For the next decade, to make ends meet he
also worked periodically as a sheriff and a scientist when surveying
work was unavailable.

Marston journeyed to London in 1787, hoping to find redress for
his petition for the property, worth at least a thousand British pounds,
that he had lost during the Revolution. The government Claims Office denied his appeal, however, and for the next five years Marston
struggled to make ends meet. "Sometimes," according to Philip Beaver, "he was whole days without bread, and for weeks together his
daily expenditure amounted only to three halfpence—a penny worth
of bread and a halfpenny worth of figs. Too noble to beg, yet willing
to work, but unknown and friendless in England, no one would employ him." Marston spent months depressed by the thought that he
was being punished, Job-like, for backing the Loyalist cause, and that
his decision to oppose American independence had resulted in a curse
that might never end.[36]

Marston was living in abject poverty when the opportunity appeared to move to Africa. The Bolama Association offered him a
position as a surveyor. While details of how he attained this offer remain unknown, his response was unbridled joy. "I have at length
waded through the slough of Despondency," he wrote his sister, and
"I am now landed on the opposite side, and shall go on my way re-
joicing."[37]

The pioneering nature of the job was another reason to rejoice.
The upheavals of the past sixteen years had awakened in him an in-
nate love for adventure. Like Philip Beaver, Marston craved the challenges ahead, including, he supposed, the thick jungle, wild animals,
and savage inhabitants. "No expedition could have hit my taste and
humor more exactly than such a one as this promises to do," Marston

wrote excitedly. Like Beaver, he compared himself to a popular fictional character of the day: "It is so much of the Robinson Crusoe kind, that I prefer it vastly to any employment of equal emolument and of a more regular kind that might have been offered me in this country." Marston recognized in himself "that rambling humor which was born with me—and which has never yet been fully gratified"; he prophesied that, "being now unrestrained by any local connections, [it] will be yet prompting me to engage in adventures which will carry me to new scenes, especially while I have vigor of body and mind of fatigue and application."[38]

By this time, Marston had become part of a group of radical thinkers. He envisioned the Bolama enterprise as a crusade against slavery. To him the colonization effort meant a chance "to cut off by the roots that most wicked traffic, the slave trade which all Flesh in this country are strongly setting their faces against." He also wanted to spread the Christian gospel, a more common desire of European civilizers, and to promote free trade. In this respect, Marston subscribed to the philanthropic fervor that engulfed many Britons during the late eighteenth century, even if their philanthropy was sometimes based in profound misunderstandings of the world beyond the British Isles.[39]

His noble intentions notwithstanding, the money from the new job surely swayed the impoverished Marston. He was to receive a salary of sixty pounds sterling per annum, plus subsistence. Along with this came a generous allotment of five hundred acres on the island colony, a perquisite that exceeded his most hopeful expectations. He was so excited about the land that he began to dream about it even before he laid eyes on the island. In a few years, he imagined, his property would increase in value to more than five hundred pounds, and he would reap enormous profits from selling off portions.

Marston also expected to establish a commercial business similar to the one he had had during his days in Marblehead, but on a far grander scale. The company was dedicated to establishing a reciprocal trade relationship between Bolama and other parts of the Atlantic trade circuits. Raw materials in the form of commodities, rather than people, would be shipped from the African settlement to Europe and

North America, and finished goods would return from these areas to West Africa. Although determined to perform his surveying job efficiently, Marston was confident that he could play a prominent role in this new trade system.

Marston's eagerness to join the crusade against slavery was also rooted in his desire to compensate for the "wrongs" he had committed by remaining loyal to the crown. Over the years, Marston had begun to question the stand he and a quarter of the American colonists had taken during the American Revolution. By the time of the Bolama expedition his thinking had evolved, as indicated in the remarks made in the final letter he penned to his sister before embarking on the trip to Bolama:

> There is not remaining the least resentment in my mind to the Country [United States] because the party whose side I took in the late great Revolution did not succeed, for I am fully convinced it is better for the world that they have not. For it [the Revolution] is the foundation—the first step to what has since followed in France and of many others yet in Embryo in the other European kingdoms, in almost all of which the fermentation is already begun. And it will proceed till all Usurpation, all Lording of one over many, both in Spirituals and Temporals, will be entirely wrote off and ended, and man be left master of himself. . . . To be aiding in bringing about such events, though confined to the humble station of Surveyor of Lands, is more eligible, and in fact more meritorious than to be at the head of 100,000 disciplined cutthroats, murdering one's fellow creatures, to gratify the ambition, malice and avarice of some Great Scoundrel and Rascal, called King or Emperor.[40]

In the seventeen years before his voyage to Bolama, Marston had struggled. Now, although only an employee with limited benefits rather than a full-fledged Bolama Association member, he was thrilled about sailing toward a new life of prosperity and redemption. He did experience new adventures, but he had not made much money before he died of a fever in Bolama within a year.

By all accounts, Paul Le Mesurier was suave, debonair, and personally agreeable on every level, although he was not physically handsome. A British Huguenot and Bolama Association subscriber brought into the organization very early, Le Mesurier was an ardent supporter of the plan. In 1792, he was a Member of Parliament and soon to be lord mayor of London. In that official capacity, he worried about how to dispose of criminals sentenced to transportation. British officials had sent lawbreakers to their North American colonies before the American Revolution. (Benjamin Franklin once suggested, satirically, that the colonists should send rattlesnakes to Britain in return.) Le Mesurier believed that Bolama might be the answer. Indeed, some judges in London had already begun specifying Africa as the destination in their transportation orders.[41]

Le Mesurier belonged to the East India Company when the *Hankey* departed for Bolama. Chartered by the crown, this enormously powerful joint-stock company—its highly lucrative import business was partly responsible for the Tea Act that stirred the Bostonians to dump tea into their harbor—enjoyed a monopoly on British trade with the East. The company's reach stretched across India, Southeast Asia, and China, and it lobbied successfully for commercial policies that would bring more profit to its directors. Establishing a British colony in Africa that emphasized wage labor and free trade might be turned into a promising enterprise for the East India Company and, Le Mesurier assumed, profit himself as well. He appealed personally, if unsuccessfully, to Britain's secretary of state to approve the expedition. Le Mesurier's membership in the East India Company also put him into contact with naval men like Philip Beaver and Henry Dalrymple, who sought his advice and support as they organized the Bolama Association.

Le Mesurier was a noted philanthropist who served on the boards of London's Eastern Dispensary, the Huguenot Hospital, and the Asylum for Female Orphans. When he became mayor, he tried to stop merchants from hoarding bread and firewood to drive up the cost. At the same time, he dealt harshly with several demonstrations waged by workers and poor people protesting the forced transportation of petty thieves and the widespread kidnapping of men into the British navy. The act of impressment was carried out by detachments of sailors empowered by the military command to force men into the services, which spawned the hated term "press gang." (In 1795, after months of famine in London and dispiriting defeats of the British by Napoleon, Londoners would again take to the streets, even threatening the king as he drove by in his coach. Le Mesurier did not waver in his loyalty to the crown despite the hard times for the poor.)

Still, the African slave trade disturbed Le Mesurier's conscience. He was among the first subscribers to purchase a former slave's autobiography, *The Interesting Narrative of the Life of Olaudah Equiano, or Gustavus Vassa, the African,* and he was deeply moved when reading it. Published just three years before the Bolama expedition, the antislavery book and Equiano's speaking tour in Britain undoubtedly were familiar to the colonists who set out for Bolama.[42]

The seafaring nature of the new venture also must have appealed to Le Mesurier. Born in 1755 on the island of Guernsey in the English Channel, Le Mesurier was the son of the governor of Alderney, the northernmost Channel Island. He moved as a young man to London, where for several years he tried to create a trading firm connected to his native island, with little success. When the American Revolution began in 1776, Le Mesurier's fortunes changed. He entered into a partnership with Noah Le Cras, and they made a fortune selling supplies to both sides in the War of Independence. Le Mesurier married the daughter of a wealthy silk merchant in 1786, and that same year became sheriff of the city of London.

When the trio of ships bound for Bolama departed on April 13, 1792, Le Mesurier was not aboard, but he had put up a large bond to insure the finances of the enterprise. Despite his support of the Bolama Association and investment as a subscriber, Le Mesurier's responsibilities in London kept him home. Those duties saved him from almost certain death in Africa.[43]

Men like Dalrymple, Beaver, King, Marston, and Le Mesurier assumed primary leadership roles in the Bolama Association for a variety of reasons, including their idealism, humanitarianism, self-interest, love of adventure, and patriotism. Their money, connections, technical education, and gender all worked in their favor as well, enabling them to assume lead roles in the colonial venture.

Whether poor or rich, all the participants in the Bolama adventure were caught up in the swirl of the revolutionary era. The expedition emerged from a ferment of radicalism and reform that typified much of the transatlantic world during the last quarter of the eighteenth century. In North America in 1776, in France in 1789, and in Saint-Domingue in 1791, millions of people engaged in violent rebellions that transformed their societies fundamentally, with the general goal of making all people more equal.

At the heart of this turbulent period was the American Revolution. It produced political independence for the thirteen former colonies and led to the establishment of the Western world's first major republic in more than seventeen centuries. It also unleashed a flood-tide of desire for freedom among many dispossessed and marginalized peoples. Poorer American white males, for instance, demanded and gained greater political rights in the new nation. Revolutionary Pennsylvania and Vermont granted all adult male white taxpayers—not just property owners—the right to vote. The same two states became the first to end the legal sanctions of slavery.

Americans of African descent, who accounted for one of every five people in the new country, seized upon the possibilities trumpeted by the radical rhetoric advocating individual independence. Some pressured their owners, others petitioned state legislatures. Especially sympathetic were the slaves who had fought in the war. (Of course, the British Army had offered the greater inducement, with the promise of freedom from their American masters.) Other slaves simply ran away amid the chaos of the fighting. In total, tens of thousands of slaves claimed their liberty during the 1770s and 1780s.[44]

The French Revolution carried ideas about equality even farther. By attacking hereditary privilege and decapitating the king, queen, and numerous nobles, radicals also aimed to expand the political rights of ordinary men and women. They extended their ideas about liberty, equality, and fraternity to slaves as well, ending racial bondage, at least temporarily, in France's West Indian colonies in the early 1790s. Slaves and free people of color did not hesitate to take advantage of the fervor, staging sporadic rebellions and a bloody revolution in those colonies that quickly mushroomed into a race war. For fifteen years, former slaves and *gens de couleur libre* (free people of color) fended off three of the best European armies and navies, achieving the only successful slave uprising in the modern era and creating the nation of Haiti. Yellow fever carried by the *Hankey* would give the revolutionaries crucial assistance.[45]

Radicals and reformers engaged in less violent efforts to democratize Britain during the first half of the 1790s. Crowds of men and women marched through northern England chanting, "No King! Liberty! Equality!" Sailors staged strikes and riots, occasionally forcing unsympathetic officers to parade naked through the streets. Weavers, laborers, tailors, and cutlers demanded human rights not only for themselves but also for other laborers. Thousands of industrial workers in Manchester, sympathizing with the plight of bound people, signed petitions to end the slave trade. Simultaneously, middle-class artisans and tradesmen formed a host of political societies to advance their reform agenda. Some went so far as to advocate revolution.

In many respects, 1792 was the British equivalent of France's 1789 and America's 1776. Artisans and workers in the London Corresponding Society sent an address to the French Convention praising the "defenders of the Rights of Man" and claiming that the Britons were "preparing to be" as free as the French people. The Sheffield Constitutional Society held pro-French demonstrations and advocated the expansion of the right to vote to the middling and lower classes. Industrial strife occurred in cities in the northeast and ports in East Anglia. Perhaps more frightening, many Britons recognized a radical voice from the past. Tom Paine—the revolutionary gadfly who encouraged radicals as he moved from North America to France to England—published the second half of *The Rights of Man,* a manifesto that advocated equal rights. It reverberated through the British Isles much as *Common Sense* had ignited the North American colonies sixteen years earlier.[46]

Men of property grew fearful that revolution might spread across the Channel from France. Government leaders like William Pitt the Younger, who had once supported modest parliamentary reform in the 1780s, clamped down on the protests. In response to rumors of an insurrection scheduled in London, Pitt sent hundreds of troops into the city, strengthened the defense of the Tower of London, and called up local militias. He also ordered constables to jail hundreds of Londoners, supposedly for plotting to destroy Parliament and Buckingham Palace and even to assassinate the king. During the next few years, Pitt's government suspended habeas corpus and passed the Seditious Meetings Act and the Treason Act, all designed to dampen the ability of radicals and reformers to spread their messages.[47]

The *Hankey* set sail for Africa in the spring of 1792 within this political context. The idea for the expedition had grown out of the radical and reformist movements, but the conservative governmental backlash had set in by the time the ship sailed. Even if the British government did not support their venture, many of the Bolama colonists were still proud of their nation and its ideals. Some of their antislavery motivation emerged from the notion that "British liberties" should be extended to the entire globe. Yet as part of their humanitarian spirit, the Bolama migrants intended to impose their political, cultural, and religious ways of life on African peoples. Unfortunately for them, most Africans had little desire to have their lives transformed by outsiders, even well-intentioned ones.[48]

CHAPTER 3

West Africa

ฉณ

W hile the *Hankey* and *Beggar's Benison* were sailing from port to port searching for the expedition's missing third ship, Henry Hew Dalrymple, the original organizer and governor of the colony, and 148 other passengers on the faster *Calypso* were enduring a much rougher voyage along the European and African coasts. After the *Calypso* had sailed ahead, smallpox scythed through the ship's passengers, killing some and terrorizing all. When the ship finally anchored at Tenerife to await the rest of the expedition, the captain initially lied to port officials, claiming the vessel carried no contagion. However, Dalrymple, the moralist, could not stand dishonest dealings, so he went ashore to inform the Health Office about the smallpox. The authorities promptly ordered the ship into the standard two-week quarantine. Otherwise, they threatened, the fort's cannon would blow them out of the water. The *Calypso* snuck off in the middle of the night, without leaving word of its next destination.[1]

Dalrymple's problems were just beginning. Like Philip Beaver, he now came to the realization that the Bolama Association had neglected to find out precisely where Bolama was located, who owned it, or how to buy it for their planned colony. Dalrymple made a hasty decision, ordering the ship to the nearby port of Gorée, where he hoped to find someone who would know how to find the island.[2]

Gorée, though a tiny island, was an important hub of the Triangular trade. If the interaction in the Canaries established the initial pattern of invasion and occupation of new lands by Europeans, Gorée was among the first outposts established by Europeans to facilitate the transportation of material goods and human slaves around the Atlantic. It became one of the principal French slave factories of coastal West Africa during the fifteenth and sixteenth centuries, supplying unfree laborers whose toil helped enrich much of Europe and North America in the eighteenth century. As in the international battles over the control of oil today, European nations struggled for centuries for control of the slave trade. In the process, the Portuguese, Dutch, French, and English captured and recaptured Gorée a half dozen times.[3]

From his months serving in Gorée, Dalrymple knew that the island had a reputation for laxly enforcing health regulations. It was also an easy port to enter, even for ships with known diseases aboard. After fighting through violent surf to reach shore, however, he realized that the island contained neither a water source nor much extra fresh food for incoming visitors. The few available supplies, imported from France or purchased from the neighboring continent, barely kept alive the African captives held in chains at the fort awaiting sale to the next passing ship.

Because the French Revolution had sharply curtailed imports in recent months, the colony's governor could offer Dalrymple and his fellow pioneers only one small chicken and a few loaves of bread for dinner. Enterprising locals swam out to the *Calypso* pushing barrels of water in front of them to sell to the ship. But Dalrymple located neither a pilot guide nor an interpreter willing to accompany them. The disappointed voyagers sailed south, toward what they hoped was Bolama.

The *Calypso*'s wayward journey lasted several more days before the ship made landfall. Along the way, the death of four passengers did little to boost morale. The passengers committed their dead to the sea and continued subsisting on dried peas and salted meat for a little longer. Then the ship began to leak badly, and the crew had to work overtime, pumping water out of the bottom deck. The *Ca-lypso* entered the channel of the Bijagos Archipelago on May 24, a little more than six weeks after its departure from England. This group of thirty islands forms a cluster that extends nearly eighty miles westward from the coast. By sheer luck, especially given the treacherous tides that swirl around the area, the pioneers reached Bolama, the easternmost of the islands, located very close to the mainland, a few days later. The *Calypso* anchored on the western end of the island, as far from the prying eyes of Portuguese officials at Bissau as possible.[4]

Shortly after their arrival, Dalrymple sent several boatloads of armed men ashore to explore what he believed was an uninhabited island. The appeal of solid ground and a chance to see their new home was too great for the colonists, weary of confinement on the ship. Dalrymple initially pleaded with them to stay on board, but discipline quickly broke down as eager pioneers swarmed ashore to search for water, escape their cramped quarters, and find fresh food. Dalrymple was an easygoing dreamer rather than a hard-driving disciplinarian, and he could not control his passengers.

During their first "jovial day" on the island, they rejoiced in their good fortune, hoisted the British flag, and, disregarding their constitutional pledge to purchase Bolama from the Africans, took possession of the land for the British king. The future of their enterprise seemed worth celebrating. Each male settler, as one of them wrote, "flattered himself with the pleasing idea of acquiring, by his industry, a sufficient fortune to enable him, in a short time, to return to his native country in a state of independence."[5]

On the same day they claimed the island, the settlers spotted a small craft in the distance. Rowing furiously in their jolly boat to catch it, they came even with the craft, which contained six Africans, who informed them in a Portuguese Creole language that this was indeed the island of Bolama. However, they cautioned, the British should not stay there until they held a palaver with the owners, Canabacs, "who were very hostile to Europeans." The Canabacs lived on a nearby island and belonged to the larger ethnic group of Bijago inhabiting the archipelago. The colonists—actually invaders at this

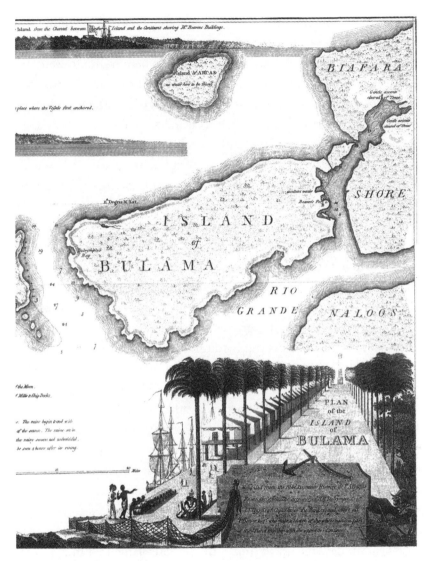

Plan of Island of Bolama. Detail of the "Nautical Map Intended for the Use of Colonial Undertakings" (1794). Note the vision of a colony containing an impressive wharf for trade, where Africans and Britons would work in harmony. From Philip Beaver, *African Memoranda . . .* (London, 1805), frontispiece. Courtesy the Library Company of Philadelphia.

point, since they were occupying somebody else's land—understood neither the African men's language nor their own personal danger.[6]

The pioneers found mangrove swamps, where mosquitoes flourished, surrounding most of the island. The land rose gently from the sea to fifty feet in height. Woods covered much of the island, and monkeys occupied virtually every tree. Natural savannas as well as areas cleared by humans dotted the landscape. The colonists also discovered elephants, a creature they had heard about but never seen, along with gazelles, antelope, hyenas (which some mistook for wolves), and hippopotamuses (which they took to calling water horses). Freshwater springs, a lynchpin for any successful colony, and meadows suitable for agriculture existed across much of the four-hundred-square-mile island. A few of the more ambitious pioneers immediately set about transforming their new, exotic environment, so different from the places they had left. To clear land for planting on one side of the island, they set the long, dry grasses of the fields afire. These fires soon grew out of control, burning through nearby grasslands and jungle trees for days. The residents on the nearby island of Canabac, who claimed Bolama as their own, could easily see the smoke.

The servants and laborers started to gather brush and strip branches, in order to assemble crude huts near the shore. They also began construction of a shelter to store their armaments. Largely unsupervised by Dalrymple, the new arrivals were carefree. They fished, gathered oysters and crabs, chased butterflies, watched wildlife, strolled through the woods, and snoozed in the shade. The place seemed to resemble the paradise they had imagined.[7]

"On Sunday, the 3d of June," Beaver later lamented in his diary about Dalrymple's failures as a leader, "instead of assembling the colonists at prayers, and taking that opportunity of pointing out to them their precise situation, the difficulties they had to encounter, the necessity of order, regularity, sobriety, and industry; in short, the virtues that would ensure the prosperity, or the vices that would tend to the destruction of the colony; instead of doing this, which their situation imperiously called for, everyone was wandering about the island in pursuit of some favorite amusement."[8]

As more than one person has observed, history makes fools of us all. The Bolama colonists could have served as models for that aphorism. Even when three dozen armed African men appeared the next day offshore in a canoe, the colonists were not upset, at least not sufficiently to take precautions. Despite British engagement in the slave trade for more than a century, the colonists knew virtually nothing about Africa or the peoples who lived there. No one in the expedition except Dalrymple had ever set foot on the continent.

In stark contrast, Canabacs and their fellow Bijago across the archipelago knew Europeans all too well. They had been among the first Africans kidnapped and enslaved by white foreigners in the fifteenth century. They had a long history of interactions with British, continental European, and American ship captains and merchants. During the first century of contact, European traders often were powerful enough to seize what they wanted by force, and they had no scruples about kidnapping free people and selling them into slavery. Many of the foreigners had routinely plundered and destroyed Bijago villages if their efforts to obtain slaves were thwarted.

However, Africans gradually began to take control of their interactions with the new intruders. Unlike the Vincheai in the Canary Islands, the Bijago had the immense benefit of adjusting to Europeans over a long period. They learned important lessons from the frequent incursions. They kept all but the most aggressive intentions of the visitors at bay through trade and alliances, and they waged war with those who could not be appeased. The Bijago developed a reputation for considerable military prowess, which they employed against both Europeans and Africans on the continent as they deemed necessary. As a result, they were able to maintain an independent homeland well into the nineteenth century.[9]

The people on Canabac Island grew alarmed when they saw the fires raging on Bolama, and they set off to investigate. They discovered a peculiar tribe of white people cutting down trees, constructing huts, burning grasses, damaging rice fields, and disrupting wildlife—all on an island where Canabacs had hunted and gathered food for generations. It required no great leap of imagination to conclude that these strangers had come to take their land. Canabacs knew very well how to respond to white predators. They would repel the intruders from their shores.

A week after the settlers occupied Bolama, according to colonist Joshua Montefiore, they "were surprised by the arrival of a war canoe full of armed *Indians*" (a term the British used indiscriminately for indigenous peoples around the globe). Montefiore described the encounter:

> I was deputed with a flag of truce to parley with them. When I arrived at the canoe, which was not until I was up to my middle in mud and water, I found near forty men on the beach, and in the canoe, armed with muskets and cutlasses. These men were stout and tall, but had very disagreeable features, their lips being exceedingly thick, and their noses remarkably broad and flat. Their complexion was of a coal black, and they had no sort of clothing, except a small leather apron behind, which was brought forward tight betwixt the thighs, and tied to the middle.[10]

Shouting from their canoes, the Canabacs warned the settlers to leave and then quickly paddled out of sight around the end of the island. The pioneers might not have understood every word of the Portuguese Creole commonly used along the coast, but this warning was unambiguous. After several hours of deliberation, the migrants decided against taking action other than retreating to the protection of their ship that night.

When they went ashore in search of water the next morning, the colonists found that during the night the Canabacs had carted off every article left on the beach, from kitchenware to linen. The Canabacs had given their second notice to the invaders.

After the seizure of the colonists' goods, Montefiore urged his shipmates aboard the *Calypso* to abide by the pledge they had made in Britain to locate the local people and offer to purchase the island. After some discussion, and again proving himself an ineffective leader, Dalrymple demurred, deciding to wait instead for the arrival of the *Hankey* and the trade goods it carried before approaching the Canabacs about selling some of their land. The decision to delay was a serious mistake.

The settlers remained remarkably blithe about the risks, continuing to send out unarmed people to survey the island. Several of the explorers brought back "two elephant's teeth [tusks] that had been dropped." Their report was very encouraging:

> They found the island clear of wood in many places, and covered with high grass; the soil rich and fertile; several large rivulets of wholesome water, and good lofty timber of various qualities, fit and convenient for every purpose. . . . The country is somewhat flat, except in the middle, which is mountainous; in many places the land had been cleared, and cultivated for rice. The party met with large droves of buffaloes, deer, antelopes, and wild hogs, with flocks of Guinea fowls and pigeons. Of fruits, they observed, wild plumbs, grapes, and the sour pap.[11]

They also reported spotting thousands of monkeys, one in "almost every tree." The colonists killed several and found them good to eat. What they did not know, and what would not be understood for another century, was that these monkeys harbored a vicious strain of yellow fever, circulated among them by mosquitoes that infested the mangrove swamps of Bolama.[12]

A few days later, on a hot sunny afternoon, the Canabacs launched a preemptive strike. Having reconnoitered for several days, they devised a clever strategy. Landing on the other side of the island, they surprised the British invaders during their daily nap, when only a few were on shore. Combatants equipped with guns fired an initial volley into the hut containing the armaments, then rushed the blockhouse, seized the sixty firearms stored there, and turned them against the settlers. They killed the tailor Aaron Baker and wounded Henry Gardiner, a member of the Bolama Council.

Meanwhile, a second group of Canabacs, armed with four-foot rapiers, sprinted down the shore to intercept colonists retreating toward the ocean hoping to reach the *Calypso,* anchored a few hundred yards from shore. As the injured Gardiner stumbled into the sea, pleading for mercy and raising his arm for protection, one of the adversaries slashed off his hand. In a shocked, bloody daze, Gardiner walked up to his chin in the water, where he stood for several hours until he died. Ironically, considering the colonists' aim of introducing Africans to commerce, the Canabacs cut off Gardiner's hand with weapons that came from expert blade makers in Solingen, Germany, evidence of Africans' established trade patterns with Europe.

The Canabacs dispatched four more colonists in equally bloody fashion, hacking them to bits on the beach within sight of the ship. They then fired their weapons at the *Calypso* itself, although it was out of range of their muskets. This was far from the triumphant arrival the colonists had envisioned. "The noise and confusion that reigned on board our ship is not to be imagined," wrote Montefiore. "Some bewailed the loss of their husbands, others of their fathers, and some of their wives and children, a scene too shocking to dwell upon." Eventually, the passengers and crew regrouped, hauled their guns out of the hold, and mounted four cannon on the ship's decks. Realizing they were no match for Bijagos in canoes, the men decided not to lower any boats to aid their compatriots. It was too late for that, in any case, for the would-be colonists' bodies that lay sprawled on the shore.[13]

The Canabacs spared most of the women and children on land, taking them as prisoners. They dragged into their canoes five adults and three children, including Susan and Julia Baker, two of Aaron Baker's daughters, who had collapsed in tears at the sight of their father's death. When the wounded wife of Henry Gardiner could not keep up with the retreat to their canoes, they shot her. All told, the Africans killed eight people, wounded a number of others, and took seven captives. Since the laborers and servants had been assigned to start work on shore, they suffered the highest number of casualties.

Not all the settlers on shore died in this initial hostile exchange. Some hid among the rocks, while others fled into the forest. When the group of Canabacs decamped with their prisoners, the remaining survivors waded neck deep into the ocean, waiting for a jolly boat from the *Calypso* to rescue them. The frightened people on the ship, however, responded warily, sending out assistance only after dark, and then refusing to land a boat on shore. The settlers were too terrified to retrieve the bodies of the dead. Keeping watch on deck that evening, the colonists could hear something rustling in the trees near the bodies.

The following morning, a group of heavily armed colonists went ashore, intending to retrieve both the human remains and the filled water casks, essential to any voyage. They found nothing but skulls and bones. In a sure sign of their savagery, the British thought, the local Africans had eaten the bodies of their friends and loved ones. The pioneers could easily believe the rumors about cannibals that circulated in Europe. They had not seen the hyenas and other scavenger animals that had surely been responsible for devouring the corpses during the night. The sight of the picked skeletons so disconcerted the landing party that they fled in terror.[14]

Fear enveloped the passengers on board the *Calypso*. The ship winched up its anchor and unfurled its sails, heading for anywhere *but* Bolama. As the canvases filled with wind, the "Indians came down to the beach, attired some in men's, and others in women's apparel, belonging to our people whom they had murdered or taken prisoners, hallooing, hooting, and treating us with contempt and derision," wrote Joshua Montefiore. A few feinted chasing the *Calypso* in their huge canoes. From the Canabacs' perspective, they had merely protected their lands and won another victory over European invaders and slave traders. From the standpoint of the settlers, their initial view of Bolama as paradise had turned into a conviction that Bolama instead was a hell, but at least they were safe from "savages" for the moment.[15]

The settlers had learned that Africans could be formidable foes, and they believed that they had witnessed evidence of cannibalism. The colonists' only hope was to retreat to the more "civilized" precincts populated by Europeans more like themselves: the slavers at Bissau.

With hindsight, it is easy to wonder how Dalrymple could have been so inept as a leader and the colonists so heedless of danger. The crew and pioneers on the *Calypso* seem to have given every appearance of trying to steal the Canabacs' island; how could they not have expected to be attacked in return? In a scenario repeated often during the centuries of European imperial "explorations," the colonists saw little reason not to move onto and reshape the land that they anticipated would be theirs. The Bolama pioneers, though, at least intended to buy the property rather than seize it by force. But the local West African people, who had long had to resist European encroachments on their land and their freedom, were unwilling to wait for the colonists to declare their peaceful intentions.

On June 5, 1792, the *Calypso,* in full flight from the Canabac attack five days earlier, encountered the *Hankey* and *Beggar's Benison.* The two smaller ships had just left Bissau, the nearby Portuguese colonial capital. They were headed for Bolama when the three ships spied one another. Hauling to the wind, the seamen on the *Hankey* and the *Beggar's Benison* brought their vessels alongside. Rather than celebrate a joyous reunion, however, the passengers on the *Calypso* spilled out horrifying tales of murder, cannibalism, and kidnapping.

Many of the passengers were suffering physically as well, enervated by months of subsisting on dried foods. Moreover, a mysterious fever had broken out on board. They did not yet know it, but yellow fever had sneaked onto the *Calypso.* In their brief time on Bolama, some of the colonists had caught the disease. In addition, when they refilled their water barrels, they brought the infectious mosquitoes buzzing around the casks onto the ship. Yellow jack was preparing to make its vicious tour of the Atlantic Ocean.

Recognizing the possible contagion of the new fever, the leaders on the two uninfected ships decided to keep their distance from the *Calypso.* The resolution contradicted previous Bolama Association policy, in which people were free to move among the vessels, mixing together with friends and family. The exasperated passengers on the infected ship responded by berating their fellow colonists. "Nothing was heard but mutual reproaches from the people of the *Calypso,*" Beaver complained, along with arguments urging everyone to return to England immediately. Beaver believed that their complaints resulted from being "tired with the length of the voyage, irritated with sickness, their loss of their associates, and the disappointment of their hopes." Consequently, they "became extremely dissatisfied with their situation." Beaver urged the colonists to band together while maintaining the temporary quarantine. He then took the jolly boat to Bissau to see if he could find some assistance.[16]

The horror created by the Canabacs' attack swiftly circulated to the other ships once they made the decision to send Beaver to the Portuguese slaving port. "When I quitted the *Hankey* on the morning of the 5th to seek help in Bissau," Beaver noted, "I had left a quiet, clean, healthy, and orderly ship, the colonists contented and in good spirits." However, when he returned just two days later, "I found a noisy, dirty, disorderly ship, the colonists dissatisfied and dispirited. That such a change could have been operated in so short a time was scarcely credible, but such was the effect of the *Calypso*'s rejunction."[17]

The colonists needed to address several pressing problems. A number were dead, their bodies strewn (and eaten) on the beach at Bolama, and their remains needed recovery and interment. In addition, the four women and three children held hostage by the Canabacs had to be rescued. Dalrymple, Beaver, and other council members debated their next course of action. Tellingly, and setting a future precedent for how power would be exercised in the colony, these men ostensibly committed to democracy found it hard to share decision making. Without consulting the rest of the colonists, the council chose to retreat to Bissau. It was the closest safe harbor, and there they could regroup, resupply, and obtain assistance to redeem the hostages. A few of the leaders wanted to immediately abandon Africa altogether. Others, like Beaver, still held out hope that they could buy Bolama from its owners and continue with the colonial venture. The three ships weighed anchor at noon on June 8 and set off to Bissau.

The glorious ideals of the colonists aboard the *Calypso* had already run up against harsh reality. From this time on, they would need to employ practical if mundane means of making their dreams come true. Fortunately for the Britons, a hardheaded individual by the name of Philip Beaver was ready to wrangle with Portuguese authorities in nearby Bissau and find ways to negotiate with the Canabacs. Beaver's journals provide the major source for information about what happened on Bolama. When the three ships of the expedition finally reunited, the prosaic work of setting up their colony would begin in earnest. Many colonists were ready to give up the enterprise at this point, but Beaver and a number of others insisted that the colonial enterprise was still feasible.

CHAPTER 4

Cross-Cultural Negotiations

ဘဝ

I ronically, and certainly unknown to them, the antislavery colonists had chosen an island that lay at the heart of the region where the Atlantic slave trade had begun. After the Portuguese tried unsuccessfully to conquer the Vincheai in the Canary Islands, northwest of the Bijago's homeland, they established an outpost on an unoccupied island of the Cape Verde archipelago south of the Canaries. In 1446, two Portuguese ships, commanded by Gil Eannes and Nuño Tristão, became the first European vessels of record to sail down the West African coast as far south as the Bijagos Archipelago. They were equipped with the new technology of the movable lateen sail, which they had picked up from Arabs. These sails would enable them to tack into the strong northern headwinds on their return to Portugal. Eannes and Tristão landed at the Bijagos Islands to buy ivory, pepper, and gold—commodities (along with a few slaves) that West Africans and Europeans had been trading overland for centuries via caravans across the Sahara.[1]

After exchanging goods with Africans in the region, the two captains attacked a Bijago village, kidnapping a handful of individuals and carrying them back to Portugal as slaves. It was a suitably brutal beginning for one of the greatest crimes in world history.[2] Hundreds of European explorers around the world, including Christopher Columbus, would continue this tradition of kidnapping indigenous peoples to take home to display, present as gifts to kings and queens, or use as bound servants.

As early as 1526, slavers began to sail regularly between Africa and the Americas. Portuguese and Spanish slavers initially bought Africans from the Upper Guinea coast, the region encompassing Bolama. During the seventeenth century, the slave trade expanded substantially to meet the labor demands of the plantations in the West Indian sugar islands and Portuguese Brazil. Slavers transported the largest number of captives from Upper Guinea in the seventeenth and early eighteenth centuries. At the same time, they started to work more intensively south of Bolama, especially in the Bight of Benin and the Bight of Biafra. The number of enslaved people forced across the Atlantic Ocean by the two Iberian powers rose sharply from the end of the eighteenth century until the end of the slave trade in the second half of the nineteenth century. However in total, only 4 or 5 percent of Africans transported as slaves across the Atlantic came from the regions near Bolama.[3]

Both the Bijago and the colonists were compelled to conduct their lives within the framework of imperial expansion, industrialization, and, crucially, the slave trade, striving to maintain their communities and cultures against a vast array of forces, both local and international. The British colonists, pulled to Africa by altruism and avarice, were also pushed from their homeland by a variety of problems that afflicted their communities, the region, and the larger Atlantic world. Over the centuries, the Bijago had developed creative strategies to deal with the growing importance of buying, selling, and slaving, while at the same time resisting capture and transportation themselves. One mistake might condemn an individual or an entire village, along with all their future offspring, to a lifetime of slavery. Neither the Bijago nor the British were able to act completely independently of the intermeshed economic, political, and social networks that framed their choices. In that sense, the struggles of the two groups had parallels, even as there were also vital differences.

The colonists did not have to fear the brute power exercised by well-armed slavers in Africa. The Bijago had the home-field advantage, local knowledge, an advantage that they successfully defended for a long time. If measured by sheer longevity, the Bijago held their own against the Europeans who initiated the Atlantic slave trade in the region, certainly for a far longer period than the Vincheai. The Bijago were able to control many of the aspects of their existence for more than four centuries. In stark contrast to the Bijago's local knowledge and centuries of dealing with Europeans, the colonists knew nothing of the region or its history, which played no small part in their inability to found a successful settlement. The changing nature of commerce, cooperation, and strife with their neighbors on the nearby African coast played a significant role in the Bijago's ability to manage their affairs.

When their ships entered the harbor of Bissau following the *Calypso*'s disastrous experience on Bolama, the pioneers saw an island covered with woods, on which small mountains sloped like an amphitheater from the shore to their peaks. The island lay a short distance from the African continent, but just far enough away to be defensible against nearby coastal residents. Defense of their slave factory, from both interior attack and hostile European ships, was a key consideration for the Portuguese. Bissau's governor and merchants were organizing the selling and shipment of thousands of slaves to the coffee plantations of Brazil when the *Hankey* arrived. The Portuguese were purchasing mostly Mandinka slaves from north of Bissau, Nalu slaves from the south, and Papel slaves from the east.[4]

The fort at Bissau was impressive. Philip Beaver estimated that it contained fifty cannon and three hundred soldiers, though he dismissed most of the military men as worthless since they were criminals sent into forced exile (the British had been manning their own African forts in the same way since the early 1780s). Yet the Portuguese governor and army were still strong enough to handle the Bolama colonists, if need be. The governor had imprisoned Beaver on their first meeting, and he subsequently used the threat of further jail time to keep Beaver from interfering in the established trade between Bissau merchants and local peoples.

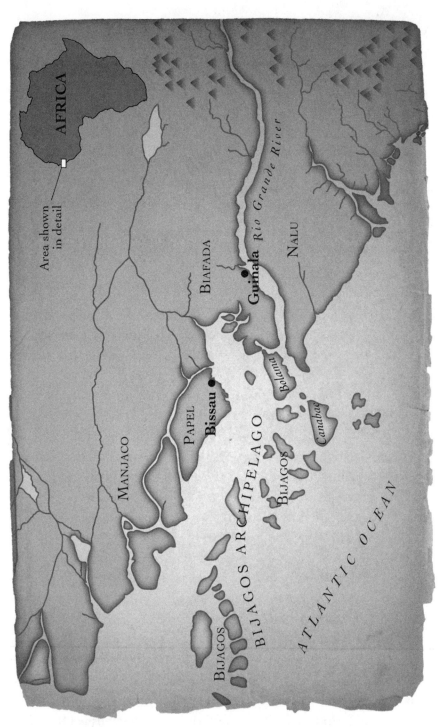

Bolama region, 1790s. Map drawn by Michele Angel.

The world the Bolama colonists stumbled into was already governed by long-established trade and power relationships. The Portuguese had been unable to move inland after founding Bissau. The Kaabu state had governed the area around the major rivers of Guinea when the Portuguese first arrived in the fifteenth century, and the Kaabu's military strength, assisted by tropical diseases, was still keeping the Europeans from moving up the nearby rivers. Over the centuries, as the Portuguese took slaves and African wives back to their Cape Verdean colony, a European and African mixed-race population had emerged. These people became intermediaries between Europeans and Africans, as well as traders who interacted with the various ethnic groups of the Guinea-Bissau coast, since they had many friends and kin among the various communities.[5]

The Portuguese called this West African coastal section Guinea, a name that came to define the region between the Sénégal River and Cape Palmas. (At the time, the British used it indiscriminately to describe all of Africa.) Though the Portuguese were never able to conquer local Africans or dictate terms of trade with them, they did encourage dissension among the numerous groups in the region. This policy enabled them to buy captives seized in local wars and ship them across the Atlantic. Yet West Africans exerted considerable control over the commercial and cultural networks that linked the Cape Verde Islands, the slave fort named Bissau, and the surrounding areas, including the Bijagos Islands. Some West Africans benefited from the Atlantic trade, acquiring not only new material goods but also the innovative ideas that circulated widely. While European nations were rivals but had a sense of shared culture, West Africans shared many elements of their cultures but simultaneously redirected their rivalries into an evolving economic system in which the slave trade played an increasingly greater role over time.[6]

The Bijago tried to manage the commerce in slaves so that they would lose as few of their own people as possible.[7] From the beginning of contact, the inhabitants of the Bijagos Islands had pursued an even more hostile strategy than the Kaabu to shield their lands from European encroachment. Early European explorers and merchants both feared and grudgingly admired the Bijago for their aggressive behavior, their huge canoes suited for combat, and their daring raids on European shipping and local peoples along the western coast. The violence seemingly peaked in the early seventeenth century, when Bijago combatants forced three groups of Biafada, an ethnic group living on the continent, to appeal for protection to both the Portuguese government and the Catholic pope. When the British antislavery colonists arrived in 1792, some Biafada still claimed original ownership of Bolama Island, maintaining that the Bijago had forced their ancestors to flee earlier in the century.[8]

This history of continual conflict punctuating the commerce between Africans and Europeans provides a longer-range perspective for the Canabacs' fierce response to the Bolama colonists' first landing. Most important, the Canabacs believed the pioneers to be yet another group of European invaders meaning to occupy their land. When several warnings failed to dislodge them, an attack seemed the natural next step, part of the aggressive strategy that had served the Bijago well in defending their homeland in the past. For centuries, African coastal societies had grown increasingly militarized in order to fend off attempts to enslave them. As one European ship captain recognized, "Upon the whole of the sea coast, and for a considerable distance inland, the natives are very dexterous in the use of fire-arms." Indeed, "the prevalence of the practice is doubtless to be attributed to the insecurity of person" of people who were constantly subject to capture and enslavement. (According to many abolitionists, the Africans' desire for firearms was one of the tragic by-products of the slave trade.)[9]

The Bijago, like many other West Africans (and not unlike many Native Americans), slowly grew more dependent over time on items acquired in trade with Europeans. Because they were unreliable, European guns usually were not the most important defensive weapons used by local people. Instead, iron spears and swords were crucial. The Atlantic trade became the source of most of the iron with which the Bijago and their neighbors fashioned both weapons and agricultural implements. The trade itself became a vicious circle: Africans used metal weapons to capture their neighbors to sell to Europeans for the iron, which they used to make more weapons.

As a British navy officer on half pay, Philip Beaver respected the prowess of the Bijago. "Every Bijago is a warrior; his amusement the chace, his delight war." For weaponry, the men used "a long buccaneer gun kept in the most perfect order and carried in the right hand; a solingen [German] sword, about four feet long and as sharp as a razor, is slung on the left shoulder." They also toted spears and convex shields covered in tough animal hides. Beaver admired their skill: "In the use of the broad sword they are more active and expert than any people whom I have ever seen." After the *Calypso's* disastrous first encounter, the Bolama colonists were terrified of the Canabacs, perhaps as much because of their own predisposition to imagine all Africans to be vicious cannibals as because of the Africans' weapons and reputation as fearsome combatants.[10]

The Bijago's warlike behavior would probably not have been enough to ward off all Portuguese attacks over the centuries. However, their combination of military prowess and commercial and political acumen enabled the Bijago to remain independent until well into the nineteenth century. Three centuries of European-African trade provided the basis for their success. The Bijago were among the most active slavers in the region, making raids on coastal communities from their canoes, which measured as much as eighty feet in length and were capable of carrying more than a hundred people. The Bijago supplied Africans to the Portuguese by capturing people from rival groups, especially the Biafada, and selling them to ship captains.[11]

Nonetheless, this strategy did not shield the Bijago entirely from being captured and sold into bondage themselves. While some European captains refused to purchase Bijago because of their reputation for rebellion or suicide once enslaved, a number of Bijago still ended up chained in the holds of ships sailing to the Americas; most of these were transported to Portuguese Brazil. More women than men fell victim to slavery, in part because the warrior mentality made males more difficult to capture alive. Through the centuries of struggle, the Bijago had lost so many people to war and kidnappers that they suffered a significant population decline during the decades preceding the appearance of the Bolama colonists; this may have been the reason none of them lived on Bolama when the pioneers first landed there.[12]

Supplying slaves was hardly the only way that Africans helped shape the terms of Atlantic trade. Along the western coast, from Senegal to Cape Mount, African traders defined iron bars as the medium of exchange with which to value European and local goods. The negotiations over buying Bolama Island from the Bijago, for example, would take place using this measure of exchange, although additional goods were included in the bargaining. The value of a bar fluctuated from place to place along the coast, as Africans controlled this monetary system and Europeans apparently had to adjust. As one British ship captain complained, there was no strict equivalence between bars and shillings, at least according to European measures of worth. A gun "that costs 20 shillings might sell for 6 bars, while tobacco equal to 4 or 5 shillings may also be 6 bars." Africans established their own valuation of goods, and local merchants impressed ship captains with their quick, effortless calculations in converting prices and payments among iron bars, British pounds, Portuguese reals, and American dollars. These African agents frequently were more sophisticated and accustomed to cross-cultural commercial relations than their European counterparts.[13]

Philip Beaver's experiences with African merchants, both Bijago and Biafada, convinced him that Africans were shrewd bargainers. He believed that slave-ship captains had taught Africans "only the vices" of commerce, and that, in the process, Africans "had been tutored in the arts of deceit." Beaver gave Europeans too much credit, even if negative, since Africans had been trading with other Africans for centuries. Even when white slavers used underhanded business practices such as light weights or short measures, they had difficulty imposing their own terms.[14] Africans along the coast, for instance, forbade Europeans to sell salt to people in the continental interior, since they wanted to keep the lucrative trade for themselves.

Initially, Africans provided gold, ivory, wax, ostrich feathers, and spices for trade with Europeans; they later added rice, soap, and cattle to this list. The commerce in slaves, however, eventually became pre-eminent as the demand for laborers escalated in the plantations in the West Indies and Brazil. British and French merchants became serious competitors with the Portuguese in the slave trade, especially during the eighteenth century. This competition benefited African traders, since it enabled them to bargain up the price of slaves as well as to demand more barter items in exchange.[15]

By the early nineteenth century, Africans had begun demanding a wide range of goods from Europeans. In 1807, one ship captain advised British slavers to bring a variety of specialized products from around the world, such as handmade cloth from East India. In response, factory owners in Manchester turned their workers and machines to making cheap knockoffs of the printed cotton and silk materials, and then sent them to Africa. Among other items Africans purchased were rum and tobacco from the Americas, as well as muskets, gunpowder, swords, flints, knives, pewter basins, axes, hatchets, looking glasses, and a host of miscellaneous manufactured items from Britain and Europe. This wide exchange of goods provided profits throughout the Atlantic region, at least for those who could stay free of the slavers.[16]

The Europeans' lust for the profits of this trade provided yet another means for Africans to escape slavery. South of Bolama, on the Gold Coast of the Gulf of Guinea, the British Company of Merchants controlled the infamous Cape Coast Castle as a slave factory but maintained good relations with the nearby African communities precisely to keep their private and company trade going. Problems there in the 1780s were directly linked to the unwillingness of some British to follow established African rules of barter and the consequent disruption of the trade by local Africans. The Portuguese at Bissau would remain suspicious of the Bolama colonists' intention of taking at least some of the local trade between Europeans and Africans for themselves. The colonists on Bolama would eventually find that favoring one African community over a neighboring rival in trade relations was one of their many misjudgments in their new environment.[17]

When the Bolama Association's three ships anchored at Bissau, the passengers discovered three slave vessels moored near the wharves. Each ship sailed beneath the flag of a different nation: Portugal, Britain, and the United States. Despite their repugnance for slavery, the passengers did not mind being ensconced in the nearest equivalent of a civilized European town. Initially, the prospects of the would-be settlers appeared to improve. The association hired Joseph Cordoza de Sylva, a local Portuguese merchant, to begin negotiations with the Canabac Island Bijago for the return of the women and children from the *Calypso*.

They also received a welcome of a different sort. News of the British expedition and its plans to colonize Bolama had spread quickly along the West African coast. The following day a delegation arrived from the Papel, who lived on the continent, east of Bissau, and had a long history of both trading and fighting with the Portuguese.[18] The delegation delivered a curious letter to the Bolama colonists, translated into English by a local ship captain. The Papel "king"—Europeans erroneously labeled all local leaders around the world kings and queens after their own traditions—had learned that the British wanted to establish a colony nearby. "The Portuguese would not allow you to settle here. But it is not for them to choose," complained the Papel leader, asking bluntly, "Does the country belong to them?"[19]

The Papel urged the British colonists to "settle here," among them, "though the Roman Catholics [meaning any Portuguese] with you should go elsewhere." Along with the missive, the Papel leader sent the British his cane—a common West African symbol of power—as "proof of his fidelity and attachment": "You may depend on the king's word, as he declares he is ready to take up any cause against the Portuguese." The probable motivation of the Papel is not hard to divine. They envisioned the British as a potential trading partner and ally, who would undermine the monopoly of the Portuguese. Like many other West Africans, they sought to play one European nation against another, a strategy that mirrored the Europeans' relations with different African groups.[20]

The Bolama Association leaders suddenly found themselves thrust into the middle of long-standing disputes among African peoples as well as between the Portuguese and these societies. The colonists desired friendship with the Papel, but they desperately needed assistance from the Portuguese. Dalrymple took a diplomatic approach, informing the Papel leader in a letter that he "gratefully returned thanks," but the colonists were "desirous of avoiding all occasions of offence to their friends the Portuguese that may tend to weaken the firm and faithful alliance which has long subsisted between their respective sovereigns."[21]

In addition to hiring Cordoza de Sylva, Beaver also engaged the services of Captain Moore, commander of the U.S. slave ship *Nancy*. Moore opened negotiations with the Canabac Island Bijago for the colonists' purchase of the island of Bolama. Simultaneously, Moore's *grumettas*—hired African workers (who later would play a key role in the colony)—negotiated the ransom of the three women and two children who had been taken hostage. The price was 250 bars of iron, worth approximately 40 British pounds. As collateral in the continuing talks about Bolama, however, one of the captured women, the visibly pregnant Mrs. Harley, and her young daughter remained on Canabac Island.[22]

When the female hostages were returned, they were all naked, which grated on Beaver's sense of European women's modesty. Yet otherwise the captives had received kind treatment. After the violence of June 3 at Bolama, such humane behavior surprised Beaver and the other colonists, who had feared the Africans might have raped, killed, or eaten the prisoners. Instead, "these women had been very well treated by the Canabacs," wrote Beaver. He believed that the Africans' self-restraint might have resulted from the fact that they looked upon white woman "rather as objects of disgust than desire." Indeed, marveled Beaver, "their devil is white."[23]

With the majority of the hostages returned and negotiations for the purchase of the island proceeding, the three ships sailed the fifty miles from Bissau back to Bolama. Fever continued to afflict the people on the *Calypso,* though the sickness had yet to reach the *Hankey.* Even discounting the sick, the potential colonists were slightly fewer in number. Nine dissatisfied pioneers asked to stay in Bissau, hoping to find passage back to England. Among them were two senior association subscribers, who were effectively abandoning their investment, and six servants. From this time forward, Beaver started to keep a daily tally of the loss of colonists by death, desertion, or disappearance. His scorecard over the next eighteen months would present the expedition's grimmest—if perhaps most accurate—reckoning.

The ships anchored at the western end of Bolama during the evening of June 22, in the same bay the *Calypso* had chosen. Just after dawn the following morning, Beaver and a ship's mate from the *Hankey* went ashore. They planned to inspect the area where the conflict on the beach had taken place and recover whatever they could of the abandoned dead. They found a few scattered planks from the primitive structure the colonists had started to build, but "not a vestige of human bone." "We therefore returned on board," wrote Beaver, "thinking that we had mistaken the place of attack." A group of thirty heavily armed men from both the *Hankey* and *Calypso* later returned to the shore, intending to find and inter the dead. They had limited success. Three weeks had passed since the attack, and all that remained, after exposure to hyenas and other scavenging animals, were two human skulls and a few bones. The colonists buried these in a deep grave near a tree, where they inscribed a Christian cross. They collected the few planks, climbed back into their launches, and returned to the ships.[24]

The expedition set off to explore the other end of the island, but in the receding tide the *Hankey* drifted aground, raising questions once again about Captain Cox's competence. All the ships had to wait together until the next morning to embark. Given the previous attack on the island, the overnight stay produced a great deal of anxiety among the colonists, but no combatant parties appeared. Riding a swelling tide at dawn the following day, the three ships sailed to the opposite end of Bolama, anchoring a few hours later in a pleasant, deep channel—large enough, claimed one excited colonist, to hold nearly the entire British navy.[25]

The colonists had finally arrived at their chosen destination. However, the Bijago remained perilously close, from the perspective of the Britons: only thirty miles away on Canabac Island. Moreover, the purchase of Bolama had still not been completed. The pioneers desperately needed to establish a constructive relationship with the Canabacs since they were, after all, neighbors capable of providing assistance or harm in this alien wilderness. Beaver, several colonists, and two grumettas on loan from Captain Moore loaded the *Beggar's Benison* with an assortment of goods "brought from Europe, to make presents to the native chiefs, and to purchase of them the island of Bolama," and cruised toward Canabac Island. Beaver characterized one of the grumettas, named Gillion, as "an honest, good, and valuable man," and he proved critical in serving as the mediator in the purchase of the land.[26]

Those left behind on the ships at Bolama felt a mixture of exhilaration and fear. In the next few days, their dream of transforming the world through their humanitarian colony might begin to come true. The group busied itself with examining the channel at the eastern end of Bolama, determining that it was "commodious," between seven and fifteen fathoms deep. But charting the territory was much easier than trying to discern the Canabacs' intentions. Just as the local flora and fauna struck the colonists as a sharp contrast to what they were used to seeing in Britain, the local people seemed to them equally mysterious and frightening.

The next morning on Canabac, Jalorem, a leader of one of the island villages, and a crowd of people stood patiently on the beach, awaiting envoys from the ship to come ashore. Beaver was wary: "We had learned through the grumettas, who had redeemed our women, that the Bijago were willing to treat with us for the sale of the island of Bolama, and that we should find no difficulty in purchasing it. Yet we were at the same time informed that these were a treacherous and faithless people, in whose professions no confidence could be placed and we ought therefore to be always on our guard, for they would lose no opportunity of surprising us if anything was to be gained."[27] These negative characterizations probably came from the Portuguese and neighboring local people on the continent, all of whom felt long-standing animosity toward the Bijago.[28]

"Unconnected by any ties with the neighbouring nations, whom they generally hold in contempt," Beaver wrote, the Bijago "consider the world as their own; and that what it contains they have a right to plunder." The only valid comparison among European nations, Beaver thought, was to the Algerians, who "war with everybody and always plunder the weak." Beaver had convenient amnesia about the past several hundred years of European conquest, plunder, and slave raiding in West Africa.[29]

The initial meeting between the colonists and the Canabacs went extremely well. Beaver later described Jalorem as mild and with a "peaceable" disposition. The following day, Jalorem sent his two sons, Jamber and Demiong, with the grumetta Gillion to visit aboard the *Beggar's Benison,* where they were well received, and they chatted comfortably about the ownership of the island and the return of Mrs. Harley and her daughter. After some negotiations, they decided that a party from the cutter should go ashore, while Jamber and Demiong remained aboard the ship as good-faith hostages—a custom common in bargaining between Africans and European slave-ship captains.

As the launch carried Beaver and several others toward shore, dozens of Canabacs waded into the sea to give them a friendly greeting, in their enthusiasm almost overturning the jolly boat. The Canabac leaders guided the party to a house belonging to Jalorem's wife that was set back a distance from the shore. "We entered the house, composed of three concentric circles, with six doors through one of its diameters," Beaver wrote. "In the inner circle lay [Mrs. Harley], but it was so dark that one could not see, and she knew not of our arrival." Some women lighted small parcels of long straws, "which they held upright in their hands," allowing the group to see. "On a wicker frame, supported by half a dozen posts about a foot from the ground, and covered with long grass, lay Mrs. Harley and her young child."[30]

Harley initially said nothing, only gazing at Beaver. After being a hostage for twenty-five days, she was in a debilitated state, suffering from various ailments, and wearing the same clothes in which she had been captured. "She stared upon me with such a look of hope, of doubt, of fear, and of madness, as I shall never forget," Beaver wrote. He re-created their dialogue from memory in his published book, which appeared a decade later.

"Mrs. Harley," Beaver remembered saying, "I am come to put an end to your sufferings, and to carry you back to your husband, whom I left well the day before yesterday."

"Who are you, sir?" Mrs. Harley responded. "How came you here? Do I dream? Are you a prisoner?"

"No," Beaver replied. "I am come to redeem you and your child, to take you back to your family, and to purchase of the king the island of Bolama."

Beaver explained that he needed to meet with "King" Jalorem and that she should prepare herself to return to the ship. As he turned to leave, Mrs. Harley became panic-stricken at the prospect of Beaver's abandoning her. She begged him to stay. After a lengthy discussion, Beaver convinced her that he would return.

Bijago women helped prepare Mrs. Harley and her daughter for the trip back to the launch, displaying "delicacy and feeling which, from either pole to the equator," Beaver commented, "will be generally found characteristic of their sex." Beaver's view about the unwavering nature of men and women's behavior superseded any notions about differences among people due to race or habitation. He generally ignored Bijago women, just as he ignored female colonists, although he commented that the Canabac women performed "all the menial domestic duties" that British female colonists would be expected to do. Beaver described the women on Canabac Island as being as "simple in their dress as the men[;] a thick fringe made of the shred of palm leaves, about six inches long, tied round their waist, formed their only clothing."

Englishwomen such as Mrs. Harley appeared in Beaver's narrative only when they died or required men to protect or rescue them. As was conventional among Europeans, Beaver rarely provided their first names in his narrative. The only reason he gave a rather detailed account of Mrs. Harley and her daughter was because they were hostages whom he meant to rescue. The daughter, "about five years of age, was in the same situation" as her mother: "vermin had absolutely eaten little holes in her head and neck and her shoulder-blade, the lower part of the vertebrae and hip bones had made their way through the skin and formed ulcers, from her emaciated body having lain so long."

When Jalorem released the captives, neither Mrs. Harley nor her daughter proved able to walk, and it took a long time for Beaver to convince any of the Bijago men to help transport them to the beach. "At length," Beaver wrote, "a man undertook it," helping to steady the captives as they rode on a pony, "but with evident disgust." Beaver interpreted this as the man's revulsion at touching white skin, although he may also have feared contracting a disease.

Beaver opened the formal meeting by having his interpreter Gillion assure Jalorem that it was extremely unfortunate when people misunderstood one another, "and that that had been the case with us." However, since "what had already happened could not be recalled, I should say nothing on that subject, but hope that we should hereafter live like good friends and neighbors." Beaver then offered to buy "their hunting island of Bolama." Jalorem replied that he too was sorry for what had occurred, but when the colonists first occupied Bolama, the Canabacs "neither knew who we were, nor our intentions; *we were strangers, and we took their land.*" Jalorem wanted friendly, peaceful relations, and as a show of good faith he had released the last two English hostages. As for purchasing the island, Jalorem needed to consult with other Canabacs in a nearby village who also grew rice and hunted on Bolama.

Beaver and Jalorem exchanged gifts, both at the meeting's conclusion and later, when Beaver returned to his ship. Beaver's presents included cloth from India, manufactured iron goods from Britain, and tobacco and rum produced by slave labor in the Americas. Jalorem, in turn, gave the colonists exactly the items they needed: a bullock, several goats, and a dozen fowl. Jalorem had his men fire seven blunderbusses outside his house as a way of honoring Beaver when he left. When Beaver managed after some struggles to convey the ailing former captives to the *Beggar's Benison,* the small group of colonists on board breathed easier and even celebrated that evening.

To satisfy his curiosity, while Mrs. Harley and her daughter were being prepared for transport, Beaver had strolled around Jalorem's village, "accompanied by Gillion and the king's sons, with a view to obtain, by that means, a tolerable notion of its extent and population." The village contained approximately fifty round houses, with thatch roofs and mud walls, arranged in a circle around an open communal space. This was one of two towns on Canabac Island, and it numbered among several dozen villages dotting the thirty islands in the Bijagos Archipelago. According to another European report, the Bijago "adorn their houses with the scalps of their enemies." Yet whites often used these kinds of stark images—including cannibalism—to justify their own brutality toward Africans. Beaver discovered no scalps either outside or within the homes. Instead, he was favorably impressed with the Bijago's way of life.[31]

Beaver's visit coincided with the Bijago's decades-long turn toward increased isolation, including a decline in their raids against peoples on the continent. As they continued to lose their own people through warfare and slavery, the Bijago focused on cultivating rice and palm oil and engaging in fishing and hunting. As in many West African societies, gender determined the types of work people did. Females grew rice and males pursued fish and game. Indeed, the knowledge that transplanted slave women possessed about rice cultivation may have been a factor in its adoption as a crop in the New World.[32]

Women exercised a great deal of independence and power in Bijago society, especially within the realm of the family. The Bijago had developed a matrilineal society, where property and prestige passed down through mothers rather than fathers. Like most Europeans, Beaver and his fellow colonists embraced ideas of male superiority and found gender arrangements among the Bijago perplexing. (Europeans sometimes responded in a similar fashion to some Native

American societies, where women also often exercised a good deal of power, if not full equality.) For many whites, the "unnatural" order of women's power over men was another sign of the "savagery" of indigenous peoples.[33]

From the time of their first contact with Africans, the British had expressed negative views about the darkness of their skin, and that prejudice had grown more intense during the centuries of the slave trade.[34] The Canabacs harbored similar dislike of Beaver's lighter skin, feeling it cautiously, "as if it was the skin of a snake." They also "lifted my hat and touched my hair, and clapping their hands together, expressed their astonishment by calling out *Hoo-oo-oo-oo*." Perceptively, Beaver realized the similarities of their negative views: "The repugnance which some Europeans feel to touch a black," he claimed, "will give but a very faint notion of what these people feel at the idea of touching a white person; for besides the dislike of the color, common to both, the Africans couple with it the notion of disease."[35]

Bellchore, the leader of the other nearby Canabac village, arrived early on the morning after Mrs. Harley's return to the ship. Beaver tried to provide his readers with objective descriptions of the Canabacs, although how accurate he could be depended on a number of factors: Beaver's ignorance of their languages and the linguistic skill of the translator Gillion; the Canabac leaders' self-representation in negotiations; and Beaver's presuppositions about Africans. In Beaver's words, most likely exaggerated for his readers, Bellchore was "the greatest warrior the Bijago nation ever produced." He was six feet tall with large, penetrating black eyes, "the fire of which seventy rains have not yet extinguished." Like most Bijago men, he powdered his hair with red ochre. The same characteristics that made him preeminent among his own people—a reputation for understanding, courage, restless activity, and daring enterprises, plus his love of war—earned him the "hatred and detestation all those nations that lie within the reach of his lawless expeditions." Bellchore boasted of having once set fire to the town of Bissau despite its fort and garrison. He was the "dread of the neighboring people" and would prove to be a terror for most Bolama colonists as well.[36]

Jalorem, Bellchore, and the leaders of the Bolama Association, along with most of the Canabac villagers, convened on the beach after Bellchore arrived. In the pouring rain of July, the group haggled for hours. The villagers—men and women alike—all exercised a voice in the negotiations, making their decisions far more democratic than those in the colony under the dictatorial power that Beaver would soon wield. The power of the "sovereign," both among the Canabacs and "like all others on the coast," Beaver was surprised to learn, "seems trifling." These societies appeared relatively egalitarian, since the leader "cannot be known [distinguished] from his subjects by any external mark of dress or respect shown to him, and he eats out of the same calabash with any of his people."[37]

European traders frequently complained about the patience of Africans in bargaining: they could go on for hours, if not days. Beaver finally made an offer of a variety of goods, ranging from cloth to knives to umbrellas, worth approximately 473 iron bars (roughly the equivalent of a British ship captain's annual income), for the island. Even more important than the value of the goods, several Canabacs argued, was the advantage of having another colony of Europeans in the nearby vicinity. "As long as white men lived near them," Bellchore proposed to the villagers, "they should want nothing" in terms of access to trade goods.[38] Ideally, the Canabacs would enjoy the advantage of competitive bargaining with both the Portuguese in Bissau and the British in Bolama. For some Africans along this part of the coast, trade was becoming more a necessity than a luxury. As one slave-ship captain observed, "The natives, no doubt, wish for our goods. Near the beach, they are always clothed from Europe. Guns, powder, spirits, and tobacco, from habit, may be reckoned necessaries."[39]

The colonists drew up a deed of cession and, in typical British bureaucratic fashion, copied it in quadruplicate. The grumetta Gillion translated it for the Canabacs, with "particular pains taken that they should fully comprehend every part of it," Beaver wrote proudly in his diary. However, the deed still included the foundation for misunderstandings after each party signed it. The British colonists believed they had bought the island permanently. Like most European settlers, they envisioned that this land would now officially become a part of Great Britain in the domain of the British king. The Canabacs envisioned the treaty more as a rental agreement, similar to those at most European slave factories along the coast. They expected the colonists to pay a similar amount of rent periodically. The Canabacs also stipulated that elephant tusks and anything else of value found on Bolama belonged to them. These differences in interpretation would help to sour the deal as time passed.[40]

As he was concluding his negotiations, Beaver was unaware that Mrs. Harley had "departed this life" a few hours before the colonists and Canabacs signed the agreement. When he returned to the ship and learned the news, he and the others refused to allow themselves to be discouraged by her death. They performed "the last friendly office" for the woman, committing her body "to the deep." Harley's daughter "followed her mother," succumbing to some unknown ailment the next morning, and her body likewise followed her mother's into the ocean.[41]

The visit changed Beaver's opinion about the Canabacs in ways not experienced by most of the other colonists. Seeing their village firsthand, enjoying the warm hospitality of the villagers, impressed by their treatment of the captives, and engaging in friendly, successful negotiations all lessened his fear about the colonists' supposedly savage neighbors. He also better understood their reasons for attacking the first party of colonists. All this helped Beaver overcome his fears of the Canabacs, at least temporarily, even as terror of their new neighbors intensified among his fellow colonists.

Beaver and the other negotiators were filled with hope and enthusiasm about the new treaty when they rejoined the other two vessels. To announce the good news, they called a special meeting of all the colonists. They intended to make July 2 a day of celebration, marking the establishment of the new colony. To their surprise, they found that many settlers had lost heart. Most were still unnerved about the imagined cannibalism of the Canabacs and uneasy about the deaths of their friends and families a month earlier. Indeed, few ever conquered their mistrust and fear of their African neighbors, attitudes that would greatly hinder the establishment of the colony. The settlers had also begun to realize the enormity of the task that confronted them. They had to build an entire colony on an uninhabited island. In addition, it never stopped raining—every day, incessantly— and they were appalled to learn from the locals that the showers were likely to last for months.

Beaver was eager to begin clearing the land and constructing shelters along the beach. The fears the colonists voiced about leaving the ships and going ashore stunned him. "I was astonished, I must confess, at no intention being shown or even thought of, to avail ourselves of the right which we had now acquired," he wrote. "Not a word was mentioned, nor the least idea discovered of landing and commencing with our labors; and the council and colonists separated, as if the written instrument itself was to create them a town." Frustrated by their apathy, Beaver rounded up a dozen men to go ashore. They worked all day, cutting trees, preparing the ground, and walking the land with a long-term survey of the colony in mind.[42]

When the group returned in the evening, they proposed a plan to the council for transforming the island into a place fit for human habitation. A working committee of two-thirds of the pioneers would depart each dawn for the island, where they would clear ground and build the town. Meanwhile, six armed men would guard the workers at all times. Three exploration parties would set out daily to examine the island more thoroughly. Beaver and his group further suggested that the *Calypso* and *Hankey* should be more heavily moored in their present location. Colonists could construct wooden roofs above the decks to protect against the continuing rains. For the time being, the settlers would live on the ships rather than on shore.

The settlers had owned the island for exactly one day, but instead of adopting the proposals for colonizing it, the council voted to abandon Bolama, at least temporarily. The leaders decided that the three ships would sail several hundred miles south to the newly established British colony of Sierra Leone, where they hoped to find water, food, shelter, and assistance. It will be recalled that Henry Hew Dalrymple had briefly been connected with the Sierra Leone expedition, and was thus proposing that they seek out a place where he could expect to meet people he knew. Once in Sierra Leone, the Bolama colonists would decide whether to return to England or to Bolama. Given the present state of fear about the Canabacs, everybody knew what the decision would be.

Incensed, Beaver fought back: "Accustomed as I had been to the weakness, folly, and absurdity of the measures hitherto pursued by the directors of this enterprise, yet I was astonished. What, in the name of common sense, did we come here for?" What had happened, Beaver wondered, to "their avowed motives for having undertaken the expedition? Those motives could not have been very strong." The council argued that they feared more deaths among the colonists if they stayed. Beaver acknowledged that probability but argued that to some degree it "must be expected in such an enterprise. When was a colony settled without it?" Since a number of people wanted to leave, Beaver urged, "let them go in one of the ships" rather than send all three vessels away.[43]

Fear of the Canabacs was palpable as the council argued these points. Most colonists believed they had fetched up next to a savage, cannibalistic race. They dreaded the prospect of living near people who feasted on human flesh. All the rumors about cannibals in Africa, they felt, had been proven true.[44]

After vigorous debate, Beaver decided to make a personal stand. "I informed the council that I should remain on the island with my servant," James Watson, "though everybody else might leave it, and I expected, therefore, that one vessel would be left with me."[45]

His personal courage helped sway others. Given the option of staying or leaving, 91 people, including 4 sailors and a cabin boy, chose to continue the colonization effort at Bolama. The council declared that the *Hankey* and *Beggar's Benison* would remain at anchor, while the *Calypso* and nearly 150 passengers—some of whom had not even set foot on Bolama—would set sail as soon as possible for Sierra Leone and after for England. Along with most of the council members, even the association's president, Henry Hew Dalrymple, wanted to abandon the enterprise. Beaver dismissed Dalrymple as a "dreamer of dreams" who was incapable of accomplishing anything difficult.[46]

Two weeks of shuffling provisions and belongings between the *Hankey* and *Calypso* followed these discussions, as the majority of the colonists prepared for the return voyage to England. Meanwhile, six colonists died of puzzling ailments. On July 19 the *Calypso,* containing numerous passengers with fevers, cruised away, honoring the *Hankey* and *Beggar's Benison* with a three-cannon salute. The *Hankey* returned the signal with seven cannon blasts of its own.

Dalrymple and the disgruntled former Bolama colonists would not find a warm welcome at Sierra Leone. His arrival created tension with the leaders in Sierra Leone, who had dismissed him as governor six months earlier. When the Bolama colonists landed at Freetown, the inhabitants, mostly African Americans who had freed themselves during the American Revolution, greeted the newcomers largely with cold contempt and suspicion. The colony was already encountering problems of insufficient food and supplies; the exhausted, hungry Bolama colonists disembarking from the *Calypso* threatened to consume too many of its limited, precious resources.[47]

Compounding the problem was illness. While in port, an increasing number of the Bolama colonists came down with the now long-running mysterious fever. According to one member of the expedition, people on board were very sick, and five or six were dying each day. The Freetown residents, fearing the spread of the disease, quarantined the passengers on board the *Calypso.* The deadly combination of poor planning and bad luck was bearing fruit: of the 146 passengers who boarded the *Calypso* to leave Bolama, at least 60 would perish before the ship reached England months later. Several years later, ironically considering the antislave-trade ideals of the Bolama group, the *Calypso* made one more trip to and from Africa, this time as a slave ship carrying humans in chains to Barbados.[48]

CHAPTER 5

Death in Bolama

ಬಲ

W
ith the band of hopeful pioneers of the Bolama Association torn asunder by the departure of the *Calypso,* the
rump council recognized Philip Beaver's energy and
leadership qualities by voting unanimously to make him their new
president. Beaver, in return, demanded nearly unlimited authority.
His conditions were not unprecedented. As Beaver was aware, John
Smith had used dictatorial power nearly two centuries earlier to save
the Jamestown colony in Virginia from starvation and failure.[1]

The council agreed, perhaps because many of them were planning to return to England, perhaps because the mostly affluent councilors had never fully embraced the radical constitution they had
signed in Britain stipulating that every adult male, regardless of race
or property ownership, should have a vote in the colony's affairs. The
council made its decision without even consulting the other migrants,
abandoning the colony's democratic ideals at the first sign of difficulty.
The settlers' attempts to treat Africans fairly, if not as equals, would falter
as well when hardships overwhelmed them.

A disappointed but still idealistic Beaver complained bitterly
when the *Calypso* sailed away: "Thus vanished the schemes and plans
which had been formed in England, without even making an attempt
to succeed." Even as he penned these words, however, he retained a
measure of empathy for those who had chosen to depart. The passen-

gers aboard the *Calypso* had endured a far more difficult journey than those on the *Hankey*. While Beaver's ship had regularly restocked its stores during the voyage from England, the *Calypso* had not received fresh food since departing the Isle of Wight. Many aboard the ship, Beaver reminded himself, "not having eaten a fresh meal since their leaving England, their comrades slain and made captives, their ship infected with fever and the scene of discontent, their irritation against their leaders could not fail to be increased."[2]

Beaver, no stranger to giving orders from his days as an officer in the navy, began to take charge immediately. "Since our arrival on this island," he complained, "there has been, hitherto, little or no order, no work done, every one going whither he pleased and returning when he chose, whence the idleness and licentiousness of every description of persons have arisen to an intolerable height." Like John Smith in 1607, Beaver decided to institute "the severest discipline. It is high time that they know whom they are to obey and what they have to do."[3] For security purposes, all men would be armed, organized into four squads, and stand watch every day. The regulations of the British navy would become the basis of the new discipline imposed in the colony. As the rains continued, so torrential that nobody could work outdoors, Beaver drew up strict regulations about nearly every aspect of life in the colony. To keep the "general order," he demanded "obedience" to his commands at all times. That included extinguishing all lights at nine o'clock each night, "and that there be no singing after that hour." For the colonists on Bolama, creating a new society was going to be a test of character and a life of hard labor, and they would need to rely on the middle-class values that had led them to found this outpost of freedom.[4]

To protect the settlers' health while they lived on the *Hankey,* Beaver ordered that the ship be fumigated twice a week with vinegar, commonly used as a disinfectant, and that the animals be moved off the vessel. Every morning the pioneers were required to fill the water barrels from the island streams and hoist them on board the ship. Unknown to the settlers, in the process they would also renew their supply of yellow fever–carrying mosquitoes each day.

Beaver apportioned tasks to himself as well as telling everyone else what to do. "No man can object," he reasoned, "to public prayers being read to the whole community every Sunday morning." He assumed the responsibility of reading prayers once a week, although he frequently canceled the service because of inclement weather. While many abolitionists, such as the Quakers, drew inspiration from Christianity, the Bolama colonists were less committed to religion. In addition to Christians, the colonists included deists, a few Jews, and several atheists. Over time, as conditions worsened on the islands, public worship became observed less frequently.[5]

On Saturday, July 21, the colonists began their first full day of work. Beaver first sent the *Beggar's Benison* to Bissau for new provisions. Then he ordered one group to begin building a protective roof atop the decks of the *Hankey* while others went ashore to cut timber for the ship's housing. Rain was pelting down so hard by midmorning that everyone had retreated belowdecks. Within an hour, both a council member and a Mrs. Rodell, wife of one of the servants, died of fever. Regardless of the unrecognized health threat of close confinement with yellow fever virus–carrying mosquitoes, the colonists had to huddle on board the *Hankey* for the next six months as they laboriously constructed quarters on the island.

The purchase of Bolama was also turning out to be more complicated than the colonists had realized. One day a Mr. Bootle, a "mulatto man" and slave-ship captain whose vessel had anchored nearby, sought out Beaver for a discussion. He was an "intelligent man," Beaver noted, and "I asked him to stay and dine with me, so that while dinner was being prepared I might converse with him alone." On the pretext of inspecting the progress on the island so far, Beaver and Bootle took a walk on shore. Bootle knew about the Biafada living on the mainland across the channel from Bolama. Then came the shocker. He said that the Biafada, "a quiet, inoffensive people that would never attack us," were the real owners of Bolama. Since "this island belonged, in right, to them and not to the Bijago of who[m] he had heard that we had bought it, the Biafada would expect to be paid for it."[6]

If it were not for bad luck, the Bolama Association would have had no luck at all. They had already paid for the island of their prospective colony once. Now, seemingly, they had to buy it again. Wanting to keep conflict with local peoples to a minimum, Beaver initially offered gifts of hogs and wine to the Biafada. Then he went farther, hiring Bootle to bargain with them to sell both Bolama and the island opposite it. Beaver's geographical knowledge of the region was so limited that he later discovered that what he thought was another island was in fact a peninsula that jutted out from the continent. Bootle sailed off in the evening to open negotiations.

Meanwhile, the British transferred almost all their animals from the ship to shore during the next few days. They left the two oxen, four donkeys, eight sheep, and dozen goats on their own overnight, imagining that they would wander about the island and graze. The colonists apparently had not thought to inquire about the wild animals they were likely to encounter on Bolama. Disaster struck quickly. Going ashore the next morning, the settlers discovered nothing but scattered bones. Beasts of prey, most likely large cats and hyenas, had devoured the hapless livestock. The settlers had once again compounded their poor planning and bad luck through ignorance of their new environment.

The colonists started felling trees, planting seeds brought from England, building the skeletons of shelters, and exploring the island during a brief break in the rains. Getting lost on one expedition, several men encountered an elephant, which lumbered away into the forest. Another group made a valuable discovery: four potable springs of water in the island's interior, a necessity if they hoped to establish a successful settlement.

They received some reassuring news as well, when a letter arrived from Mr. Bootle. The negotiations with the Biafada had moved forward. If Bolama's leaders visited them with "a proper assortment of goods," they might strike a deal. On July 30, Beaver and John Paiba— the adult son of a council member and one of the few people who would survive the entire trip on the *Hankey*—left for Guinala, a Biafada river port on the Rio Grande, to negotiate with the Biafada. As the *Beggar's Benison* sailed north past Bolama's headland, the team met a slave schooner, the *Experiment;* its captain lay very ill in his cabin. Beaver kindly sent him back to the *Hankey* for medical treatment, a compassionate decision, but one that also introduced yet another person with a possible communicable disease aboard the ship.[7]

The *Beggar's Benison* navigated thirty miles up the nearby Rio Grande (present-day Rio Grande de Buba). The waterway, Beaver marveled, was "the most beautiful river I ever saw, indented on either side the whole way, but more particularly on the northern shore, with deep and large bays, and many creeks." At Guinala, the cutter encountered two more ships engaged in buying Africans, a reflection of how busy slave vessels were in the region. Bootle escorted the hopeful colonists to meet Matchore and Niobana, leaders of nearby Biafada villages. The negotiations proved long and arduous. While the conversation started well enough, "after the usual ceremony of giving drams" of rum, the embattled history of Bolama began to emerge. Niobana claimed that his ancestors had long lived on the island, and that the Bijago "had always been at war with them," forcing them to abandon the island. However, the Biafada still claimed Bolama as their territory.[8]

The following day, the negotiating party traveled to Niobana's village. Beaver offered rum and tobacco to the two men, explaining that his organization "had never intended to take possession of another person's land without the free consent of its owner." The Africans countered that they wanted the British colonists to settle closer to them, since such proximity would assure them easier access to trade for Western goods. "If white men live here," Matchore was reported to have said through the interpreter Bootle, "we shall want nothing, but if white men do not live here, we shall want everything." After many hours of getting to know one another and bargaining, most of the participants were drunk. The next morning, Niobana was too ill to meet. "But he sent his head woman with his cane, to represent him," Beaver noted, adding that the cane she carried was representative of official power.[9]

The August 2 *palavra* (the Portuguese word for "talk," commonly used in the region) for ownership of Bolama Island and "greater Bolama," the peninsula off the African coast, occupied the entire day. Although both sides agreed upon a rough price in trade items, Matchore "kept me from 11 o'clock, the time these things were produced, until sunset, changing sometimes one thing and sometimes another. At one moment he would have six or eight guns, and the next I must take them back again, then he would re-demand them; and so it was with every separate article." This shrewd strategy was often employed by Africans. If they bargained long enough, white captains, anxious to close a deal and set sail, tended to give in. Beaver and the Biafada finally agreed on a payment of twenty-six different commodities, ranging from cloth to flints to guns, worth about twenty-six pounds sterling. In the deal the colonists also acquired claim to a small slice of land on the African coast opposite Bolama. To seal the agreement, Niobana spit in Beaver's hands and said they were brothers. "To be called the brother of Niobana, I had no objection." However, Beaver offered in a rare touch of humor, "I would willingly have dispensed with the ceremony by which I was made so."[10]

Having bought the land yet again, Beaver returned to Bolama, but not before anchoring overnight as a strong tide surged up the river. The group discovered on arriving home that a baby had died, four more people had contracted a fever, and nineteen of the eighty-three colonists were ill. Still, they found progress as well. Workers had completed the *Hankey*'s deck cover and built a pen for cattle (if they ever got any more) on the beach. Heavy rains resumed, and the colonists could neither work nor hold Sunday prayers.

At dawn the next day, "a boy named Coggins, who had been ill of a fever some days, fell overboard. He could not swim, but the boat picked him up just as he was sinking. In two hours, he died—buried him. Everybody employed in cutting down and burning wood. Thermometer at noon 76—wind S.W." This entry in Beaver's diary, tersely recording a death along with the kind of work done and the weather, would become all too common.[11]

Not surprisingly, a number of settlers began to grow despondent about the wave of sickness in their new home. As Beaver prepared the *Beggar's Benison* to go to Bissau to collect new provisions, vegetables, and fruits, eight colonists approached him, asking to be allowed to return to England. Among them were John Paiba the younger, who had recently accompanied Beaver to Guinala, and laborer Henry Rodell, whose wife had died a week earlier. "What a farce!" Beaver fumed. "Can anything be more ridiculous? Is it not odd that these people could not have made up their minds sooner? It is only 19 days since the *Calypso* sailed. Had they gone then, it would have been better." Moreover, Beaver moaned, "it greatly dispirits those who remain." Nevertheless, when he set off in the cutter for Bissau, he took with him four men and one child who wanted to leave the colony.[12]

At Bissau, Beaver headed directly to the house of their negotiator, Joseph Cordoza de Sylva, in another downpour. After playing a central role in the rescue of the Bolama hostages, he had promised Beaver regular fortnightly supplies of fresh food for the colony. Beaver ran into Owen Williams at Cordoza de Sylva's house. Williams had originally signed on as one of the doctor-surgeons aboard the *Calypso* but had quit the mission several weeks earlier and stayed at Bissau, where he had recently buried his wife. Now he requested passage for himself and his son to Sierra Leone, where he hoped to catch up to the *Calypso* and return to Britain. Beaver agreed, if bitterly, to the request, "merely out of humanity, and on account of his little boy, for he [Williams] is a miserable wretch, destitute of every good quality." Beaver never hesitated to write harshly about the people who abandoned the colonial enterprise. Planning to find a way back to Bolama by other means, probably on one of Cordoza de Sylva's trading vessels, Beaver ordered his cutter to sail for Sierra Leone with all the colony's refugees. Beaver was clearly prepared to get rid of anyone who was not committed, body and soul, to the Bolama mission.[13]

After the *Beggar's Benison* left for Sierra Leone, perhaps as a pleasant diversion from the stresses of the last month, Beaver and his host took a walk through the countryside on the mainland, across from Bissau. Since Beaver's first visit to the Portuguese slave factory, the

Papel had repeatedly expressed a desire to trade openly with the British colonists. Beaver had always declined, since the Portuguese regarded the overture as a threat to their own commerce with local peoples. Now, as Beaver and Cordoza de Sylva walked through the farms and rice plantations, Beaver began to reconsider the idea.

Papel culture fascinated the colonists. "The natives of Papel mark their bodies in various forms, called tattooing," wrote Joshua Montefiore. Their skin under the tattoos was "jet black." They "also plait their hair in a very curious manner. They appeared a very inoffensive people, and very desirous of an intercourse with the English. The clothing of the Papels consists of different kinds of St. Jago [Cape Verdean] cloths, tied round their middle, some of which sell for 60 bars of iron"—a substantial value for clothing. The Papel, according to Montefiore, demonstrated "remarkable sophistication and hygiene, bathing at least twice a day in moving water," quite startling to Europeans who usually did not even bathe twice a year.[14]

The Papel cultivated fruits, such as plantains, yams, limes, bananas, and "kola fruit" (which tasted bitter but possessed medicinal qualities), as well as rice, which they ate with palm oil. They husbanded livestock: oxen, pigs, goats, and fowl. They constructed canoes as expertly as the Bijago, and their houses were large, supported by wooden posts, roofed with palm thatch, and lined with grass floor mats. When trading with Europeans, at least in the late eighteenth century, they wanted muskets and cutlasses. These helped them kidnap or acquire prisoners in warfare with neighboring peoples to sell to ship captains.

As Beaver chatted with a few Papels, he noticed their obvious good health and prosperity—a sharp contrast to the current lack of vigor among his own people on Bolama. He also realized the advantages that might accrue in buying products from them, especially food for the colonists and goods to sell to England. Beaver's interest did not escape the notice of local Portuguese officials, who immediately began to block his commercial schemes. "The governor, with the collector, who by the bye manages him, came this evening to Mr. De Sylva's, where it was debated whether or not they should put me in prison," Beaver wrote. "Had it not been for the remonstrance of De Sylva, I believe that would have been the case. They however wished to put a guard over the house to prevent my having any communications with the natives." Just like Africans, Europeans bickered with one another about controlling trade.[15]

Beaver came down with a serious illness shortly thereafter, probably yellow fever, malaria, or dengue fever, the first of many illnesses contracted during his sojourn in Africa. He suffered for a few days, then "finding myself no better," he "resolved to go back while I was yet able." He returned to Bolama on Cordoza de Sylva's provision-laden boat, which also carried "a cow, a calf, and three dozen fowl." For much of the short trip, he rested belowdecks. When they reached the island, he received bad news. Two more of the association members had died, including Benjamin Marston, the former Loyalist and surveyor. Marston elicited one of the few lines of praise that Beaver made after a colonist's death. He was "a good man, [who] lived respected, and died regretted by all."[16]

Meanwhile, heavy downpours continued to trap the remaining seventy-one colonists on board the *Hankey*. Thirteen were sick. Few of the settlers worked during the next ten days while Beaver lay ill. From his bed, he ordered pipes and tobacco issued to all the colonists to help prevent disease. Sailors commonly believed that smoking belowdecks would fumigate a ship; in addition, the inhaled smoke was thought to protect the smokers. Since smoke repels mosquitoes, the smoking did help make the ship healthier, if only marginally.

While an unidentified female colonist cared for Beaver during his infirmity, John Morse, a subscriber and surgeon, asked to leave the colony, to go first to Bissau, then by some means on to England. Beaver's irate reply to this newest request came quickly: "I have not yet asked anyone to remain with me, and I believe I never shall. I cannot select half a dozen colonists that deserve their bread. As to asking my leave, it is ridiculous in the extreme, for, were I inclined to detain them, they all know that I have no power to do it." Beaver did not mention that because the home secretary had not approved the colony's constitution when they left Britain, he actually had no official power over the comings and goings of any of the settlers.[17]

The pioneers narrowly averted a disaster in the post-midnight hours of August 14. In a strong wind and heavy seas, the *Hankey* broke free from its moorings and drifted north. With the dawn, the crew quickly realized the problem and returned the ship to order in its former site. But stabilizing the ship occupied the entire day. Sick in his cabin aboard the *Hankey,* Beaver remained unavailable to lead the colonists. During days of sliding in and out of consciousness, he experienced one heartening moment. One night as he lay seemingly near death, he overheard people talking outside his cabin, "speaking only my praise; every one said that I had killed myself by my exertions for their good." In all likelihood, Beaver, who often failed to understand how other colonists thought or behaved, misinterpreted their conversation. He probably overheard a snatch of the kind of respectful, laudatory talk people often use when discussing a dying man, rather than an honest appraisal of his leadership. After all, if he died, the colonists had already decided that "they *must* go home for there was no one left who could take care of them." Given all the difficulties during their time on Bolama, many of the settlers would have been grateful to escape fear, fevers, threats, death, rain, hard work, and wild animals, and the demise of the governor of the colony would mean that they could officially disband.[18]

Beaver was "seized with a rattling in my throat," which everyone thought to be a death rattle, and the ship's master, Captain Cox, ordered his crew to "get ready to sail for England." The two surviving council members were prepared to depart Bolama the moment Beaver perished, since "nobody would have staid" after he was gone. Then Beaver experienced a spectacular resurgence of strength and spirit. By the next morning, under "beautiful" skies, he was on his way back to good health. In celebration, he ordered the colonists to return to the island to clear more ground.[19]

After his remarkable recovery from fever, Beaver became a whirlwind of activity. Despite all of the hardship, he seemed even more determined not to be slowed in his plans to construct the colony. Five days later, Beaver felt well enough to begin setting longer-lasting goals. He unilaterally decided that instead of constructing individual small shelters, as they had been doing, the colonists should build a large, substantial blockhouse, or fort. "Knowing the indolence of most of the colonists," Beaver wrote in his journal, "the surest and readiest way to get a covering, or a house, for every individual, is by making every individual interested in making the same building." In addition, since "a blockhouse is absolutely necessary for our defense, I think it best to make the same building answer the double purpose of defense and dwelling. By these means, too, I shall have every one under my own eye."[20]

Beaver's use of *blockhouse* might have brought to mind another definition of the term. While it had a primary meaning of a fortified area for defense in the wilderness, to the Britons of that era it also carried a second connotation: prison. For those migrants who had been in or narrowly escaped jail in England, the double meaning of the term probably was not lost.

Beaver claimed to have only the colonists' interest at heart. He forcefully proposed his communal plan even while disclosing his innermost beliefs in his diary—that the colonists were lazy and self-centered. Once constructed, the fort would contain houses for groups of colonists according to their social status. Each paying subscriber would receive a large house, each married laborer a smaller one. Among unmarried laborers, four would occupy a single smaller unit. The most diligent workers would earn the first dwellings. The colonists faced a major problem regarding the planned blockhouse, however. It was far too large for the number of colonists physically able to work to be able to construct it successfully.

Illness continued to weaken them even as they began pacing off the foundation, leveling the area, and cutting and squaring timbers. On Friday, August 24, John Ashworth and his wife died of a fever. Of the original 275 passengers who had left Gravesend, only 69 remained alive on Bolama, and a quarter were too sick to climb out of bed. In addition to building the blockhouse, the pioneers continued

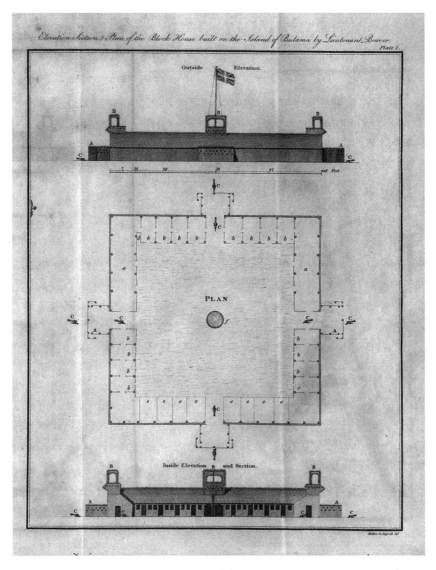

The blockhouse, or fort, that Philip Beaver envisioned on Bolama. The plan proved to be far too ambitious for the colonists. From Philip Beaver, *African Memoranda* . . . (London, 1805). Photo: Biblioteca Nacional de Portugal.

to explore the island. Particularly ominous for the colony's ultimate fate was the frequent discovery of dead monkeys lying on the ground. Today, we know that they were most likely the victims of sylvatic (jungle) yellow fever. The colonists knew only that they were an easy, tasty food supply. The Britons ate gratefully, and, Beaver confided to his diary, "All was silent, except frogs and mosquitoes."[21]

Understanding how the disease was spread among the colonists helps explain the death toll on Bolama and in the upcoming Atlantic world pandemic, so it is worth pausing to investigate the peculiar conditions of Bolama Island that made this strain of the fever's reign of terror so remarkable. Infectious mosquitoes thronged aboard the *Hankey,* where they discovered ideal breeding places in the open barrels the pioneers thoughtfully refilled every day with water and a new supply of insects from the island. The insects, spreading viruses that produced yellow fever and dengue, could feast on the colonists' bodies every time they went to have a drink. The settlers also routinely gathered scrap wood, stowing it in the ship's hold as ballast. The mosquitoes undoubtedly escorted the lumber and everything else the pioneers brought on board.[22]

To make matters worse, the colonists began to modify Bolama's environment in ways that encouraged both insects and the yellow fever virus to flourish. In the forests of West Africa, as in some tropical parts of the Americas today, monkeys served as a reservoir for the virus. Specialized types of mosquitoes, such as the *Aëdes africanus,* fed primarily on monkeys, spreading arboviruses among them. Areas of high mortality for monkeys are often regions where swarms of *Aëdes africanus* circulate diseases among the primates. Even today, native residents know to flee an area whenever they come across a great many dead monkeys. The Bolama colonists knew nothing of the transmission of disease by mosquitoes, of course—much less of any specific ecological connections among monkeys, mosquitoes, and disease.[23]

The hordes of monkeys in the forests held a particular fascination for the settlers, who brought down the simians as they felled the trees to obtain material for building the blockhouse. The colonists sometimes killed and ate them in a "delicious monkey pie." In the process, the settlers also cut down the treetop canopy where the *Aëdes africanus* liked to dwell. The insects quickly adjusted: they surely feasted on humans as well as monkeys. The severity of the disease the mosquitoes spread among the simians in the treetops was markedly different from its impact on the ground among the colonists. West African monkeys had developed over generations some resistance to the arboviruses that infected them through mosquito bites. The Bolama colonists had not. By repeatedly disrupting the African forest habitat, the European settlers unwittingly exposed themselves to a radically new epidemiological environment. They intruded on what modern scientists call the "sylvatic cycle" of a pathogen's transmission—that is, the time during which the yellow fever virus circulated between monkeys and mosquitoes. The colonists became human hosts for the disease even as they were slapping at the annoying mosquitoes that buzzed around their heads. (In addition to the *Aëdes africanus,* the colonists were also providing fertile breeding ground for a mosquito that was even deadlier to humans, *Aëdes aegypti.* It was this mosquito that would make the journey west with the *Hankey.*)[24]

The settlers had survived a variety of local diseases while children in Europe to which they were now immunized—typically, smallpox, measles, and mumps—but none of these maladies provided any resistance against tropical ailments. In many places along the west coast of Africa today, by the estimates of modern scientists, residents on average receive stings from three hundred infectious mosquitoes a year. A few hearty settlers on Bolama survived one of the diseases spread by the mosquitoes, but attacks by two or three ailments simultaneously or in sequence simply overwhelmed their bodies' immune systems. Like the AIDS epidemic centuries later, a virus that most likely had been confined to a troop of sick monkeys found that humans were an even better host, for their immune systems had no defense. The disease could proliferate wildly.[25]

Exhausted by heavy toil and sickened by unknown diseases, the colonists also faced an unwelcome surprise from the Canabacs. One day, when the weather was so foul that none of the colonists attended public prayers, a canoe materialized from the gloom along the beach and glided alongside the *Hankey.* The Canabacs on board carried a copy of the sales agreement for Bolama, which Beaver had asked them to bring whenever they stopped at the island. Bellchore, one of the Canabac leaders, had come for a visit. "Having put on over his goat skin his ceremonial dress, and changed a red woolen cap for a three corner hat, with as many buttons on each side as it had corners, and one on the crown," Bellchore stood on shore with about forty of his people. When invited aboard the *Hankey,* he and seven others came on deck. The colonists and their guests spent a day together in considerable merriment, drinking a good deal of rum to enliven their spirits. Beaver ordered his servant to make beds for Bellchore and three of his compatriots on the floor of his own cabin for the night.[26]

The following morning, Beaver saluted Bellchore and his group by firing six cannon. "To show him the distance to which I could throw a shot," Beaver wrote, the colonists "fired a four pounder directly up the river; a squall prevented his seeing the shot fall and he supposed it went into the wood five or six miles distant." Europeans had used similar techniques of intimidation for centuries, for example when Hernán Cortés sought to cast terror into the Aztecs when he arrived in Mexico in 1519. Designed to threaten indigenous people implicitly with superior military technology, the display could also be thinly disguised as enjoyable pyrotechnics. The visitors seemed impressed but not overly awed by the demonstration. They had been familiar with European armaments for centuries, and they used many modern weapons themselves. Besides, the visiting armed contingent of Canabacs already outnumbered the healthy colonists that day, diluting the impression of power Beaver wished to assert.[27]

In keeping with the day's festivities, Bellchore presented the settlers with a bullock, several goats, and nine fowl. Things were going well until they slaughtered the bullock on the deck of the *Hankey* for a feast. After butchering the bullock, a Canabac took the raw, unwashed entrails of the animal—considered a delicacy among them—to Bellchore, who sat in one of the ship's cabins conferring with several of the council members. Disgusted at the sight of the uncooked meat, one of the councilors, John Munden, "indignantly turned the poor Bijago and his food out of the cabin, and on the interference of Bellchore, he rudely turned him out also." Despite the celebration, tensions remained between the two groups, especially among colonists who were still frightened by the people who three months earlier had killed some of their friends. Munden was probably reacting to the rumors that the Canabacs had eaten the colonists they had slain, and he could not stomach having Bellchore eat uncooked meat in his presence. However, his actions were insulting and harshly undiplomatic. Even worse, he had created dissension at a time when the colonists desperately needed the Canabacs as friends and potential allies against hostile neighbors, including the Portuguese.[28]

Beaver was on shore during the incident. "When I returned to the ship," he groaned, "the expressive countenance of Bellchore immediately convinced me that all was not right." Beaver railed against Munden's prejudice: "That surly and uncomplying disposition, that contempt and intolerance of other nations, manners and customs, that uncivil treatment of strangers, which characterize the illiberal of all nations, but more particularly of ours, had greatly offended our guests." Beaver's early attempts at cultural relativity showed him to be more forward thinking than many of his fellow Britons, even though he would later fall short of that ideal.[29]

Munden's behavior broke the spell of goodwill between colonists and Canabacs. Beaver tried to smooth over the incident by giving Bellchore a tour of the leveled and clear ground that the British had created in preparation for the blockhouse and the livestock pens. "He admired much our English fowls," Beaver noted, "being in size nearly three times as large as those of the Bijago, and I gave him a cock and a hen to improve his breed." However, Bellchore and the other Canabacs retreated to sleep on the beach that night, then left precipitously the next morning, although not without another six-cannon salute from the *Hankey*.[30]

Despite Beaver's attempts to mollify his guests, the visit had not gone well, and they had left apparently feeling insulted. The already tenuous relations between colonists and Canabacs, as well as between the settlers and their hired African workers, would grow increasingly worse.

In addition to fearing the Canabacs, the majority of the pioneers were losing their enthusiasm about the future of Bolama. Every colonist suffered not just one but a series of illnesses. In their debilitated state, most found the physical tasks of building and maintaining themselves under such primitive conditions extremely arduous. After all, the original plan had been to hire Africans to perform most of the heavy work, and none of the colonists had imagined the workload Beaver would impose. Some wanted to escape the foreign jungle and return home. There were also a number of freakish accidents—like the death of one man from a wound by the fin of a catfish and the trampling of the garden by elephants—that further unnerved the colonists. Their fears, combined with their reluctance to undertake hard labor, led to serious disgruntlement with Beaver's demands.

September 1792 began with a death. A Mr. Arfwiedson, a servant, passed away early on a Sunday morning. Beaver read brief prayers for the deceased, then announced that because the rains had slowed the colony's progress, Sunday would henceforth become a workday. If the settlers did not finish the initial structures, most notably the fort, before the rental charter of the *Hankey* expired on November 12, they would be in grave trouble. The ship still served as the Britons' dormitory, and they would be without shelter once it sailed. One subscriber, Charles Robinson, complained publicly, refusing to work because of his Christian beliefs. Beaver responded forcefully to Robinson's principled stand, ordering that "if he did not work, I should take care that he did not eat on a Sunday. This was a gratification which he had no inclination to forgo, and all his scruples vanished." Beaver's orders once again resembled John Smith's, in this case his "no work, no food" policy.[31]

This conflict over the Sabbath highlighted several issues. Most of the migrants were not deeply devout and apparently had no religious objections to working on Sundays, but a handful of the pious pioneers were in such desperate straits that although the order meant a breach in their religious practices, they went along. Beaver's victory in what was for some a matter of conscience demonstrated that he had assumed nearly complete control of the Bolama endeavor. In promoting the colony's survival at all cost, he was prepared to become a tyrant.

The day Beaver made his announcement, those well enough to work went ashore, where they found Mr. Hood, a colonist who had disappeared the day before, awaiting them in a recently built tool house. Hood's story of survival was a dramatic one. Walking into the woods the previous day, he had grown frightened by the growling of an animal, which he took to be a wolf, and climbed a tree. There he encountered a troop of monkeys that tried to drive him back down. He lacked a firearm, but he did have a knife. He quickly cut away a branch and used it to defend himself against the monkeys. After he had fought off the more aggressive animals, the remainder left him alone on his branch, where he spent the night. The next morning he returned to the beach and found shelter in the tool house. Hood's experiences reminded everyone that illness and torpor might lurk aboard the *Hankey,* but dangerous animals inhabited the land the colonists hoped to remake.

The rains subsided for a few weeks, and every colonist who was healthy enough to work helped build the fort or construct a new, small boat that could be used to trade with Africans on the continent. Aided by several grumettas from Bissau and Sierra Leone, the colonists cut down trees and stripped their bark. Once they had dug out the roots, they filled in the holes to create new, arable cropland. The workers flattened and graded the earth around the fort's foundation to assist in rainwater runoff. They then proceeded to burn away the jungle underbrush.

After several weeks of arduous toil, a growing number of colonists chose to stay aboard the *Hankey* when roll call came each morning. Some clearly were feigning illness, while others openly plotted to challenge Beaver's authority or even to leave the colony.

John Curwood grew "exceedingly dissatisfied," and he began "taking pains to make every other person so." His objective was to convince the settlers to leave when the *Hankey* departed in November. If the colony failed completely, then the association would be responsible for providing them with free passage back to England. Otherwise they would have to find their own way, at considerable personal expense and difficulty since few ships in the area sailed directly to Britain; all the slave ships navigated westward. Not long after Curwood started complaining, the colony's physician, Mr. Rowe, began questioning Beaver's power. In his journal, Beaver described Rowe as "a daring and turbulent man, difficult to be governed, [who] takes every opportunity of sowing dissention and creating disgust among the colonists. What his end or aim be, I cannot divine, unless to force me to abandon the colony."[32]

Down on his luck in England, Rowe had been a reluctant colonist from the start. A few days before the expedition departed from London, a judge had found him guilty of stealing a few articles of clothing and sentenced him to either six months in jail or banishment from Britain. He chose the latter, signing on as the physician for the colonization effort. He probably would have lived longer had he chosen jail.[33]

An unsettling event occurred a few days after Curwood and Rowe had made one of their scenes. A sloop arrived from the coast, anchoring not far from the *Hankey*. Inexplicably, the sloop's topmast suddenly exploded from a lightning strike, even though no storm cloud was in sight. The bolt's blast "shivered the mast to splinters." Beaver granted the sloop's crew of Manjaco, a group notable for their skill at sea, the freedom to go ashore and cut down a tree for a new mast. The colonists and grumettas joined them in the task.

Meanwhile, Beaver noticed "a man on shore, sitting on the beach, who had been burnt by the lightning. His left side from a little above the hip, all the way down the outside of his thigh and leg, as far as the ankle was perfectly raw." To help the sailor, Beaver retrieved from the *Hankey* a bottle of sweet oil and a large feather, which he used to distribute the oil across the burned portions of the man's body. Beaver advised him through an interpreter to repeat this treatment three times a day to ease the pain and speed the healing. "He took the bottle and the feather with the greatest indifference," Beaver wrote, "without altering a muscle in his countenance, without showing the least symptom of being pleased, or of gratitude, and without uttering a word of reply; to what can such indifference be attributed? He did not even look at me when I went away." It seems likely that the wounded Manjack was suffering from the shock of the lightning strike, or perhaps he just didn't like Europeans. Seemingly senseless and wholly unexpected events like this added to the colonists' alarm at an environment they did not understand.[34]

By mid-September, every single person aboard the *Hankey* lay abed, too ill to work despite a stretch of good weather. Richard Reeves expired on September 18. He was the third of four children of William, a laborer who himself had already descended to a watery grave. Hugh Mears, another laborer, whose infant son had been the first to die on the *Hankey* shortly after it left Britain, also died of a fever. The next night, after another day of lovely weather, fever claimed both James Box and his son.

A handful of grumettas and a few colonists who could drag themselves out of bed managed to accomplish a few important tasks in late September. The grumettas dug up tree roots and further flattened the earth around the fort's foundation. (Since no rocks were available in the muddy, silted alluvial area, Beaver planned to use the roots for ballast to steady the *Hankey* when the ship sailed.) Through the intermittent rains, they completed building their small trading boat and then floated it successfully. In a nod to the construction still required on Bolama, Beaver took the initiative and called the colony's new boat the *Perseverance*. And the settlers surely needed to persevere to survive these months of continuing difficulties and death.

On October 1, Beaver made another executive decision. The fort would be *smaller* in size, so that the colonists would at least have a chance of finishing it before the *Hankey* sailed. Beaver's earlier plan for a large fort had always been too ambitious for the number of workers available. Besides, the shrinking number of immigrants meant that less housing would be necessary.

Beaver also struck back at the grumbling among the colonists, as some became more vocal about abandoning the settlement. Tired of the arguments, Beaver posted the following announcement between the ship's decks:

Finding myself obliged to curtail the space at first intended
for the site of our blockhouse, and consequently reduced to
the necessity of contracting the dimensions of the different
rooms which it may contain, I wish that all those subscribers,
agents, labourers, or servants who intend returning to England in the *Hankey,* whose charter will expire on the 12th of
November next, would be obliging enough to communicate
their intentions to me by letter, before 11 o'clock tomorrow;
in order that I may avoid the unnecessary labour of building
more houses than will be occupied, and of too much contracting those that will.[35]

Two days later, most of the remaining colonists once again fell
ill with fever. "Not a Carpenter able to lift a tool," Beaver moaned.
"Myself with a little assistance continue the logging; everybody seems
much depressed; not a soul among them capable of exertion." Beaver continued to supervise the grumettas in cutting down trees and
clearing the land. In the meantime, the colonists began to deliver
their letters of intention to abandon the colony.[36]

Their letters did not stop the steady procession of deaths. William
Mears and William Reeves, both fully vested members of the association, perished on the *Beggar's Benison* as it returned from Sierra Leone
with more free African workers on board. On October 9, with so few
healthy workers available, Beaver decided to hire several of the remaining mariners on the *Beggar's Benison* to speed up construction of
the fort. This increased the workforce by a third, good news for the
colony. The bad news was that Richard Johnson, one of the cutter's
seamen, and Matthew Beck, a sailor on the cutter who had deserted
his ship at Sierra Leone, were the next to go. Fever claimed their lives
within a week. Beaver and two other settlers dug the graves and carried the bodies to them, tasks that they performed all too efficiently
because of long practice. The grumettas, as usual, were too disgusted
by the corpses of white people to even touch them.

That evening about ten o'clock, in yet another dark portent for
the colony, the *Hankey's* cook fell overboard and drowned. "We heard

a great splash in the water," Beaver recounted, "and ran instantly from the cabin on deck, but having examined all round the ship without either seeing or hearing any noise in the water, we returned again, and it was morning before the man was missed." The following day, perhaps to reinforce his own optimism about the future of the colony, Beaver penned the following: "Weather as before, with a tornado, generally, once in 24 hours, which increases in violence. With my blacks [grumettas] and sailors, I get on rapidly at the blockhouse, but scarcely a colonist at work. . . . Died and was buried, Sarah Reeves, aged 10."[37]

Beaver began to receive more colonists' letters of intention to depart with the *Hankey*. John Rowe, the physician and perpetually disgruntled colonist, presented Beaver with his resignation letter: "Gentlemen, from the declining state of my health, occasioned by disease brought on by the extreme fatigue I have gone through in the service of the association, I find it impossible for me to perform the functions of my duty in this debilitated state. I therefore beg you will consider this as my *formal and official resignation* of my appointment." Beaver whipsawed between compassion and indignation. Rowe "has never been out of the ship but once or twice," he complained, "and then for his own amusement." Moreover, Beaver added, he was so incompetent a doctor that many of the colonists would not allow him near them, despite their illness. With no other outlet to express his anger, Beaver seethed as he wrote in his journal. He felt increasingly on his own, "following my Robinson-Crusoe-like kind of life on the Island of Bolama."[38]

In two days, the *Hankey* and the Bolama Association had lost its cook and was about to lose its physician. Now another howling storm arrived, and its force broke the anchor cables on the *Hankey* and drove the ship aground. Captain Cox, finding that the ship had sustained little damage when coming to rest on the silt and mud beach, decided to allow the *Hankey* to remain there. In that position, his crew could more easily load the ballast into the hold. The following day a succession of three violent and squally "tornadoes" plus a day of steady rains kept the colonists confined aboard the *Hankey*. When the weather finally improved, several members of the group went ashore and continued working. They also buried the wife and infant child of the younger John Paiba, who had elected, in the end, to stay.

William Banfield—who had "long since shewn symptoms of insanity"—had earlier disappeared into the jungle. He reappeared on the morning of October 14 in an empty weapons chest. Why he chose to spend the night alone inside the strongbox on the island was any-one's guess. Perhaps the pressure of being surrounded by death had mentally unbalanced him. In the coming days, Banfield grew more dangerous to others as well as to himself. One day he smashed a three-cornered scraping tool across the skull of the ship's steward, laying open his head. Shortly thereafter, several colonists recalled that Ban-field was the only other person on the *Hankey*'s top deck at the same time the cook had gone overboard. "We have very strong grounds to believe that the ship's cook, who was drowned on the 2d of this month, was rolled over board in his sleep by this Mr. B., at that time insane," Beaver wrote. "We know that the cook was lying asleep in a tarpaulin great coat, stretched along the rough-tree [rail], just before the accident happened; at that time Mr. B. was then on deck, and the only person there, and when asked what splashing that was in the wa-ter replied 'nothing but one of the cook's old kettles.' " Beaver finally took decisive action. "For his own, as well as for our safety," he wrote, "I thought it necessary to keep him in irons."[39]

Burials continued, as did disagreements. Mr. Rowe sent Beaver a second letter specifying not only his personal grievances but also those of the other colonists. He criticized Beaver directly for disregarding the mounting number of deaths. "You sir," Mr. Rowe wrote, "ought to be conscious that the lives of his majesty's subjects, and our fellow creatures, are not to be so frittered away. There can be no plea in vin-dication."[40]

While Beaver had acknowledged the deaths, he frequently blamed the victims: "It is melancholy no doubt, but many have absolutely died through fear. More courage, and greater exertions, I firmly be-lieve, would have saved many of them. When taken ill, they lie down and say that they know they shall die."[41] Blaming the poor for their own plight, whether physical or financial, characterized the thinking of many affluent Britons like Beaver. Joshua Montefiore, the wealthy lawyer who had bailed out of the enterprise early, displayed a similar class bias. "The climate here, though hot, appeared to me fine and healthy," he noted. Thus, "I attribute their [the poorer of the colonists'] sickness and dying so fast, more to a want of cleanliness and attention to their health."[42]

Mr. Rowe's accusations that Beaver was frittering away the lives of the colonists made Beaver apoplectic. He copied the letter in its entirety into his diary while dismissing Rowe as an "unprincipled villain" and claiming that he was "as mad as Banfield." Several days later, Beaver challenged Rowe in front of a group of colonists, asking who among them agreed with the indictment. Rowe interrupted him, claiming that no one should be compelled to answer the question. Because the British government had never approved the colony's constitution, the colonists were not living under "military discipline," and Beaver possessed "no authority" to ask for names.[43]

Beaver then read Rowe's letter aloud, refuting claim after claim, and asking why, if these allegations were true, no one had complained before. Finishing his rant, Beaver warned Rowe "in the presence of the whole colony that if he did not quit the island before the 23rd day of December, I should on that day stop his provisions and turn him out of the blockhouse." Moreover, "if, before that day, he gave me any more trouble by forming parties and cabals in the colony, I would put him in irons and chain him, like a bear, to a tree."[44]

The five-month rainy season finally seemed to be ending. The weather in the last weeks of October remained mostly clear and warm, and only occasional storms interrupted the construction of the fort. Yet the more favorable weather did not bring better health. The colonists continued to perish at an almost metronomic rate. On October 23, William Smith—a full subscriber of the association—died of "complications." Two days later, John Hargrave, a sailor on the *Beggar's Benison*, died, as did the three-month-old son of servant James Reeves. The child's mother, Sarah, died the next day, along

with John Venus, a seaman on the *Beggar's Benison*. Fever then claimed
the insane man, William Banfield, who by then had been released
from his irons. The colonists began to hail one another each morning
with the morbid greeting: "How many died last night?"[45]

Although Beaver never mentioned discouragement in his journal,
the constantly declining number of colonists had to be disheartening.
Having started with 275 people six months earlier, the Bolama colonists were reduced by disease and desertion to 58 settlers. Beaver
seemed to be in a state of denial about the high mortality rate suffered
by the pioneers, dismissing it as a phenomenon common to all new
colonies. "Mortality in some degree must be expected in such an
enterprise; when was a colony settled without it? Not that of New
Plymouth, Rhode Island, New Hampshire, nor Connecticut, not
that of Maryland, Virginia, the Carolinas nor Georgia. And why are
we to expect being exempt from what is the necessary and inevitable
attendant in the clearing a new country?" Beaver was right that all of
those North American colonies had suffered high death rates in their
early years, mostly from famine or from the new disease environment
into which they had entered. He did not know, however, that the
odds of his colony's survival were so much worse because of tropical
fevers.[46]

Beaver and the grumettas, along with a few remaining reasonably
healthy colonists, stalwartly pushed ahead with building the fort,
though the process remained agonizingly slow. Beaver often worked
alone with the grumettas since so many colonists, either planning to
leave or discouraged by the prospects of ever finishing the project,
refused to pitch in. As construction continued, two more colonists—
John Frasier and Thomas Sparks—wrote letters outlining their intention to leave.

Anticipating the sailing of the *Hankey,* the settlers and grumettas
started to transport the colony's provisions from the ship to the island,
securing them in a large, if leaky, room on the east side of the blockhouse. The pioneers, for protection, moved several "carriage guns" to
strategic positions atop the blockhouse walls. On November 8, even
though the shelters were still crude lean-tos, the colonists began to

sleep on the island for the first time. Two of the laborers—Thomas Lister and Joseph Riches—had to be carried to the fort, so ill they were barely alive. The following day, removing the last of their belongings from the *Hankey,* the colonists took heart that their efforts had produced solid evidence of a new British community in Bolama.

Any feelings of achievement dimmed, however, when Beaver fell seriously ill once again. For a full fourteen days he barely moved from his bed, tended by one of the few surviving women. Somewhat recovered during those two weeks, Lister, accompanied by the disgruntled Frasier, took advantage of Beaver's illness to surreptitiously catch a ride on a small vessel headed for Bissau. Lister did not survive this attempt to escape Bolama. Seven other colonists died of disease during Beaver's illness.

Beaver finally recovered, and the *Hankey* set sail on the morning of November 22. With its usual ill luck, the wind that would bear it away died immediately. Mariners used the jolly boat to tow the ship back into the bay for an additional night. Sailing on the vessel the next morning were twenty-six former colonists and several sailors; they left behind just twenty-eight people. Those remaining on the island were now truly on their own. For the first time in two weeks, an agitated, despondent Beaver was well enough to write in his journal. "Everybody seems low and depressed, but the ship is gone and our own exertions must decide our fate."[47]

By remaining on Bolama, Beaver escaped responsibility for spreading the island's malignant new strain of yellow fever. The fainter-hearted colonists—almost all of whom would perish from yellow jack themselves—were the agents of that disaster. Each day they would descend into the hold of the *Hankey* for fresh water. Swarming around the kegs, laying their eggs on the scum on top, were the epidemic's vectors of death.

Meanwhile, the colony was entering a new, even deadlier phase. The toll exacted by fatal fevers would grow ever more fearsome. At the same time, the settlers would encounter new problems, especially in conflicts with the African workers and neighbors.

CHAPTER 6

Grumettas and the Final Days of the "Canabacs' Chickens"

ฌ

Remarkably, after all their setbacks, twenty-eight colonists had remained on Bolama rather than flee on the *Hankey*. Twenty-three of them were ill (a handful too sick to make an informed decision about staying or leaving). Some, like Philip Beaver, remained committed to the ideal of establishing a successful settlement. Others still clung to the hope of a bright financial future in the new outpost. Some did not want to go home to a life of servitude in England. One or two had no choice: if they returned to Britain after being sentenced to transportation, they would hang. These remaining colonists were no match for their healthy West African neighbors. Once the *Hankey* left, on November 23, 1792, the settlers took on a new role: that of the "Canabacs' chickens," as Bellchore labeled them, defenseless creatures to be nurtured or harvested at the whim of the residents of the nearby island. The colonists struggled on for another year, growing ever fewer in number, before Beaver finally admitted defeat and declared the colony ended.[1]

Focusing on the dwindling days of the settlement makes it easier to assess the colonial enterprise from the perspectives of both settlers and Africans. The stories of a handful of colonists still left on Bolama—James Watson, James Johnson, and Peter Hayles—help us understand their circumstances, conditions, and decision making as they coped with many of the historical forces that shaped life in the Atlantic basin.

The local peoples had to make choices as well; while some of their difficulties resulted from the decisions made by the pioneers, Africans still wielded the bulk of power over events. But how did they view and experience these efforts from an uninvited cluster of British migrants? Did the colonists' neighbors know or even care about the settlers' goals? What did Africans want from the colonists?

The *Hankey* had sailed away, but its legacy remained. The fates of the survivors on the island, both African and British, are vital to the larger story of how individuals and their societies coped with the forces that had brought these groups together. The lives of the grumettas— the free-floating (often literally) workforce who lived along the coast of West Africa, usually near slave-trading forts, where jobs were available—were also intertwined with those of the peoples whom the colonists had come to "save" from savagery.

Unfortunately, historical records about the grumettas and Canabacs are scant indeed. British men left virtually all the surviving written accounts concerning the interaction between the colonists and the Bijago. To gain an understanding of the perspectives of the local Africans is therefore extremely difficult: we must read those accounts cautiously, "against the grain," in the words of historians, to try to pierce through the biases of the authors. It is likewise important to place the Bijago within the historical context of the African coast—an area that, fortunately, has received a great deal of study from scholars. This assessment of the motives and behaviors of the Canabacs must therefore be more tentative than that of the Bolama colonists, yet it is based on the best evidence available.

The chronicle of James Watson, Beaver's personal servant and the only surviving black man among the original colonists, illustrates why some settlers stayed. He had few other promising options.[2] Conditions for blacks were far from easy in Britain. Lord Mansfield's verdict in the Somerset case prevented owners from using force to seize runaway slaves or sell them abroad, but the decree did not legally halt racial bondage since slaves brought into the country did not automatically become free. The number of slaves declined precipitously in the final decades of the century, primarily because bound workers undermined the system. Many simply fled, leaving their masters to find and retrieve them without the full support of the law. Still, most Britons did not consider either slaves or free blacks entirely human. Artists of the time, for example, depicted black servants and slaves aligned with domestic animals at the bottom of the great chain of being. The abolitionist movement of the 1770s and 1780s had only begun to challenge those stereotypes.[3]

While a number of white Britons, especially idealistic reformers and members of the working class in London and Manchester, supported abolition, racism remained strong. Black veterans who had fought on the British side during the American Revolution flooded into English cities in the 1780s, intensifying racial tensions. Lacking skills appropriate to their new setting, and facing widespread discrimination, these blacks experienced considerable difficulty in earning a living. Some worked as personal servants for white masters—work they had escaped by taking up arms a few years earlier. A good many were unemployed, languishing in poverty, with little hope for a secure financial future. James Watson made his decision to migrate to Africa, and to stay there regardless of the conditions, within this context.[4]

Peter Hayles's very different tale was also typical of the era. He had signed onto the *Beggar's Benison* as a sailor when it stopped at Tenerife. In his life before Bolama, Hayles had been a pirate, capturing ships and cargo out of Honduras—a profession he acknowledged after the *Hankey* left Bolama and it was no longer possible to ship him back to England. Piracy was not as unusual as it is today or even regarded as necessarily morally corrupt. After each major European war—and there were many in the seventeenth and eighteenth centuries—national navies decommissioned ships and cut sailors free as a way of saving money. Piracy provided one way for these jobless seamen to survive. In addition, since the same nations commonly commissioned privateers to operate lawfully as little more than pirates, the line between legal and illegal operations was a thin one. The golden age of piracy had been over for half a century, but European buccaneers still operated in parts of the Atlantic Ocean.[5]

Hayles was a typical pirate—that is, he was not the anarchy-minded individual depicted in the popular culture of our own times. Many pirate crews viewed themselves as akin to sovereign nations. They sometimes elected their captains, wrote constitutions in the form of articles of piracy that established an orderly and equitable distribution of spoils among the officers and crew, and even specified acceptable behavior and punishments aboard ships. Given the rise in self-governance at the time, the act of becoming a pirate, sailors sometimes maintained, was a positive step toward exercising the independent rights of humanity. Hayles may well have agreed with the radical democratic constitution approved by the Bolama colonists and its laudable goal of ending the slave trade. For the next six months, he was one of the hardest workers in the colony.[6]

On the day that the *Hankey* cruised out of the bay, filled with discouraged colonists hoping only to make their way home, a small boat from Bissau passed it on the way to Bolama. It carried James Johnson, who proved to be a remarkable addition to the colony. Working for wages, Johnson became "exceedingly useful" to the settlers as their chief interpreter and procurer of grumettas. He drew high praise from Philip Beaver for his many talents: "He is a good hand at an axe, understands caulking, is a tolerable sailor, a good servant, an excellent hairdresser, and an admirable cook"—all skills precious to the struggling settlement.[7]

Like James Watson, Johnson was a former slave. Born into racial bondage around 1755, probably in Virginia or New Jersey, Johnson began early to develop his impressive talents as a jack-of-all-trades. He started as a blacksmith and then became a carpenter. When the War of Independence began, Johnson seized the opportunity to free himself by enlisting in the British Army. It was a strategy fraught with risk since he would have suffered whipping, castration, or even execution if captured and returned to his owner. He may have been a member of the Black Guides and Pioneers when they occupied

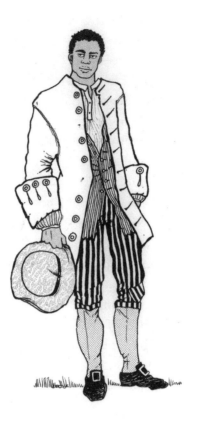

Artist's rendering based on descriptions of runaway slaves at the time of the American
Revolution. The vast majority of the *Hankey*'s colonists and the other people in this
Atlantic world are faceless in the historical archive. James Johnson, a former slave
who freed himself and later contributed greatly to the colonial effort, was one such
colonist. Drawn by Adrienne Mayor.

Philadelphia. At war's end, Johnson traveled with other black and
white troops to be mustered out in Nova Scotia. The British government had promised to provide land there for veterans, but it failed to
make good on its pledge for most black Loyalists. Johnson eventually
made his way, working as a ship's steward, to England. He then spent
several years as a gentleman's personal servant, traveling extensively
in Ireland, Scotland, and England.[8]

Johnson fetched up in London in the mid-1780s, where he struggled with poverty and racial discrimination. He joined with other
black Londoners, mostly former slaves from North America, to establish the Committee of the Black Poor in London. With funding from
wealthy gentlemen like Granville Sharp, the lawyer who had been
involved in the Somerset and *Zong* cases, and permission and encour-
agement from the British government, the Committee of the Black
Poor in London signed an agreement in 1786 to establish a colony in
Sierra Leone, which they called the Land of Freedom. (This was the
precursor of the group that in 1792 would hire and quickly fire Dalrymple as governor before he joined the Bolama expedition.)[9]

Johnson and 459 other passengers, mostly black, boarded ships
bound for West Africa in 1787. Mary Jones, a white woman whom
critics of the adventure described as a prostitute, accompanied Johnson as his wife. They had pawned their clothes to raise money for the
trip, but things went badly from the beginning. Eighty-four passengers died as the vessels waited in the English Channel for official approval of the enterprise. After witnessing the poor organization of the
colonial project, Olaudah Equiano, the black abolitionist, pulled out
of the expedition at the last minute.[10]

Johnson and Jones sailed on the *Atlantic,* which embarked for
Sierra Leone on February 16, 1787. On reaching Africa, the settlers
founded the colony of Free Town, which survived for a few years, suffering a high number of deaths due to tropical diseases. (Mary Jones was
among the hundred settlers cut down after their arrival at the beginning of the rainy season.) Angered by a dispute with an English ship
captain, perhaps over his right to buy slaves, local Africans eventually
ordered all British settlers to leave. The pioneers dispersed in 1790 but
then formed a new settlement, Granville Town, nearby. Nearly twelve
hundred free blacks living in Nova Scotia, most of them refugees from
the American Revolution, took advantage of the British government's
offer to move them to Sierra Leone a few years later.[11]

In 1790, when the colony briefly fell apart, Johnson took up work
as a grumetta, wandering along the coast as a temporary laborer. He
married an African woman, fell into financial difficulties, and landed

in jail as a debtor in the Portuguese slave-trading port of Bissau. Most likely fearful of suffering the common fate of debtors there—being sold into slavery—Johnson absconded to Bolama.

Johnson typified a group that scholars have since labeled Atlantic Creoles, free blacks and people of mixed race who lived on the margins of society. Without a strong national identity, often moving from place to place, they lived on the boundaries, from the coast of West Africa to the cities of North America and Europe. They frequently served as ships' crew. Speaking a myriad of languages, they could communicate with virtually anyone.[12]

After the departure of the *Hankey,* Watson, Hayles, and Johnson proved providential for Philip Beaver, who was still recovering from a fever that had lasted two weeks. They were self-directed, energetic, disciplined, and capable of taking initiative, like Beaver himself. Watson's dedication to the colony was particularly impressive. Beaver prized his loyalty until the end. Johnson had learned Creole, comprising Portuguese and local languages, that served as a common commercial patois for many of the grumettas along this part of the coast, and he was valuable both as an interpreter and as a go-between to hire other grumettas.[13]

"That Peter Hayles had been a notorious pirate in a small schooner, in the bay of Honduras," Beaver confided to his diary on November 23, "that he had also run away with one vessel, in which he had sailed, and sold her; and that he had set fire to another, and then plundered her, for which he had been tried, but escaped—I was sorry to learn all this, for he is certainly the most useful man in the colony." Because of Hayles's hard work during the period before the *Hankey* departed, Beaver tripled his wages, from one to three pounds sterling a month.[14]

The colonists endured several weeks of hard labor, sickness, and death following the *Hankey*'s sailing. Anybody healthy enough to walk had to work; the number of relatively able-bodied colonists varied but was never large. On most days, only Beaver was vigorous enough to work with the grumettas, who did the most difficult jobs.

Disease took the lives of three more colonists during the first few days of December, and digging graves was seemingly the most common chore performed by the pioneers.

On the morning of December 5, Beaver and the colonists faced another round of negotiations with the Bijago living on Canabac Island—this one the most threatening yet. Bellchore and thirty Canabacs came around the head of the island in a trio of large canoes. Beaver immediately beat to arms, assigned two guards to each gate of the uncompleted fort, and ordered them to fire on anyone trying to enter. James Johnson gathered the seven grumettas into the dubious safety of the fort. After anchoring, Bellchore came ashore with a few of his men and spent the evening dining with Beaver in his quarters. Beaver believed that he was conducting a scouting trip to assess the state of the colony, since the number of colonists was diminishing rapidly. When Bellchore requested a tour of the fort, it only heightened the colonists' fears.

All the Bijago camped out near the huts where the grumettas lived. One of the hired men brought back disturbing news, which Beaver was quick to record in his diary: "He had overheard Bellchore tell his people, 'that most of the white men were dead, and that the living were all sick but the captain (meaning me), that he had put us here and that *we were his chickens';* therefore, said the grumetta, he means to attack you." The Bolama colonists armed the fort in the dusk, keeping their weapons loaded and their cannon ready near every fortress entrance. "I laid down, wrapped up in a cloak," Beaver remembered, "with a brace of pistols under my head. Rather than be taken by these people, I would blow them all up. There was about a ton of gunpowder a few feet only from my cot in the store room." Five sentinels were obliged to stay awake, loudly shouting "all's well" to the group inside the fort, as well as the nearby Canabacs, every five minutes during the night.[15]

The colonists and the grumettas—partly a mix of Biafada, Papel, and Manjaco, peoples who had long histories of conflict with the Bijago Islanders—all feared the Bijago from Canabac Island. Their trepidation proved to be unfounded this time, however. After exchanging presents, Bellchore and his followers left the next morning. But during the first week of January when Beaver was briefly away from Bolama, the colonists were terrified by another visit. Bellchore returned with 150 men in seven canoes, and landed quietly in the night within fifty yards of the fort. The grumettas were engaged in high-spirited play—singing and making loud noises—inside the fort that evening, and Bellchore reportedly called off the assault, saying, "I hear too many tongues." The next morning, while Bellchore planned his next move, a British ship sailed into the harbor, and all the Bijago men slipped away. Beaver noted at the time, "The colonists thus almost miraculously escaped the greatest danger they have ever yet been in."[16]

Fevers remained more deadly for the settlers than did hostile African neighbors. On December 9, Jane Harwin died. She had recently nursed Beaver back to health from his own illness. Peter Box, Henrietta Fowler, and an infant all followed Harwin to the grave on the next day. Virtually everyone was sick. Only the grumettas, local people who possessed some immunity to yellow fever since they probably contracted it in childhood, continued to work.

In one of the many ironies of this colonial venture, Africans that the British colonists had come to save by introducing them to Western civilization instead had to save the settlers. Most grumettas were Africans, although some were mixed-race Creoles, characteristic of a newly emerging Atlantic world tied together by the trade routes. While on Bolama, Beaver hired almost two hundred of them, usually by the week or month, to carve the colony, physically, out of the uninhabited island. They performed most of the backbreaking work. They also did much of the hunting required to obtain meat for the table. In addition, they planted a garden, but the colonists' cattle broke down the fence and trampled it.[17]

We know little about the grumettas except the names that Beaver recorded, many of them seemingly of Portuguese or Spanish origin: Antonio Lopez, Jose, Tonga, Francisco, and Lysander. Others gave Beaver names from Britain or North America: Liverpool, George, Lawrence, and James Johnson. Most were men, though he also listed a few women: Christiana, Esperanza, and Maria.[18]

The grumettas became by default the dubious recipients of the colony's civilizing efforts in West Africa. Rather isolated on Bolama Island, with frequently hostile Bijago neighbors rather than the anticipated Africans who would be eager to work for the colonists, Beaver availed himself of a group of workers from a well-established system that had been supplying labor to both local Africans and European slave traders for centuries.

Beaver employed the colony's grumettas to construct the various buildings, among other tasks, thereby proving one of the founding principles of the colony: employing Africans for wages rather than enslaving them was effective and economically viable. Complicating this principle, however, was the fact that Beaver had hired some of the grumettas directly from captains on passing slave ships (the rest were obtained through merchants in Bissau). The threat of permanent enslavement made these grumettas' decision to work for the colony less a matter of idealism than pragmatism. But why should Beaver quibble? He needed healthy workers, he found them within the large pool of grumettas, and he never bought or enslaved any Africans, true to the colony's principles.

Peter Onsfield's role in the colony illustrates how grumettas created niches for themselves in the midst of these complex race relations. "An intelligent man," according to Beaver, Onsfield escaped bondage during the American Revolution, fled the country, and, by means unknown, made his way to Africa. He had recently joined the ranks of the grumettas, having worked as a servant for a merchant in Bissau. Quickly earning Beaver's trust, Onsfield took charge of the colony's small boat to buy provisions. He visited the Papel, trading successfully for fowl, goats, and rum in addition to grass for thatching the colony's huts. Beaver then sent him farther afield, requesting that he buy cattle and goats in Guinala. Beaver and Onsfield continued to work together for months, despite the short tenures of many other grumettas employed in the colony. Onsfield's success in trading parallels the stories of other former slaves like James Johnson.[19]

One evening in December, the now respectable Peter Hayles, whom Beaver praised as the only person on Bolama who was not terrorized by their Canabac neighbors, sought Beaver out during dinner, informing him that the grumettas were "dissatisfied and meant to leave." The news grabbed Beaver's attention. "Greatly astonished, ill as I was," he wrote, "I sent for them all, and told them that I had learned that they were not pleased with their situation, and begged that they would tell me the cause of their dissatisfaction." One by one, Beaver asked each hired worker why he was unhappy. Most simply said they wanted to leave, although a few were more specific. Antonio complained that he had never received any new trousers even though he had been working in the colony for a month. More important, he needed to leave to pay a debt of rice in his hometown. Lysander was sick and needed to see his own doctor. Another worker wanted to visit two relatives who had recently been captured by the Portuguese and were about to be sold into slavery. "I told them," Beaver wrote, "that every man on this island was free to leave it whenever he pleased, that they all had voluntarily come to work for me, and that I would not detain them a day longer than they wished." After all, the major purpose of the colony was to demonstrate the feasibility of hiring rather than enslaving Africans.[20]

Johnson later reported that the grumettas were more fearful of attacks from Canabacs than dissatisfied with their work conditions. Nonetheless, all the grumettas except Johnson left. He ferried them to Bissau in the colony's small boat, and then hired twenty-three new grumettas: eighteen men, three women, and two boys. Beaver was happy to have married men among his workers: "Their wives will be found useful in washing, cooking, and beating of rice, and their children also in many ways. They will much more than repay their sustenance, which in this country is very cheap." That was the good news; the bad news was that five of the men had fled the Portuguese outpost under suspicion of murder. Desperate for laborers, Beaver and the other colonists overlooked the accusation and hoped for the best. Johnson also brought back yet another warning that the Canabacs planned to attack Bolama.[21]

Beaver, the grumettas, and the Canabacs all helped fashion what we might today call race relations among the British settlers and African peoples. Beaver's writing shows that he did not equate British colonialism with claims that all white people were superior to all black people. He criticized the white Bolama colonists in his journal for their lack of middle-class values, considering the *colonists* rather than Africans lazy. Beaver also condemned the Europeans who trampled on humanitarian principles in the brutal slave trade and ignored their own societies' rules of fair dealing when selling and buying goods of all kinds from Africans. Europeans, according to Beaver, had taught Africans dubious business practices that amounted to cheating, so it was little wonder that they didn't trust whites.

The way Beaver wrote about the Africans he met suggested how someone of his background could treat black workers as equal to white workers. That bar was not very high, of course, since his attitudes toward the white people in his company were shaped by hierarchical views of class and gender. Beaver extended these attitudes to the Bijago from Canabac Island and other neighbors. He would have found inexplicable later racial stereotypes that contrasted the good qualities of all white men, regardless of class, with the negative qualities of all black men. Similarly, European women escaped his scathing comments about the poor work performance at Bolama primarily because he rarely mentioned women at all except when they were engaged in their proper work as wives, mothers, cooks, and nurses. Besides, their sex disqualified them from displaying the "manly virtues" that Beaver associated with hard physical labor.[22] Grumettas who did their duty were thus seen as more admirable than colonists who did not.

Such notions of equal standing did not extend to a democratic political ideal, though. Once Beaver decided that the colony was foundering, he abandoned the principles of political equality written into the Bolama Association constitution. He reorganized the outpost under the British naval model of absolute obedience to one commander. In his account of the settlement a decade later, Beaver focused on the concept of duty to justify his own behavior, and it became a favorite nineteenth-century British rationale for most colonial endeavors. Beaver often appealed to his own sense of duty to the British crown as well as his duty to the humanitarian goals of the association when he wrote about his decisions as leader of the colony.

During the final weeks of 1792, most of the colonists, including Beaver, were so sick that many fell into a state of delirium. Hannah Riches and the female grumettas, probably the three women who had accompanied the new male workers, performed most of the nursing and cooking for the ill. The majority of the grumettas continued to work on the fort. Believing that the end of his own life was approaching, Beaver summoned two of the remaining council members, George Fielder and John Hood, to record his last will and testament on December 13. The following day, Mr. and Mrs. Freeman—a couple that Beaver had recently married—died and were interred in the same grave. Twenty-four hours later, George Fielder lost his life to a fever. Robert Harwin, a servant who had recently witnessed his wife's demise and was one of only three men among the colonists who was "working and well," announced his intention of taking his son to Bissau and seeking a boat back to England.[23]

The situation on Bolama had deteriorated from extremely bad to unimaginably worse. A month after the *Hankey* had left, twenty-nine grumettas were effectively operating the colony. On December 18, fever claimed two more colonists. After three more days of general illness among the group, a council member gave up the ghost with a "mortified face." One of the subscribers to the colony passed away later that same day. On Christmas, the surviving British numbered only thirteen, nine of whom couldn't get out of bed. The end seemed imminent.

Beaver rallied to deal with a different kind of problem—accusations of witchcraft. On December 28, several of the grumettas grumbled about Francisco, who "was not a good man," saying that "he wanted to eat one of them [John Basse] who had been taken ill." Speaking for the group, James Johnson explained to Beaver that Francisco was a "witch, and that he was the cause of John Basse's illness by sucking his blood with his infernal witchcraft." The grumettas asked

Beaver to allow them to tie Francisco to a tree and "flog him, after they had finished their work."[24]

By accusing Francisco of wanting "to eat" one of them, the grumettas probably meant that he had tried to consume Basse's health, soul, or body, and this had resulted in Basse's sickness. Belief in witches was common among most African peoples in Upper Guinea, and Johnson's explanation to Beaver resembled other statements recorded at the time. Accusations of witchcraft were serious charges along the coast. Most societies attempted to identify witches in their midst and put them on trial. If found guilty, they were often sold to European slavers or sentenced to death. Witchcraft "was never forgiven," according to Johnson.[25]

Unwilling to give up his right to discipline the grumettas, Beaver refused to grant permission for them to flog Francisco. A man of the Enlightenment who rejected common British "superstitions," Beaver likewise dismissed African beliefs about witches. One of the colonists claimed that "like all uninformed nations," the Africans are "strongly addicted to superstition," but Beaver did not single out Africans. Not only did he know that many Europeans and Americans still believed in supernatural spirits in the 1790s—some had recently rioted against scientists who wrote rational explanations of the world and proposed alternatives to such beliefs—he scorned European Christian missionaries for preaching to Africans that if they did not abandon their own beliefs and embrace Christianity, they would "roast like yams, yet never get done" in the fires of hell. Such preaching was not, Beaver felt, the way to help Africans become civilized.[26]

Johnson had helped Beaver sort out many previous problems with the grumettas, but this time he sided entirely with them. Johnson claimed that Francisco was "well known to be a witch, that he has killed many people with his infernal art, and that this is the cause of his leaving his own country, where, if he should ever be caught, he would be sold as a slave." Indeed, Johnson said, he had barely been able to prevent the workers "from throwing Francisco overboard on their passage from Bissau hither." Beaver was not persuaded. Johnson sharply reminded him that "it was the custom of the country for *white men* never to interfere in these cases, and that at Bissau the governor never took notice of their thus punishing one another according to their own country fashion, and that they expected the same indulgence here."[27]

Francisco was not the only one. Johnson added that "there was another witch among the grumettas," a man named Corasmo, "who had the power of changing himself into an alligator to devour people, and that he also had killed many people by his witchcraft, and was consequently obliged to run from his country." Beaver asked Corasmo, through Johnson's translations, what he thought of the accusations. As recorded in his later written version of the episode, Beaver inquired:

"How say you [Corasmo], did you ever say to any of these people [that you could convert yourself into an alligator]?"

"Yes," Corasmo answered.

"What do you mean? Do you mean to say that you ever transformed yourself into any other shape than that which you now bear?"

"Yes," Corasmo replied, "I *can* change myself into an alligator, and *have often* done it!"

Once Beaver heard Corasmo's boasts, he gave in, allowing the grumettas to flog both Corasmo and Francisco, though he wrote in his diary that he "desired them to be merciful." The grumettas apparently ignored his request, and Beaver subsequently regretted having turned over the men: "From ten till twelve at night their cries were most piteous and loud, and though distant a full half-mile, were distinctly heard. This morning they cannot move."

Slaving and witchcraft went hand in hand in the Guinea-Bissau region at the end of the eighteenth century. Africans who got too close to Europeans or people of mixed race risked being accused of witchcraft. Predatory "whites" were those who turned African people into slaves, and "white" skin color was less important than a person's identification with Christians or Europeans. "Whites" bartered for African people with iron, tobacco, alcohol, cloth, and the like, all of which could be interpreted as a form of witchcraft. When the grumettas repeatedly said that "all white men are witches," they may well have been thinking that whites used witchcraft to turn Africans into slaves.[28]

The settlers still living on Bolama at the end of 1792 found their days filled with fever, delirium, and exhaustion. Would the new year bring better times? Life on the island did start to improve slightly, even if it remained turbulent. On January 1, 1793, having finished the outside of the fort and several storage buildings inside, the grumettas and a handful of healthy colonists began plastering the walls. The grumettas then set the first timber posts for housing inside the fortress. They worked beneath open, sunny skies, cooled by a refreshing, brisk breeze—a dramatic change from the rainy season and violent storms of the preceding half year. The few colonists left alive had survived bouts of the local diseases, giving them some immunity, and the tide of death receded. The settlers had plenty of provisions and livestock, with more coming all the time from Bissau. In addition, the Britons' fears of attack from either the Bijago or wild animals diminished once they started living within an enclosed fort.

A month later, the state of affairs on Bolama had become so much more settled that on Sunday, February 10, Beaver felt comfortable rescinding his order that all able colonists work on the Sabbath. As a celebration, they slaughtered a goat for the evening meal. The colonists and the grumettas continued building both inside and outside the blockhouse fortress and even began preparing a garden by grading and burning the earth around the encampment. They hunted, going deeper into the forest, where they shot doves, pigeons, owls, Guinea hens, monkeys, gazelles, "goat of the woods," and deer. Even the weather cooperated, with sunshine and cool temperatures nearly every day. About the island and its bounty, Beaver marveled, "A more beautiful and luxuriant country I never saw." Bolama was starting to resemble the paradise originally dreamed about by the colonists. "To live here," Beaver wrote to the colony's supporters in England, "a man has nothing to do but to plant yams and be a good marksman."[29]

The relationship between the grumettas and colonists remained problematic. One worker, Domingo Swar, pulled a knife on Beaver. To his credit, Beaver tried to understand both Swar's frustration and his culture. "They all carry knives in their girdles [belts]," he wrote, "and the instant they have any quarrel the knives are directly drawn. If this is not stopped, at least towards white men, I know not what may be the consequences." Beaver threatened to have Swar executed as punishment. He tied a knot in a rope, threw it over a tree branch, and threatened to hang him and any other grumetta who tried to harm one of the colonists. He then banished Swar from the colony. It was the kind of theater commonly practiced in Britain and North America as a way of demonstrating authority and intimidating poorer people and would-be criminals. Even more theatrically (though perhaps less convincingly), Beaver also boasted to the workers that they were incapable of wounding him. "They thought that I was a very great one and that few things were impossible for me to do. This idea I, of course, was desirous to strengthen, and therefore wished them to think I was invulnerable." After they had witnessed so many Britons becoming sick and dying, it is unlikely that Beaver's declarations of invincibility deceived the Africans.[30]

Beaver's treatment of Domingo Swar was a minor reenactment of the efforts of other Europeans, starting with Columbus and Cortés, to overawe indigenous people and protect themselves from local retribution for incursions on their land. Technology was a favorite means used to aid these ruses. Beaver had earlier demonstrated to some Bijago that the colonists possessed cannon capable of blowing apart a tree a long distance away. He also proudly showed off his compass, telescope, watch, and quadrant, using them as daunting displays of power. West Africans had been in contact with Europeans for centuries, however, and were probably less impressed than Beaver imagined. They had used firearms from Britain, dressed in clothes from India, and wielded swords from the Palatinate for generations. They were not by any means the isolated "savages" that most Europeans, including the more liberal Beaver, considered them. The Bijago and grumettas were, however, overwhelmed by one thing about whites—

their offensive odor. This was not too surprising since Europeans bathed infrequently. In March 1793, for example, Beaver mentioned in passing that except for when ill, he had slept in his clothes for over eight months. One can only imagine the aroma he exuded.[31]

If most of the West Africans Beaver encountered seemed suspicious of Europeans, it was for good reason. Their peoples had endured centuries of abuse from slavers, often among the most duplicitous, despicable, and dishonorable people in the world, so it is little wonder that, as Beaver reported, the local people believed "all white men [are] rogues." As a matter of course, grumettas and the Bijago would fear the motives of any slavers that came to Bolama. The following incident demonstrates that they had good grounds for their fear.[32]

An American slave ship, the *Nancy,* commanded by a Captain Moore, docked at Bolama in March. Months earlier, Moore had helped start negotiations to buy Bolama and ransom the captives from the *Calypso.* Beaver warmly welcomed him to the fort and invited him to dinner that night. Beaver's antislavery beliefs did not prevent him from being hospitable, but his entertainment of Moore flew in the face of strong objections by three men who worked closely with Beaver. James Johnson, James Watson, and a lascar settler, Thomas Dowlah (an original colonist on the *Hankey* from Britain, who was probably of mixed African and Asian parentage), all wanted to rebuff Moore. The three feared that the captain might forcibly enslave them, a sentiment shared by most of the grumettas. Beaver discovered later that Moore had in fact secretly sought out Johnson, Dowlah, and Hayles and proposed that they kill Beaver, enslave the grumettas, and turn the *Beggar's Benison* into a slave ship. Johnson and Dowlah refused to participate in the plan, although Hayles, who had not objected to entertaining Captain Moore, may have been interested in the proposal.

When Captain Moore remained overnight in the fort, Thomas Box, a colonist and white laborer who was deeply concerned about the possible enslavement of his friends, grumbled along with Johnson, Watson, and Dowlah about the unseemliness of an antislavery colony hosting a slave ship—especially one with a crew that had just

killed some Africans and kidnapped others into bondage. They con-
spired to stage a rebellion. While Watson, Dowlah, and Box dis-
tracted the other colonists, Johnson pulled a gun on Beaver. But
Hayles took Beaver's side, sneaking up on them and leveling his own
pistol at Johnson. After several minutes in a standoff, Johnson gave in,
throwing his firearm down and declaring that he could not shoot
Beaver.

The rebellion quickly crumbled, and Beaver set Johnson in irons
and locked him in one of the storerooms. In some ways, this brief
insurgency embodied the original spirit that had set the colony in
motion—the desire to end the slave trade and, ultimately, racial
bondage itself. Several weeks later, Beaver acknowledged that he had
come to understand the rebels' fear of losing their liberty during
Moore's visit. Beaver needed workers, and his self-interest must have
dictated that he try to comprehend what motivated Johnson. He soon
released him from chains and restored him to a position of leadership
among the grumettas. As for his "savior," Beaver subsequently became convinced that Hayles would have shot Johnson to keep him
from reporting Hayles's own interest in plotting with Moore to kill
Beaver.

When Moore left Bolama on March 13, the only additions to his
ship were colonists who had decided to quit, including Thomas Box—
the man who had just staged a rebellion against the ship captain!—
along with his young daughter Mary, Thomas Griffiths, and Mrs.
Riches, the last adult white woman on the island. Box and Griffiths
most likely earned their passage as sailors during the voyage. The
historical record does not reveal whether any of them survived the trip
to the West Indies. Captain Moore and the *Nancy* appear only one more
time, gathering a human cargo in the same region the next year and
conveying the slaves to Barbados.[33]

Only nine colonists remained on Bolama. Although they were in
better health physically, their memories seemed to be failing,
perhaps owing to the hardships, stress, and regular bouts of high fever
they had endured, which can cause short-term amnesia. A "wonder-

ful stupidity" had taken hold, reported Beaver. "Whether it arises from sickness, or from fear, or from both, I cannot tell," he marveled. "But the fact is evident: their minds, if they ever had any, are annihilated, some to such a degree as to render them almost idiots. Dowlah is a fool, Mr. Hood is half stupid, and Watson much the same."[34]

During this season of stupidity, Hayles and Johnson—the two most valuable workers in the colony—decided to leave. In Hayles's case, his one-year contract signed in Cape Verde had expired. Beaver pressed him hard, offering to raise his salary, and in the end convinced him to stay a bit longer.

Perhaps still angry for having been chained in irons, Johnson took a different path. He had joined the Bolama venture six months earlier because he was in debt to a merchant in Bissau and liable to be sold into slavery. Now, Johnson told Beaver, his wife's relatives on the coast owed him a considerable amount of money. If he could collect the funds, he would use the money both to pay off his debt to the merchant and to purchase a small boat and trading goods from Beaver. Johnson said that he could live in Bolama and "make his fortune, by trading" if Beaver would sell the boat to him. Because "he was a most useful and valuable man, and I was inclined to do everything that could attach him to me," Beaver agreed to the plan. He allowed Johnson to take the boat and two hundred bars' worth of trading items for a fortnight, with a promise to return and pay for both.[35]

Johnson never returned. The last Beaver heard, several months later, was that he had been thrown in prison in Bissau. "A proper reward for his ingratitude," Beaver noted bitterly. More than likely, as a prisoner for debt, Johnson ended up on a ship and became, once again, a slave in the New World.[36]

The settlers worked steadily through the summer and early fall despite the continuing disgruntlement of both the neighboring Bijago and the grumettas. For several months, the colonists had not been dying with such depressing regularity. Work became once again the routine of daily life. The pioneers and grumettas built housing inside the fort, cleared more land, and planted more of the seeds they had purchased on their voyage from England.

In mid-July, Bellchore and thirty Bijagos from Canabac Island again arrived on an unexpected visit. While the colonists and grumettas feared a possible attack, the Canabacs seem to have wanted only to trade rice and poultry for rum, tobacco, firearms, and gunpowder. Bellchore had promised his people that they "should want nothing" in terms of access to European commercial goods with the British colony nearby. He had arrived to fulfill that promise.[37]

The colonists had resisted doing business with the Canabacs, most likely because of lingering bad feelings from their initial encounters. In addition, Beaver had found sufficient trading partners in Bissau and with Biafada on the continent. By awkward happenstance, after the Canabacs' arrival several Biafadas gathered with their goods on the beach across from Bolama, firing muskets to signal that Beaver should send a boat to pick them up. Bellchore, quickly realizing that the colonists had been dealing with his long-term enemies, was not pleased.

At the same time, a Canabac spied several ivory tusks lying about in the colony. The settlers had gathered some of them from the forests of Bolama and sawed off others from elephants they had killed. According to the terms of the treaty, Bellchore demanded that the colonists turn these over to the Canabacs. Beaver refused, and the situation grew tenser.

Bellchore tried to calm the waters, inviting Beaver to visit him on Canabac Island. According to Beaver, Bellchore tried to inveigle him by claiming that "his women do nothing but cry to see me," and that Beaver "must come and satisfy them or they will die." Bellchore belabored the point all day. Beaver dismissed him as a "cunning old rascal" who wanted to get Beaver in his power to hold him for ransom. This offer could have been a figment of Beaver's fevered imagination. Certainly Bijago women had been very reluctant to touch him during his previous visit. Beaver declined both the visit to Bellchore's women as well as the invitation to trade.[38]

Beaver's refusal to have sexual relations with Bellchore's women, it should be pointed out, did not stem from racial prejudice. At one point, he suggested, quite radically for the times, that there should be interracial sex. "Whatever rigid moralists may think of me," he wrote, "I would encourage as much as possible a connection between the colonists and native women."[39] In reporting Beaver's words, C. B. Wadstrom, a staunch abolitionist and perhaps a rigid moralist, added, "I have no doubt that Mr. Beaver means here an orderly or social connection."[40]

The original discussions of the sale of the island and the documents for the purchase of the land had not produced a common understanding between the colonists and the Bijago. Residual ambiguities concerning who owned what on Bolama can be traced partially to the Bijago's assumption that the Britons would follow common business practices between Europeans and Africans along the coast, customs about which Beaver was wholly ignorant. The Bijago believed that items found on the island, such as ivory, were not part of the land deal; Beaver assumed that both parties accepted the European notion that land ownership included salable goods discovered there. Beaver negotiated the sale at a time when most Europeans denigrated indigenous beliefs about ownership of assets and imposed their own rules, often by force. Beaver did not have enough colonists or the trained soldiery required to impose his will; he continually had to improvise other solutions to disagreements with his stronger African neighbors.

Bellchore and his men left Bolama unsatisfied after this visit, and the colonists became ever more uneasy. Unspoken among them was the fear that the nearby Canabacs might turn violent again at any moment.

July 19, 1793, the first anniversary of the *Calypso*'s abandoning the colony of Bolama, was a convenient benchmark for taking stock of the enterprise. The nine remaining pioneers were far from robust, their "shriveled carcasses" and "yellow skins" probably a result of the jaundice produced by one of the tropical diseases. The colonists' physical weaknesses belied Beaver's boast that the fort could withstand thousands of attackers: a few dozen Bijago could have overrun them with ease.

The heightened strain with the neighboring Bijago exacerbated other conflicts between the grumettas and the colonists. Most proponents of the Bolama expedition had taken it for granted that Africans would recognize the superiority of Western civilization and try to adopt European ways. It might take a while for Africans to learn to become both consumers and paid laborers, but their transformation would be inevitable. According to this argument, as the colonists taught local peoples how to fulfill these social roles, Africans would become "civilized" and abandon their state of "savagery." What they failed to take into account was that the Africans had for centuries been negotiating with Europeans as traders, consumers, and paid laborers without adopting European culture. The colonists soon discovered that local people, far from ignorant of European civilization, were often uninterested in it. Their "ingratitude" astounded the Europeans, whose paternalism was often matched only by their self-righteousness.

Beaver and the other Bolama colonists eventually turned to the preferred solution among European nations to problems with local people—violent correction and punishment—despite their original humanitarian intentions. Without James Johnson, who had acted as the intermediary between the two groups, using his language skills to translate people's behavior as well as words, misunderstandings mushroomed between colonists and their African workers. During the recent Bijago visit, one of the grumettas, John Lopez, had pulled a knife on the black colonist James Watson. Lopez had wanted to bring a Bijago into the fort despite Beaver's orders to keep the Canabacs outside, and Watson had raised his gun and refused to allow them to enter. Beaver ham-handedly attempted to mediate the conflict between the two men, but without success.[41]

Next, Beaver held a palavra with the other grumettas, first laying "a brace of pistols on the table," clearly meant to intimidate the workers. He tried to convince them of the "enormity" of Lopez's "crime," arguing that the Bijago would enslave them all if they were able to kill the colonists. The African workers understood his point, but insisted that they should be the ones to reprimand Lopez for his poor

judgment. The power conflict lay at the heart of colonial relationships, and had governed relations between Puritans and Pequots, and
between Britain and its North American colonies—interactions that
had ended in violence.[42]

Beaver refused to give the workers the authority they demanded,
insisting that "I only could punish on this island." With his pistols
backing him up, he kept two grumettas, a Manjaco and a Papel, as
witnesses while he tied Lopez to a tree and administered "lashes with
a cat-o'-nine-tails," the same kind of brutal penalty that British ship
captains employed against sailors. Perhaps he regarded his action as
part of the naval discipline of this training. Or perhaps he thought
that the grumettas would accept it because they had earlier used
whipping against the "witches" in their own group. Yet when a
white man flogged a black man, it conjured different images—those
of the slave masters in the Americas and on slave ships who literally
whipped their slaves into line.[43]

Nineteen grumettas, outraged by Beaver's punishment and determined to leave Bolama, all tried to crowd onto a small trading boat
headed to Bissau. Beaver allowed seven to leave, though he refused to
pay wages to any but those who had fulfilled their full month-long
contracts. To retaliate, the fleeing workers stole some cloth, killed a
few fowl, and freed the cow from its pen. Many slave communities in
the Americas exacted a similar sort of retribution. The grumettas
subsequently explained to authorities in Bissau that by stealing, "they
had paid themselves"—a moral understanding also common among
New World slaves. From his perspective, Beaver claimed, "I am always
to be surrounded by villains."[44]

Beaver's ill-chosen corporal punishment of Lopez intensified
the colonists' already acute fear of Africans. Beaver maintained that he
was exempt from racial dread, although his claims came well after the
fact. Since he directed all the work on Bolama, when the settlers constructed sturdier huts for the grumettas *outside* the blockhouse fortress
it can be assumed that they were following Beaver's orders. By treating the grumettas as inferiors, the colonists had broken a central trust
with their workers and splintered the earlier solidarity the two had

maintained against Bijago threats. Although they had armed the laborers to help protect the colony against attack, times had changed. From this point on, the grumettas remained outside the barricade, where they posed less threat to the colonists.[45]

The pioneers had migrated to Bolama with incredible confidence, even arrogance, in their ability to convince Africans about the virtues of Western civilization. Simply by living side by side with the Britons, Beaver believed, the grumettas "would in a short time become so attached to good masters that I question whether they would ever leave them." The reality of life in Bolama first tempered, then transformed the colonists' noble notions. The environmental difficulties they encountered as well as the deterioration of their health awoke their worst instincts. When the Africans did not respond as the Britons had planned, Beaver's dictatorial behavior led him gradually to employ violence to enforce the behavior he demanded of the grumettas. (Beaver played the tyrant with the colonists as well, but if he ever flogged any of the white pioneers, he did not record it in his diary.) Because the colonists' position was so precarious, the increased separation into two camps did not augur well for the future.[46]

From the outset, the white settlers had seemed unable to overcome their terror of both the real and the imagined dangers of living among Africans. They had not forgotten that a year previously armed Africans had slaughtered their friends and kin. Their dread of what the Canabacs might do in the future spilled over to their relationships with the grumettas. The settlers, including Beaver, lost whatever ability they might have had to understand that their own behavior helped shape whether the Canabacs would treat them as neighbors or interlopers, and whether the grumettas would treat them as allies or enemies. Racism, even if consciously resisted, probably underlay the colonists' fears. Beaver claimed he was above racial prejudice, but as the colony's end approached, the comments in his journal grew much more negative about all Africans, especially those living on neighboring Canabac Island.

The dozen grumettas forced to remain on Bolama became sullen, idle, and insolent. One pioneer, William Bennet, claimed that a grumetta tried to stab him. The key to the wine cellar mysteriously disappeared, as did a number of bottles of alcohol. One day Beaver returned to his room to find it robbed of all of his shirts and silk handkerchiefs. He discovered the thief and then ordered the other grumettas to give the burglar severe corporal punishment. (He was too ill to administer it himself.)[47]

Further outraged by the second flogging, as well as for not being paid, the grumettas now stole cloth and muskets from a trading boat arriving from Bissau. They also passed along news of their mistreatment to their former employer in Bissau, claiming that Beaver "not only punished his grumettas severely, but gave them low wages and starved them." The governor of Bissau sent a message imploring Beaver not to chastise the grumettas, but simply to send them away if they were troublesome. At least one of the grumettas, he added, was Manjaco, a group that "never forgets or forgives an injury." The governor feared that the man might retaliate by killing one of the colonists.[48]

Beaver, the man who had prided himself on trying to understand local cultures, now denigrated all Manjaco as "deceitful, thieving, lazy, treacherous people," easily falling back on European stereotypes about Africans. He was also stung into justifying his own behavior. To the charge that "I flogged them all most severely," he responded that he only punished two grumettas, the man who had pulled a knife on one of the colonists and the man who had stolen his shirts and handkerchiefs. Beaver admitted that he had withheld wages, but claimed that he always fed the workers well. Fewer grumettas would sign contracts with Beaver after these incidents, however, and the ones who did come to the colony were often hostile and engaged in work slowdowns.[49]

The nightmarish rounds of death that had earlier plagued the colony now returned, terrorizing the colonists anew. After months without a death, a Mr. Scott fell ill and died of the black vomit. Even worse in terms of the colony's day-to-day continuation was the loss of Peter Hayles, who stole the launch from the *Beggar's*

Benison and deserted the island under cover of night. Hayles left behind a letter asking Beaver to let him go and to pardon him for running away. William Bennet, who had earlier quarreled with a grumetta, also absconded in the night, "having taken all of his things, and some of mine," Beaver grumbled. The remaining survivors blamed the men's desertions on their fear of another Bijago attack. Now there were only six colonists left.[50]

Beaver, waiting desperately for a ship with supplies and additional colonists that had earlier been promised by the Bolama Association in London, kept pressing the five settlers to keep working despite the setbacks. More weeks passed, during which most of the Britons were too ill to work, while the grumettas did less and less. By the end of October, the remaining colonists were talking openly to Beaver about leaving. "Last night," Beaver wrote in his diary, "Mr. Hood told me that he did not like to desert me, but that he thought it not safe to remain any longer upon the island."[51]

Following this conversation, John Williams, James Watson, Thomas Dowlah, and John Hood sent a strongly worded letter to Beaver: "We are at all times ready and willing to do everything in our power under our worthy governor's direction for establishing the colony." However, the death of Mr. Scott and the desertions of Hayles and Bennet had left the colony at only half strength:

> Not having any reinforcement from England which was ex-
> pected, we find ourselves in a very dangerous situation, not
> only from fear of the Bijago but of our own grumettas. As a
> small vessel will be here in a few days, we think it our duty to
> make this public declaration, in order that you may be pre-
> pared for our departure by the first vessel that comes. It is not
> out of disrespect for you, sir, far from it, we are all very sorry
> to leave you. . . . We therefore beg you will value your own
> life for the sake of ours, and embrace this opportunity to
> leave the place before it is too late. If it is once known how
> weak we are, by the Bijagos, you and all of us shall have our
> throats cut in a short time.[52]

Beaver, having grown increasingly paranoid by this time, was unable to recognize the untenable state of the colony. Instead, he accused the other colonists of "cowardice and treachery," arguing that their actions would "inspire my enemies with confidence." Beaver vowed to stay. If everybody left, he would bring Portuguese soldiers from Bissau to keep the colony functioning—a notion the Portuguese would never have endorsed and an indication of his state of mind. [53]

Everyone save Beaver could see that the end of the Bolama colony was at hand. The colonists' earlier fears of the grumettas increased. The most recently hired group seemed particularly untrustworthy, no longer performing the hard labor that previous grumettas were willing to do. Colonists and grumettas maintained a sort of grudging coexistence. The grumettas did whatever work they felt like taking on and shrugged off the rest. Cultivation suffered, as did the care and feeding of the livestock. The looming presence of the Bijago was felt constantly; they were envisioned as hovering just out of sight in their war canoes, waiting for an opportune moment to attack. Bolstering the colonists' fears, several warnings came from Bissau that they should arm the grumettas against the anticipated aggression. For months it had been a foregone conclusion that Bellchore would return with a large war party to collect his British "chickens." Although for nearly eighteen months of enormous human effort and suffering the colonists had managed to hide from themselves how hard it was to establish an African colony, now the truth was starkly apparent. The lofty ideals hailed long ago in London had been damaged beyond repair.

On November 13, James Watson, Beaver's personal servant, informed him that he would catch the next available boat out. Uncharacteristically, Beaver accepted Watson's resolution calmly. Perhaps he understood that the continuing passive resistance on the part of both the grumettas and the settlers meant that no more work would be done. "So panic struck are these people at the idea of being attacked by those treacherous islanders [Bijago]," Beaver complained, that "not one of them will even go to work in the day, though in sight of the blockhouse, without having his musket loaded and primed, lying by him." He might even finally have realized that disease had killed almost all his colonists, and the rest were too few to keep a settlement going. He finally began to waver.[54]

The next day, the remaining colonists submitted yet another appeal to Beaver. "We have informed you in a former petition about the dangerous situation we conceive ourselves to be in. We therefore beg leave to remind you for your own sake, as well as ours, to consider the danger which so alarms us." Whatever Beaver decided, the men wrote, "we are determined to see [to] *our* safety by quitting the island as soon as possible, for the preservation of our lives."

Beaver finally acquiesced on November 14, with one condition. Because they should "not leave anything behind," the pioneers could not depart the island for "some time." He wanted to dispose of the equipment, provisions, blockhouse, and livestock before leaving.

Beaver acknowledged the failure of the colony in his diary: "Having done everything in my power to prevail upon the colonists to alter their resolution, and to remain on the island; having offered to each individual one hundred acres of my own land, if they would remain only till succors arrived; and having endeavored, on Sunday last, to prevail upon them through their ruling passion, fear, to remain on the island, by pointing out the danger of leaving it, but all to no effect, I this morning finally determined to quit it; and therefore ceased clearing the ground of stumps."

The work of colonization stopped completely.

While the settlers began packing materials onto the *Beggar's Benison,* Beaver contacted merchants at Bissau, offering a quick sale of larger items. The traders were happy to buy cannon and provisions at a cut rate.

With no experienced sailors other than Beaver, with torn sails and worn rigging, and with everybody sick, the colonists boarded the *Beggar's Benison* and headed south toward Sierra Leone. They towed the surviving livestock in the *Perseverance,* the small boat they had built on Bolama. All the animals perished within a few days. A week out, the winds died. The cutter was becalmed, and the waves almost wrecked it on the rocks. After a few dangerous days, they rode the tide up the Rio Nuñez to a slave factory, where they sold their small boat and bought some ivory to take back to England. The refugees finally reached the British colony at Sierra Leone after two weeks. In a last exclamation point to a disastrous trip, the *Beggar's Benison*'s boom broke and a strong wind carried it away just as the ship dropped its anchor.

Now that they had escaped Bolama, Thomas Dowlah and James Watson decided to remain in Sierra Leone. Life in the free colony was better than returning to London for a person of mixed race and a former slave. Beaver sold the cutter for a thousand British pounds. He then succumbed to a fever and jaundice, which incapacitated him for two weeks.

While still in the harbor in Sierra Leone, Beaver upbraided himself and the entire enterprise of Bolama. "I feel a great reluctance at being obliged to abandon a spot which I have certainly very much improved, and to see all my exertions, my cares, and anxieties for the success of this infant colony entirely thrown away." But he still felt pride at having done his work and his duty. "I do feel an honest consciousness that everything that could be reasonably expected from me has been done, to secure, though without success, its establishment." He ended the entry: "Myself, very far from well."[55]

If Beaver concluded that everything "that could be reasonably expected" of him was done, he had to find another explanation for the disasters on Bolama. In his published account of the expedition, he leveled most of the blame at his fellow colonists, especially the members of the lower classes, who lacked, he felt, the virtues of hard work and discipline. He censured the Bolama Association's original organizers for their extremely poor planning, conveniently forgetting that he was one of the planners. He accused Henry Dalrymple and the passengers on the *Calypso* of "invading" Bolama at their first visit, without contacting its owners, as planned. The *Calypso* colonists had brought the violence on themselves by appearing to steal the island.

The one group who drew no censure from Beaver was the Africans themselves. Probably Beaver, like most Europeans at the time, no matter how humanitarian their impulses, could not fully recognize the military power of the indigenous people. The initial Bijago attack had unnerved the colonists sufficiently for many of them to flee immediately. Their continued threat provided the final tipping point in the decision of Beaver and the handful of survivors to abandon the enterprise. Moreover, the grumettas—some of the "uncivilized" people Beaver wanted to save—paid no attention to the Britons' claim of superiority. They resisted, rebelled, and ran away. The truth of the matter was that the departure of James Johnson, the grumetta who acted as a mediator between the workers and the colonists, spelled the doom of Bolama.

John Hood and Philip Beaver eventually caught a berth on the *Harpy* to Plymouth, arriving on May 17, 1794. They had been gone more than two years. Beaver returned the few hundred British pounds in his pocket to the Bolama Colonization Society; subscribers had lost virtually all their original ten-thousand-pound investment. Yet Beaver went on to have a distinguished career in the navy. As for John Hood, he disappeared from the historical record.

The Bolama disaster soon became infamous. The major reason was because the pandemic that the *Hankey* spread throughout the Atlantic world originated in the failed settlement. But the downfall of the colony had another impact, serving to solidify arguments that West Africa was too dangerous for white people to settle. Previous British colonies there, such as the one in Senegambia of the 1760s, had ended with similarly tragic results; two-thirds of the Senegambian garrison died within the first year. Though British authorities were still hoping to use Africa as a dumping ground for undesirables, the deaths in Bolama convinced them of the folly of their plans. If any of the transported criminals were to survive, they would need to be deported some place other than Africa. Thus was born the forced migration to Australia.[56]

One way to understand the Bolama expedition is as an adventure tale: a band of white pioneers boldly moving into an uncivilized, unknown territory. That is certainly how most nineteenth-century Britons interpreted the event. John Stuart Mill, the great philosopher and advocate of individual freedom, was one of the avid readers of

Beaver's book, which became a best seller. But Beaver's account provides only one side of the story, a perspective steeped in his standpoint as a self-made British naval officer. Even though the colony
failed, he still represented himself as a hero in the saga of the British
Empire, and many Britons agreed with his assessment.[57]

Another way to construe the story of Bolama is as a narrative of
well-meaning but naive colonists filled with hubris, supremely confident in their own capabilities, in the superiority of their culture, and
in their ability to transform the world in their own image. In this
reading, the colonists chose to be ignorant about virtually all aspects
of the societies and environment of West Africa because they considered them irrelevant. The incidents at Bolama were a stark reminder
that much of European and subsequently American expansion, even
in our own times, has operated in a similar vacuum, with more tragedy than triumph. Nineteenth-century Britons boasting that the sun
never set on their empire ignored disasters like the one on Bolama, a
colony where the sun had set decisively before the nineteenth century
even began.

The Bijago perceived the story of the Bolama colony from a different vantage point. For them, the Britons must have seemed inept,
unimpressive, struggling, and physically and militarily weak. They
could not defend themselves—they could not even feed themselves,
but instead bought their food and hired Biafada hunters to bring down
game.[58] Moreover, the Britons had repulsively light skin, strange eat-
ing habits, and foul-smelling bodies, and they lived in cramped quarters
on a ship. They also seemed willing to trade with everyone except the
Bijago. Since the promise of commerce was a primary reason why
they sold (or leased) Bolama to the colonists, the Bijago eventually
lost their patience. Bellchore finally asserted his superior position,
commenting that the Bijago had permitted the settlers to stay on the
island, but that ultimately they "were his chickens." Surely he believed that he could collect them at any time he chose.

The grumettas hired by Beaver warned him about Bellchore's aggressive intentions. Comprising people from many different ethnic
and racial backgrounds, they were the most reliable and hardworking

people on the island, quite an irony given that the Britons had moved to Bolama to teach middle-class values to Africans. They were crucial to whether the colonists would hold out long enough to establish a permanent outpost. They also were just one of the unresponsive targets of the colony's efforts to "civilize" Africans.

But the influence of the Bolama adventure was not confined to the Guinea coast or Britain's ventures there. Bolama's role as the origin of a virulent strain of yellow fever that would ripple across foreign lands led to consequences far beyond place and time. Every time the *Hankey* dropped anchor at ports in the Atlantic world, its infectious mosquitoes would fan out to find new hosts. As the colony slowly withered away, the ship of death was sailing on to new shores, carrying what soon became known as the "Bolama fever."

CHAPTER 7

Yellow Jack
Comes to the Caribbean

ᘛᘚ

Afterwardleaving Bolama, the *Hankey* crisscrossed the Atlantic for six months, disgorging sick passengers and infectious mosquitoes wherever it went. In addition to the ports at which it landed, the *Hankey* liberally spread yellow fever to other ships, widening the scope of the virus exponentially as the newly contaminated vessels visited dozens of ports in the West Indies, North America, and Europe, dropping off their own infected insects. The result was a pandemic that killed hundreds of thousands of people around the Atlantic Ocean. And the death toll did not end with the *Hankey's* last call. The ship of death's terrible endowment returned annually for the two decades following its 1792–93 voyages.

For residents in the Atlantic world, these plagues posed enormous challenges to their lives and their communities. Soldiers and sailors sent to the West Indies from Britain and France found yellow fever spread by the *Hankey* and its tentacles, other infected ships, to be more dangerous than warfare. Yellow jack also visited port cities surrounding the Atlantic, challenging inhabitants to reclaim and reconstruct their urban centers following the swath of death cut by the fever.

At the same time, this plague born of the slave trade played a part in ending it in one corner of the Atlantic world: with the assistance of the contagion spread by the *Hankey,* revolutionaries were able to end

slavery in Saint-Domingue. The successful Haitian Revolution offered hope to millions of oppressed people in the Atlantic world. But
it simultaneously warned white slave owners and their sympathizers
that the brutality perpetuated through generations of slavery might
one day unleash a race war of unimagined violence. Ultimately, the
Hankey's legacy of death was the legacy of slavery itself, and its consequences continue to influence our world.

When the *Hankey* set sail from Bolama in November 1792, the
colonists' lease had expired and they were fleeing for their
lives, attempting to escape the mysterious cycle of death that had
erupted there. Before leaving England, the Bolama Association had
originally chartered the *Hankey* and its captain for nine months, at a
cost of 1,350 pounds. (By comparison, a Philadelphia day laborer of
the time might earn 10 pounds annually.) Captain John Cox's initial
plan after the lease expired was to leave the colonists on the island
and pick up a shipment of ivory and other African commodities. He
would then catch the trade winds to Grenada, sell the freight, buy
molasses, and convey both the cargo and the ship back to England. In
the classic Triangular trade, merchants and captains earned tremendous profits on each leg of the voyage by buying and selling products.
In reality, relatively few ship owners and captains could pull off the
entire Triangular trade successfully on a continuing basis, simply because so many physical and fiscal risks were involved.[1]

For British merchants able to negotiate the commerce successfully,
earnings from the slave trade were remarkable. In the seventeenth
century, the Guinea coast in Africa was so important as a source of
African gold that the British named a new gold coin after it. As the
Hankey fled Bolama, slave traders in Liverpool were investing some
of their profits in building the largest warehouses in the world. Aptly
called the Gorée Warehouses, their name came from the slave factory
at Gorée (where the *Calypso* had stopped on its voyage to Bolama). A
portion of these enormous profits found its way into financing the
Industrial Revolution, which would help transform Britain into a
major global power.[2]

As the disaster on Bolama unfolded, Captain Cox changed his plans. The colonists initially pressed the *Hankey* into service as a shelter from the incessant rain. For the next few months, the ship became a hospital and refuge. Several dozen passengers and crew, many too sick to stand, were determined to leave Bolama as soon as the association charter expired in November. Under these circumstances, it was impossible to consider locating, purchasing, and loading goods onto the *Hankey,* and Cox decided to head directly back to London. Without the traditional salute when a ship left port, since both the crew and the settlers were too ill to fire the cannon, the *Hankey* finally struggled out of the bay on November 23. The colonists, at least those who were conscious, imagined that they would be on their way home after a brief stop at Bissau.

But the passengers on the ship fared little better than the settlers who remained: yellow jack and the mosquitoes that carried it had boarded the ship along with them. Few of the passengers or crew would survive the next few days, let alone what became a circuitous voyage back to England. Mister Grim, the popular slang for death, was another confirmed traveler on the *Hankey.* Two days after leaving Bolama, one of the sailors died, as did Mrs. Curwood, leaving her husband and two children behind. The Curwoods had been the last surviving intact family among the Bolama settlers. Now yellow jack claimed young Richard Curwood and another victim three days after his mother succumbed, while the vessel still lay at Bissau harbor. Then John Munden, one of the original council members, Mrs. Hancorne, the wife of another council member, and John Mitchell, the ship's carpenter, all died. Edward Fowler, a servant, expired the next day, and Charles Robinson perished two days later. The *Hankey* limped out of Bissau on December 3 with almost all its sailors too ill to work at their posts.

In yet another display of questionable competency, Captain Cox ran the *Hankey* aground on a sandbar a day after leaving port. With the ship half seas over (meaning, at the time, both a drunken sailor and a ship tilted on its side), Cox organized all the passengers who could stand to start pumping water out of the hold. He also sent the five sturdiest men off in a small boat to find help at Bissau, now a distant ninety miles away. All five grew ill from exposure and the hard work of rowing for three days and nights before reaching the port. Meanwhile, the waves continued to pound the *Hankey* as its bow stuck fast to the sandbar. The only redeeming feature was that the ship sat tight, never becoming completely swamped.

Help arrived on several boats from Bissau on December 8. The men unwound the *Hankey*'s anchor cable and pulled the ship free during the rising tide. Cox promptly ran the *Hankey* aground again. After another day of laborious effort, the colonists and their rescuers from Bissau floated the ship free once more. Four of the *Hankey*'s crew—the mate, an apprentice, and the last two skilled sailors—died of fevers during the ordeal. Patience Bates, a servant, and Joseph, a ship's boy, succumbed to sickness on the return to Bissau, as did Mr. Birkhead, the former captain of the *Beggar's Benison,* who had left his own vessel with the Bolama settlers. Captain Cox and the surviving untrained men docked the ship at Bissau to refit after the long week aground. John Rowe, the colony's dissatisfied physician, died just after they anchored.

The *Hankey* finally escaped Bissau with all the ship's mariners dead except for Captain Cox. A few sailors from other vessels volunteered to help them clear the port but retreated to their own vessels as soon as they could. Remarkably, Cox's logbook recorded no deaths or trouble of any kind for the next five days. His luck was too good to last. Cox's navigational ineptitude ran true to form when he tried to dock at Porto Praya on Saint Jago, the largest island in the Cape Verde chain. Cox mistakenly guided the badly listing *Hankey* to the wrong side of the island, finding harbor at Saint Francis Bay instead. The *Hankey* would take an entire week to beat its way back around Saint Jago. It finally docked at Porto Praya four days into 1793.

Surely, no one felt much like celebrating the new year on board the *Hankey*. Only eight colonists remained alive: John Paiba, the adult son of the council member; Elizabeth Rowe, the widow of the recently deceased surgeon; John Gandell, the secretary of the Bolama Association; Thomas Blake and Joseph Glover, both boys and laborers;

John Curwood and his daughter Elisabeth; and Captain Cox. This small number shrank even further while in port, when young Elisabeth followed her brother and mother to a berth beneath the ocean's waves.

Gandell fell victim to yellow jack while the *Hankey* laid up at Saint Jago. In the obituary later published in a British magazine, Gandell was hailed as a man of the Enlightenment who had hoped to improve the world. The son of Moses Gandell, "a respectable London citizen," John had been born in 1770. Two decades later, he and his wife and child set out on the Bolama adventure full of hope for the future. But both his "amiable wife and child fell victim to the perilous adventure of colonizing Bolama." The obituary writer lamented the loss of Gandell, whom he characterized as a young "genius" who had attempted to enrich other societies "with the treasuries of science and literature."³

Porto Praya was a modest town when the *Hankey* dropped anchor. Four decades later an unimpressed Charles Darwin, docking there with the *Beagle,* characterized it as "a miserable place, consisting of a square and some broad streets, if indeed they deserve so respectable a name. In the middle of these *Ruas* are lying together goats, pigs." Darwin's own prejudices were on view when he bemoaned the "black & brown children, some of whom boast of a shirt, but quite as many not; these latter look less like human beings than I could have fancied any degradation could have produced." In 1793, the Bolama refugees did not have the energy to write disparaging comments about the Cape Verdeans. They were busy wondering whether their ship could possibly carry them back to England.⁴

The British Royal Navy intervened at this point to save the *Hankey* and its remaining passengers. Battered physically and bereft of experienced sailors, the ship was scarcely seaworthy. Partly waterlogged, it had frayed rigging, thin and torn sails, a filthy deck, a hold reeking with sea stores and refuse that had not been cleaned out in a long while. Mosquitoes hovered in swarms about the cabins and below the main deck. Captain Dodd, commander of HMS *Charon,* had been assigned to the Cape Verde Islands to protect British merchant ships during the just-declared war between France and Britain. Dodd warned Captain Cox not to attempt to sail directly to Britain because the ships of the French flying squadrons—the fastest and most modern vessels—were actively trolling for prizes off the coast of France. The only way to return safely to England would be to cruise first to the West Indies, then sail east to London in a convoy of British merchant ships that Dodd would organize.

Captain Dodd went farther in his assistance. He sent two of his mariners on board the *Hankey* to patch up the ship and help sail it to the West Indies. But even with Dodd's help, the *Hankey* did not have enough hands to get under way. Another Royal Navy vessel, the *Scorpion,* whose captain had earlier checked up on the Bolama settlement for the association's London directors, provided two more seamen. Ship's carpenters and crew members from the *Charon* and the *Scorpion* spent a few days on the *Hankey* helping to repair the rigging. But tragedy repaid their generosity when the men caught yellow fever and carried the pestilence back to their own ships. Within a week, thirty people had died of fever on the *Charon* and fifteen on the *Scorpion.*[5]

Meanwhile, with four new mariners operating the ship, the *Hankey* unfurled its sails and left Porto Praya for the Caribbean on January 27, 1793. One of the new crew members came down with a high fever almost immediately. A few days later, two of the other newcomers grew sick and febrile. Ordered aboard the *Hankey* by their navy captains, the seamen did not stand much chance of escaping disease on board a floating container of infectious mosquitoes. Yet unlike the colonists, the sailors were at least able to identify the disease. They noticed that when the first mariner expired, his eyes took on a strange yellowish hue.

Yellow jack had gained infamy among sailors because once it broke out on a vessel, the disease easily might kill or incapacitate so many of the crew that the ship would drift unguided. (The disease may have been responsible for the many stories of legendary "ghost ships" that floated endlessly on the Atlantic, lacking master, crew, or helmsman.)[6] So feared was it in the eighteenth century that vessels were supposed to warn others not to come near when people on board were seriously ill. A yellow flag signaled to other craft that a ship carried yellow fever. Captains sometimes followed the protocol, but since it meant that the vessel was essentially in quarantine from the rest of humanity, unable to dock at any port to either sell its cargo or secure help for its crew, they sometimes neglected to fly the pennant. Popularly called "yellow fever," after the jaundiced skin it induced, the disease was known among sailors as "yellow jack," a mocking reference to the small flag (the jack) at the ship's bow that indicated the vessel's nationality.

Popular terror of yellow fever was so great that editorial cartoons of the era depicted yellow jack as a version of the Grim Reaper, a skeletal sailor who came to claim his victims. Images of yellow fever destroying port cities and even entire states became commonplace in the nineteenth century.[7]

People in the eighteenth century lacked knowledge about how to combat the contagion, but many recognized the frightening symptoms: the jaundiced, yellowish color of the eyes and skin. And though the deadly fever might kill a great many humans in an afflicted location, others would recover or be unaffected. The disease's apparent capriciousness added to people's fear of it. They knew neither how to prevent its spread nor how to help the infected victims survive. They could only watch in horror as friends and loved ones perished.

Yellow fever usually starts with a sharp pain behind the eyes, which spreads to the stomach, feet, and joints. It overtakes its victims within a matter of hours. Tears flow as the patient's eyes glaze over. First a white and then a black substance encrusts the mouth. Both the feces and the urine run red with blood. Then the vomiting begins, mostly of a pale color, and finally the skin turns a pale yellow, confirming the identity of the disease. These signs indicate that the sick person's organs are beginning to bleed internally. After a few days of very high fever, most sufferers begin to feel better abruptly; they may even prematurely rejoice that they are well. And if they do survive, most infected people enjoy some immunity to the disease for the rest of their lives. But yellow jack is unwittingly cruel. It often attacks

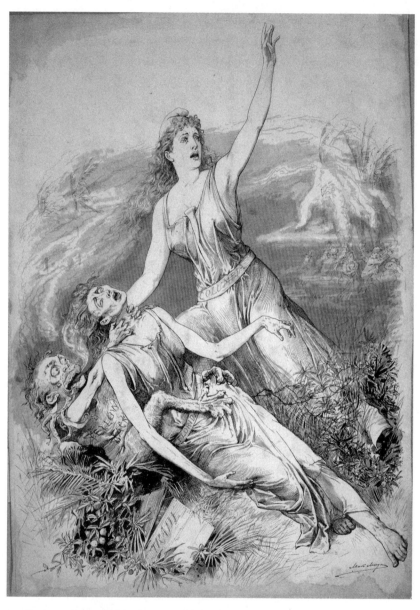

Matthew Morgan, *Yellow Fever Destroying Florida,* 1888. These types of images became common in the popular press during the nineteenth century. Courtesy the Library of Congress, Washington, D.C.

again a day after the brief respite, this time even more vigorously. Patients begin vomiting up a black substance akin to rotten coffee grounds—the blood that has leaked into the stomach. Pain courses through all parts of the body, victims start to bleed from their orifices, and the kidneys begin to shut down. At this stage, the reaper is in the room.

Today, we understand the nature of yellow fever as well as its means of transmission. Before scientists in the late nineteenth century identified how the malady spread and developed a vaccine in the twentieth century, the disease was one of the world's most dangerous pestilences. Yellow jack killed tens and sometimes hundreds of thousands of people in a single year. Even today, it accounts for an estimated thirty thousand deaths annually, and medical researchers have still not discovered a cure.[8]

Yellow fever is endemic to the coastal regions of West Africa. Recent scientific research has provided strong evidence that the disease originated on the continent thousands of years ago, and subsequently appeared in the Americas. Two strains of the virus have been identified, one with subsets in Africa, the other with subsets in South America. Although closely related genetically, the two strains diverged at some point in the mid-sixteenth century, at the same time that Portuguese and Spanish ships began carrying slaves to the Americas. Yellow fever appeared in the historical record at least as early as the 1640s in the Caribbean, almost certainly carried there by slave ships. Since then, it has been found in many warm, humid areas in Central and South America.[9]

Although the early slave vessels surely carried the disease to the West Indies, it rarely had the same explosive effect achieved by the *Hankey*'s cargo. The slave ships generally carried Africans who had acquired some immunity to the yellow fever virus. Most of them had contracted the disease either in their childhood or when they were transported from the interior to the coastal areas to be sold. Moreover, the mosquitoes that buzzed aboard the slave ships in West Africa may have been infectious and had plenty of time to lay eggs, but their own life cycles were usually too short to survive the voyage across the Atlantic. Newly hatched insects become infectious only if they feasted on infected people within the first three days of their illness, and the slave ships rarely had enough infected human passengers, as well as non-immune passengers to whom to transmit it, to act as the hosts needed to produce a major swarm of deadly mosquitoes at the end of the journey. Until the *Hankey*'s voyage in 1793, the concatenation of conditions that was to detonate the yellow fever bomb had never been present in so many places at the same time and with such ferocity.[10]

The *Hankey*'s ability to broadcast yellow-fever contagion started when the colonists altered the environment of Bolama. *Aëdes africanus* mosquitoes had long carried the virus from one monkey to another on the island. This type of mosquito typically lives in the forest canopy, often feeding on simians and circulating arboviruses among them (the so-called "sylvatic" or jungle cycle of yellow-fever transmission). As the colonists chopped down trees, they also brought down monkeys and *Aëdes africanus* mosquitoes. These insects will feed on human beings in a pinch, and they almost certainly conveyed the virus from simians to the pioneers before returning to the treetops. Possessing little resistance because they had never been in Africa before, the settlers served as spectacular hosts in which viruses could multiply and then be transferred to other bodies.[11]

While the *Aëdes africanus* prefers to feed on monkeys in jungle canopies, another mosquito on Bolama also hovered close to the colonists, since humans are its favorite source of food. Small and silvery, the *Aëdes aegypti* (loosely nicknamed the "unwelcome Egyptian" because it had caused such havoc in Egypt) also transmits yellow fever and other diseases from one person to another. These domestic mosquitoes live near people, who provide them not only with blood but also with convenient places to reproduce. After six months docked in Bolama during the rainy season, the *Hankey* was sheltering fewer and fewer people but more and more unwelcome Egyptians. Indeed, the colonists frequently complained about the swarms of insects that infested the lower decks, especially the clouds that gathered around the casks where settlers went to drink. Mosquito eggs are most successful when laid on the damp sides of containers, and the ship's water barrels, clothes-washing tubs, jugs, and drinking troughs for animals all provided ideal habitats to keep eggs moist and alive during their embryonic development. When it left Bolama, the *Hankey* continued to nurture *Aëdes aegypti* mosquitoes and provide them with free transportation across the Atlantic. Owing to Captain Cox's ineptitude, the *Hankey* was even able to supply the new hosts necessary to keep the disease strong, as Royal Navy sailors replaced the *Hankey*'s dead mariners.[12]

In ecological terms, the *Aëdes aegypti* mosquito does little besides reproduce, provide nourishment for birds, and help cull the herd of humans by spreading diseases. Each generation follows the same repetitive cycle, from egg to larva to pupa to adult—mating, laying eggs, dying. Two or three days after emerging from the pupa stage, females begin their lifelong search for blood. For the next several months, they feed primarily in daylight hours, often at dawn and dusk, finding the lower legs of humans especially appetizing. Female mosquitoes cannot reproduce without a blood supply; they metabolize the blood to create eggs. When the time comes, they lay between 350 and 700 at a time, by preference near human habitation. The somewhat hapless males do little but flit about, looking for nectar to consume and females with whom to mate. They rarely feed on people, but since the decibel of their buzzing is within the human range of hearing, they are the ones humans end up slapping. People cannot detect the sound of female *Aëdes aegypti,* which do the actual blood sucking; consequently, they whack at the buzzing, annoying males that pose no real threat.

The *Hankey* became the site of an "intermediate" transmission of yellow fever: a small-scale, second-stage outbreak that occurs somewhere between forests and urban centers. The blood supply for the mosquitoes on board the vessel was perfectly situated. Passengers remained within a relatively small space, often in the close atmosphere of the hold or their cabins, and they could not leave the ship. Moreover, they usually came to the mosquitoes, bending over the scuttlebutts to get a drink of water and waving their hands ineffectually to shoo the insects away. When a female *Aëdes aegypti* stings a person who has been infected with the yellow fever virus within the previous three days, the mosquito may in the process also ingest the virus, which will take a few days to multiply in its midgut and accumulate in its central salivary duct. The insect will then inject its saliva during the next feeding, thereby transporting the virus into a new human being. Not all stings from infected mosquitoes result in the transmission of yellow fever—the number is usually between 5 and 20 percent. If the human victim has previously had yellow fever, the new infection is relatively harmless. The ideal conditions for the speedy multiplication of the yellow fever viruses, then, are a group of non-immune humans and hordes of infected mosquitoes. The *Hankey*'s mosquitoes, carrying an especially virulent strain of the virus, were ready to find additional victims at the ship's next port of call, thereby producing the third, urban stage of transmission.[13]

Even the weather favored the insects during the sailing of the *Hankey*. Historically, yellow fever epidemics often coincide with episodes of El Niño—the semi-regular climate pattern that occurs across the tropical zones of the Pacific Ocean about every five years. Because El Niño produces wetter and warmer conditions in other parts of the world, the population of mosquitoes explodes, and so do mosquito-borne diseases like yellow fever and dengue. El Niño was in the final year of its four-year cycle as the *Hankey* sailed to the West Indies in 1793. Insects on all shores of the Atlantic were probably breeding at the height of efficiency.[14]

The *Hankey*'s voyage cut a relatively rapid and wide arc across the Atlantic, from east to west, south to north, and then back, when it returned south from the American mainland to join the British convoy heading home from the West Indies. Through terrible timing coupled with the worst of toxic luck, the *Hankey* created the first major pandemic of yellow fever in the Western Hemisphere.

The fever from Bolama was about to be unleashed in the West Indies.

The *Hankey* reached Barbados, the easternmost of the Caribbean islands, on February 14, 1793. After dropping off one of the sick sailors who had come on board from the *Charon* in Cape Verde, the ship sailed on. Two days later, it touched briefly at Saint Vincent, dropping off another sick seaman. Perhaps in an exchange of the *Hankey*'s empty water barrels for full ones on the dock, virus-carrying mosquitoes in the casks—a favorite breeding spot for the *Aëdes aegypti*—found their way to shore. Not long afterward, yellow fever epidemics broke out in the Lesser Antilles.[15]

The ship hobbled on to Grenada, one of the southernmost of the Caribbean islands. As with other possessions in the West Indies, several European nations had fought over the island. The British originally tried to colonize Grenada in 1609 but failed. The French conquered it in the mid-seventeenth century, controlling it until 1763, when France ceded the colony to Britain as part of the settlement after Britain's victory in the Seven Years' War. The *Hankey* had visited Saint George, Grenada's main port, numerous times during the past decade, usually picking up a cargo of molasses to take back to England.

On February 19, the *Hankey* arrived at Saint George "in the most distressed situation," according to Dr. Colin Chisholm, the chief physician for the British garrison on the island. The date is important because of the vitriolic debates that emerged during the next decade about whether the *Hankey* had caused the outbreak of disease in the West Indies and, subsequently, throughout the Atlantic shores.[16]

"From this period," Dr. Chisholm claimed, came "the commencement of a disease before, I believe, unknown in this country, and certainly unequalled in its destructive nature." Chisholm's accusation started a controversy that lasted for decades and grew rancorous. Each side accused the other of lying for personal and political gain. Siding with Chisholm were fellow physicians like Joseph Gilpin, who also lived on the island in 1793. "Of the infected state of the *Hankey,* I never did nor ever shall entertain the least doubt, nor do I recollect that any medical man in Grenada held an opposite opinion." Gilpin went even farther in asserting the validity of his opinion: "That those who visited the *Hankey* brought the contagion into the town of Saint George, and that it spread from thence into the country, I have as little doubt as I have of my present existence."[17]

Others strongly disagreed, claiming that the pandemic came from other sources. One of their primary pieces of evidence hinged on their disputation of the date of the *Hankey*'s arrival in Grenada. Noah Webster, the great dictionary writer who provided novel spellings and a distinct version of the English language for the new United States, became the dissenters' most prominent spokesperson. He argued that the *Hankey* could not possibly have transmitted the disease since it docked at Saint George several months after the outbreak of yellow fever.[18]

We need look no farther than the log of the *Hankey,* which provides compelling evidence for the doctors' side. The captain recorded the arrival date at Saint George as February 19. The *Hankey* was in port just before the beginning of the epidemic in Grenada, which then quickly spread to other West Indian islands.[19]

Dr. Chisholm would identify the malady as the Bolama fever, incorporating into the English language a new term for a novel disease—even if Noah Webster left it out of his dictionary. Many other reports popularized the source of the malady. "Plague, brought from Bulam [Bolama] has spread most alarmingly," according to the London *Times*. "Eighty persons died in one day at Grenada of this disease."[20] For the next century, medical men, newspaper publishers, government officials, and ordinary people used the name to describe the outbreak of the pandemic. The expression would send chills of horror through residents of towns where an outbreak threatened. In reality, the Bolama fever was not a new disease but a significantly more virulent strain of a very old one, yellow fever.[21]

After a few days anchored outside the port, officials allowed the *Hankey* to move into careenage, a section of the harbor that contained dozens of commercial vessels. In this usually safe haven, crews had attached ropes to their ships' masts, and then heeled the vessels onto their sides by ropes tied to trees on the steep shoreline. The sailors then set about cleaning the hulls of barnacles as well as patching and caulking, a process known as careening. Ships in the tropical waters of the West Indies often required this kind of cleaning, in particular to remove the worms that lived in the warm waters and did considerable damage to the hulls. When its hull grew foul with unwanted growths, a ship's speed would be considerably slowed. As one of the newer type of ships with a copper-bottom sheath, the *Hankey* did not need to undergo the process as often; the captain had another reason for wanting to move to careenage. Along with dozens of other vessels, he was waiting for the protective convoy to England being organized by Captain Dodd of the *Charon*—the Royal Navy ship that had helped out the *Hankey* in Cape Verde.

Based on his interviews with Saint George's inhabitants and his treatment of the people who fell ill, Dr. Chisholm wrote the most detailed account of how the Bolama fever spread from the *Hankey* to mariners in nearby ships and other ports:

> Captain Remington, an intimate acquaintance of Captain Cox's, was the first person who visited the *Hankey,* after her arrival in St. George's Bay. This person went on board of her in the evening after she anchored and remained three days; at the end of which time he left St. George's, and proceeded in a Drogher [small craft] to Grenville Bay, where his ship, the *Adventure,* lay. He was seized with the malignant pestilential fever on the passage, and the violence of the symptoms increased so rapidly, as, on the third day, to put an end to his existence. The crew of the *Defiance* of Blythe port, near Newcastle, were the next who suffered by visiting this ship: the mate, boatswain, and four sailors went on board the day after her arrival: the mate remained either on deck or in the cabin, but the rest went below, and staid all night there. All of them were immediately seized with the fever, and died in three days. The mate was also taken ill, but, probably from his having been less exposed to the virulence of the infection, he recovered. The crew of the ship *Baillies,* from the same imprudent civility of curiosity, was the next who suffered. These communicated the infection to the ships nearest them.[22]

Venturing on board the ship of death had immediate consequences. As the visitors returned to their own ships or stopped to chat with sailors on other vessels, mosquitoes accompanied them. After being stung on the *Hankey*, some of the seamen likewise carried the deadly virus in their bodies. Yellow fever "burst forth with all of its horrors," exclaimed one contemporary, from the cursed ship from Bolama.[23]

The port of Saint George scarcely could have furnished a better setting for enabling infectious mosquitoes to move from ship to ship. Packed tightly into the harbor, the vessels usually anchored side by side only a few feet apart—well within the hundred-yard flying distance of the *Aëdes aegypti*. Hills descending from a nearby mountain virtually enclosed the port, keeping the wind to a minimum. There was virtually no breeze to blow the mosquitoes off course in their pursuit of blood. Moreover, in the harbor, according to one contemporary account, the "atmosphere and water are commonly stagnant, while the shore of the town is remarkably low and crowded with houses and other buildings, reaching close to the wharfs." All were perfect breeding places for domesticated mosquitoes like the *Aëdes aegypti*.[24]

The fever moved gradually but inexorably from one ship to the next, "not one escaping, in succession," according to Dr. Chisholm. Nothing could be done to prevent its spread. The traditional remedies seemed powerless against this new plague. "Whatever means the captains took to prevent it, even the smell and smoke of coal tar, which is uncommonly pungent and penetrating, had no effect as a preventive." A then common belief among sailors was that ships undergoing careening were disease free, since the asphalt-like substance they applied to the hulls would guard them against most ailments. When the mysterious new fever overwhelmed the crew of the *Hope* as it was being careened, a panic ensued. Within weeks after the *Hankey*'s arrival, more than five hundred sailors—approximately one of every three mariners on the ships in the harbor—died.[25]

In early April, the disease jumped from ship to shore. It found its first foothold in the house of a merchant on the wharf, believed to have been introduced by a slave woman who took in sailors' clothes to wash. Everybody in the home perished. Sailors and dockworkers congregated in the nearby boardinghouses and inns, and the disease mushroomed among them. Many of the seamen, according to a report by a prominent abolitionist, were already ill from ailments associated with poverty and dissolution. Some were "ulcerated all over, but particularly in their legs, and their ulcers are often covered with mosquitoes." Ordinary prophylactics, like camphor stitched into small linen bags and hung around the neck, proved ineffective. The infected *Aëdes aegypti* from the *Hankey* and other ships in the harbor could hardly have found easier meals, nor could yellow jack have found bodies more defenseless.[26]

From the sailors, according to Chisholm, "the fever spread itself among the residents on the immediate edge of this inlet." Blaming poverty, the environment, and the victims, Chisholm noted that the disease took its highest toll in Saint George "among human beings enveloped in impure air, buried in filth, and devoted to prostitution and drunkenness." They lived in "wretched habitations, huddled together, exposed to the noxious exhalations and noisome effluvia of the Careenage." Higher mortality among the poor was a pattern that would repeat itself from Saint George to Philadelphia and in numerous port cities up and down the Atlantic seaboard.[27]

Simultaneously, the Bolama fever began to afflict the nearby British military base. Half the Royal 45th Regiment, Nottinghamshire foot troops who had fought well in the American War of Independence, were stationed in Grenada. Their barracks lay to leeward of the *Hankey,* meaning that any gust of wind would help carry infected mosquitoes to the post. Exacerbating the situation, several curious officers and enlisted men, perhaps egged on by their fellow soldiers, decided to visit the *Hankey* to find out if the rumors about a ship of death were true. They spent several hours on the vessel before returning to their quarters. The results were predictable. All the visiting soldiers caught yellow fever, which quickly spread to others in their regiment. "That part of the garrison quartered nearest to where the *Hankey* lay," Dr. Chisholm observed, thus "were the first of this class of men who received the infection."[28]

Yellow fever then moved up the 175-foot volcano to attack the artillery company in Fort George. A few of the gunners had stayed at the barracks of the 45th, then climbed the hill to the fort, probably taking the virus with them. Shortly thereafter, the disease took its toll, afflicting two-thirds of the men in the company.

The spread of yellow fever among the soldiers augured potentially disastrous consequences. When the *Hankey* arrived in the West Indies, Britain was organizing one of the largest invasions in history as part of the war against revolutionary France. Both sides regarded the Caribbean as an important theater. Upward of sixty thousand troops, most of them with no previous exposure to the disease, were on their way to the Caribbean. For more than a century, yellow fever had decimated invading forces in the islands. With a virulent new strain in the area, the possibilities of a severe epidemic were terrifying.[29]

Meanwhile, the disease spread to neighboring plantations and then inland. It killed a number of white people, but was less fatal among slaves, who may have enjoyed some immunity from having grown up in West Africa.[30] Overall, fully one-half of the white population of Grenada died within six months of the arrival of the *Hankey*. The death toll was staggering, and the onslaught of disease would not halt for the next dozen years.[31] Even at its first port of call, the Bolama fever carried by the ship of death had created a legend and would be regarded with awe for decades to come.

As the crews on the ships near the *Hankey* became infected by the mysterious fever, their captains began to recognize that the pestilence spreading throughout the harbor was something new, which none of their preventive measures could halt. Ship after ship unfurled its sails and fled to other islands in the West Indies, inadvertently spreading the virus to new, crowded ports. Within months, inhabitants of these islands, including Dominica, Barbados, Saint Vincent, Jamaica, and Saint-Domingue, had all suffered infection.

James Clark, who practiced medicine on Dominica at the time, tracked the spread of the disease. "Fever broke out on June fifteenth, first from an English seafaring man" who was new to Dominica. Next, "sailors on board ships in the Road" (anchored outside the harbor) contracted the disease. Within a few months, a thousand "English, including newcomers, sailors, soldiers, and Negroes," also fell victim to yellow jack. The fever declined in November with cooler weather, but then vessels from Philadelphia, where the epidemic was now raging, reintroduced yellow jack to the region.[32]

A few weeks after the fever appeared in Dominica, according to Clark, death "reached Antigua and the rest of the Leeward Islands; but all partook of its ravages." Writing in 1797, Clark made the connection between the Bolama fever in the West Indies and its subsequent transfer to the North American continent. "It broke out about the same time at Jamaica and St. Domingo, from the latter of which islands the contagious disease was supposed to have been brought to the town of Philadelphia."[33]

The islands had experienced yellow fever epidemics before the *Hankey* arrived, but the disease had not swept the region in epidemic form for several decades prior to 1793. A few outbreaks had occurred, but they were relatively rare. This was particularly true of Grenada and the Windward Islands, where yellow jack had been virtually unknown since 1763. Many of the inhabitants, therefore, especially those recently arrived from Europe, lacked resistance to the disease. Those born in the Caribbean or in environments with similar diseases, especially slaves from West Africa, had a limited immunity and were more likely to survive an epidemic.[34]

As the virulence of the disease became clear and all signs pointed to the *Hankey* as the source of the ailment, the governor of Grenada summoned Captain Cox for an interview. The issue that most disturbed the governor was the property of the people who had died on the ship, since he suspected that these belongings carried the fever. The wealthier colonists had taken many goods with them to Bolama whose value was significant. Since he would be liable to the colonists' families in Britain if he destroyed their personal property, Captain Cox refused to throw the items overboard. The governor was apoplectic, demanding that Cox either dump the goods or move the *Hankey* out of the harbor.[35]

The governor also sent an emergency message by the next ship to Britain's home secretary, Henry Dundas, the proslavery official who had denied government sanction of the Bolama expedition. Given how slowly news traveled across the Atlantic, it took weeks for Dundas to learn about the contagion linked to the *Hankey*. But when the news finally reached him, he ordered that the ship be sunk along with its cargo to end the killing spree. It took several weeks for Dundas's order to reach the Caribbean, leaving the *Hankey* and its mosquitoes afloat for the crucial months of the pandemic.[36]

Meanwhile, Captain Cox was worried about the governor's threat, and he decided to leave Grenada. Several of his seamen had jumped ship, and he had a hard time finding able sailors in port willing to join the crew of the *Hankey*. All were either already sick or so leery of the *Hankey*'s reputation that they refused to come aboard. After much searching, Cox hired a handful of sailors, including three former slaves (who may have thought they were immune since they were born in Africa) and a sailor displaced from another vessel under suspicious circumstances.[37]

The *Hankey* set off north, toward the port of Cap Français (Le Cap), on the northern coast of Saint-Domingue, where Cox and his crew must have been startled to discover the port enveloped in smoke. The area had been burning for weeks, set ablaze as part of the ongoing slave revolution. One of the largest, most vibrant cities in the West Indies, with nearly twenty thousand inhabitants, Cap Français was the size of Boston, containing some fourteen hundred buildings laid out in a modern grid pattern. The city was considered so charming that it was nicknamed the "Paris of our islands." (It was also regarded as scandalous. Though its theater, which could hold fifteen hundred patrons, was segregated by race—white, free black, and mixed—its public bathhouses were not separated by sex: a "husband and wife, or those who considered themselves as such, could go to the same bath and the same bathtub.") Now in the hands of black revolutionaries, it was in flames. Some accounts claimed that the rebels set fire to the city; others blamed the retreating French royalists for the conflagration.[38]

What had started as a slave rebellion in 1791 had become a war of liberation, as gens de couleur libres and mulattos (both groups were free people of mixed African and European descent) battled to gain equal citizenship. For French planters and other whites, it became a conflict to maintain their advantages as the master race at the top of the pigmentocracy in colonial Saint-Domingue.[39]

France had claimed Saint-Domingue, the western third of the island of Hispaniola, at the end of the seventeenth century. The colony soon became the most valuable property in the French colonial system, the richest colony in all the West Indies. At the time, it was producing half the world's sugar and 40 percent of its coffee. The island's mild climate and fertile soil also supported the production of cocoa, indigo, tobacco, cotton, and sisal. Based on the ideas of mercantilism, the French Empire's economic regulations resembled those of the British, which had triggered the revolution in Britain's North American colonies. The French demanded that all Saint-Domingue's products had to be sold directly to France at cut-rate prices. These strictures contributed to the revolt in the Caribbean.[40]

In Saint-Domingue, about a half million slaves toiled under some of the most brutal conditions in the world. About a hundred thousand West Africans (most of whom had probably contracted yellow fever during their youth) were forced onto the island between 1789 and the time the slave revolution broke out in 1791. Meanwhile, approximately thirty thousand gens de couleur libres, though laboring under less harsh conditions, lacked equality with whites. The French numbered about twenty thousand whites, consisting of planters and "petits blancs," members of the middle and lower classes. Overwhelmingly outnumbered by slaves and extremely fearful of black uprisings, the plantation owners employed excessive violence to preserve their own privileges and keep the majority of their population in bondage.

Slavery was, at heart, a system rife with violence. Yet bondpeople in some places and times throughout the Americas could devise ingenious ways to negotiate, tacitly, with their owners for some control over their lives, such as trading hard work for the right to visit their families on Sundays. Such negotiations were rarely allowed on Saint-Domingue. The power of masters and the state that backed them up was overwhelming and brutal. In part, their motives were purely economic. It was cheaper to work a slave to death and then buy a replacement from one of the ships continually arriving from Africa than to feed and clothe the slaves one had. But more than economics was at stake; the vicious treatment of slaves also stemmed from the masters' fear and hatred of Africans. Whites lived surrounded by black people whom they treated abominably; all of them, their owners believed, were savages waiting to get their revenge.[41]

Violent, degrading, sadistic treatment of slaves became accepted as part of everyday life. One observer, Francis Stanislaus, had arrived in 1788 as a visitor to Saint-Domingue. He awoke the first morning to "the cracking of whips, the smothered cries, and the indistinct groans of the Negroes, who never see the day break but to curse it, who are never recalled to a feeling of their existence but by suffering." As he strolled around Port-au-Prince, he witnessed Africans being branded by irons so they could be identified if they ran away. He also saw slave men and women slumped against a wall, waiting for their owner or overseer to use his "Arceau [whip] on their backs and shoulders." Two years later, Stanislaus was among the first refugees to flee the uprising.[42]

One man who had been in bondage for half of his life on Saint-Domingue captured the horrors of slavery on that island:

> Have they not hung up men with heads downward, drowned them in sacks, crucified them on planks, buried them alive, crushed them in mortars? Have they not forced them to eat shit? And, having flayed them with the lash, have they not cast them alive to be devoured by worms, or onto anthills, or lashed them to stakes in the swamp to be devoured by mosquitoes? Have they not thrown them into boiling cauldrons of cane syrup? Have they not put men and women inside barrels studded with spikes and rolled them down mountainsides into the abyss? Have they not consigned these miserable

blacks to man-eating dogs until the latter, sated by human flesh, left the mangled victims to be finished off with bayonet and poniard?

The man freed himself and others by fighting in the slave rebellion later known as the Haitian Revolution.[43]

It was the French Revolution, with its ideals of liberty, equality, and fraternity, that triggered the uprising on Saint-Domingue. Yet even before 1789, inhabitants on the island were becoming restless. White planters and gens de couleur libres had been tentatively cooperating to resist control by the French government. Eventually, they advocated breaking with France and establishing an independent slave-owning nation. These two interest groups tried to dominate the kaleidoscope of political and military actions in the 1790s and early 1800s, but were continually challenged by mulattos and slaves, as well as by troops sent by the governments of France, Britain, and Spain.

Although excluded from the political movement to resist France, slaves had been pushing against their bondage for years. In the 1759 Makandal rebellion, slaves poisoned water supplies and killed hundreds of masters before planters brutally crushed the revolt. By 1789, a large group of runaway slaves (maroons) had formed communities in the mountains, raiding local plantations and waging a low-level guerrilla war against whites. Maroons and slaves fighting for emancipation rallied behind Toussaint Louverture, starting in 1791, along with Jean-Jacques Dessalines. Meanwhile, the revolutionary French Assembly was sending mixed political signals to the colony, including a declaration that gave citizenship rights to property-owning gens de couleur libres and mulattos. The Assembly sent French troops to enforce the decree and to retain imperial control of Saint-Domingue. Sporadic violence and atrocities of all kinds broke out on the island. The situation changed once more when the French Republic declared war on Britain in 1793. By then the Bolama fever, on top of local strains of the virus, was already weakening the French imperial forces.

As part of its war against France, Britain decided to attack the French Empire in the Caribbean. Because of its incredible wealth,

Saint-Domingue was a key focus. A hundred thousand troops, the largest expeditionary force in British history to that time, were dispatched to put down the Revolution. In August, the French revolutionary commissioners on Saint-Domingue abolished slavery. It was a desperate move to save French imperial control and implement the ideals of France's own revolution. The maneuver was briefly successful. But it also forced yet another rearrangement of the previous alliances among whites, slaves, and the gens de couleur libres. Seeing their chance to regain control, the white French planters welcomed the invasion by the British navy in September; by June 1794 the British had occupied the southern port towns of Saint-Domingue.

Toussaint Louverture and Jean-Jacques Dessalines are the leaders generally credited with the ultimate success of the Haitian Revolution. The turning point occurred in early 1794, when France officially abolished slavery in its colonies. Louverture made an abrupt about-face, joining the French. The primary goal, which rallied the majority of slaves to his side, was now the offer of emancipation.[44]

Louverture was the British nightmare: a brilliant strategist, a shrewd diplomat, and a brave leader of men in battle. He also understood the power of the yellow jack that had invaded the island and how to use it as an ally. Louverture and his soldiers waged fierce guerrilla warfare, striking the British forces from the hills and then quickly withdrawing. When the British military followed into the mountainous home turf of the maroons, they were met with ambushes. Louverture and his lieutenant Dessalines thus kept the British Army confined to the port cities and the plains, the unhealthiest regions for Europeans. The rebels realized that when the rainy season set in, yellow jack would pose a huge threat to the British Army. Meanwhile, many of Louverture's men, who had come to Saint-Domingue directly from Africa, were immune.[45]

The Haitian Revolution created ideal conditions for outbreaks of yellow fever. Starting when the British military and naval forces arrived in September 1793, through the waves of reinforcements that continued to pour into the island over the next few years, the troops provided tens of thousands of non-immune bodies susceptible to attack by fever-carrying mosquitoes. The virulent new form of the virus introduced from Bolama combined with the local strains endemic to the Caribbean to ravage the invaders.[46]

William Pym, surgeon to a British battalion and one of the medical men who identified the presence of the Bolama fever, provided a firsthand account of the slaughter. "There were many instances of officers and men not surviving a week after debarkation." Some of the regiments, including the 82nd and the 103rd, suffered immediate decimation. They "returned to Europe complete skeletons, not having a sufficient number of men left to complete their establishment of non-commissioned officers." The devastation repeated itself with virtually every new corps that arrived. Most of the troop carriers endured tremendous losses as well, with "many of the vessels having the signal of death flying for days together, and were left at last without a single soul to haul it down." After being introduced to Grenada by the *Hankey,* the Bolama fever "naturalized itself in the different islands," according to Dr. Pym, and "continued to [do] so as long as it had fresh subjects to work upon."[47]

Infectious mosquitoes felled successive waves of British reinforcements, killing them almost as soon as they stepped off the boat. Lieutenant Thomas Howard arrived with his unit, the York Hussars, at Môle Saint-Nicolas (one of the places Christopher Columbus had landed) in May 1796. He dreaded what awaited his regiment at this naval base: "In the West Indies the Months of June, July, August, September and the beginning of October are what are called the sickly months." On average, twenty soldiers were dying every day. "It is impossible for words to express the horror that presented itself at this time," lamented Lieutenant Howard in his journal. His regiment lost almost a quarter of its men within a single ten-day period.[48]

The extraordinary losses due to yellow fever encouraged the desperate British commanders to look elsewhere to fill their depleted ranks. They impressed slaves into the army, demanding that each planter relinquish some of his bondpeople to serve in the military.

Arming slaves to fight against an army comprising people who were in the process of declaring their freedom was a bold, dangerous move. It also psychologically undermined the slave regime that the British were trying to protect.[49]

The slaves pressed into the British military were needed not only for combat but to dig new graves every day, "from sunrise to sunset"— yet still they couldn't keep up with demand. Slaves made daily rounds with pushcarts, stopping at each tent to collect the dead. After stacking seven or eight bodies onto their cart, they would wheel it to the makeshift graveyard, dump the cadavers into mass graves, sprinkle them with lime, and cover them with dirt. After a while, they ran out of lime.[50]

The capriciousness of yellow jack in selecting victims and dispatching them so quickly induced terror among the living. "Men were taken ill at dinner, who had been in the most apparent Health during the Morning, and were carried to their homes at night," where they lay abed, dying. Indeed, "death presented itself under every form an unlimited Imagination could invent," Howard moaned, and "some died raving Mad." The lieutenant continued: "The putridity of the disorder at last arose to such a height that hundreds almost were absolutely drowned in their own Blood, bursting from them at every pore."[51]

Of the nearly seven hundred York Hussars who departed from Portsmouth for Saint-Domingue in early 1796, nearly two-thirds, almost five hundred men, never returned to Britain. Only seven of the casualties resulted from combat; the rest came from disease. Their mortality was only slightly worse than average. By the summer of 1796, upward of six thousand British soldiers had expired on Saint-Domingue.[52]

The experience on Saint-Domingue was repeated on other islands in the West Indies. Sir John More led his troops against guerrilla fighters struggling for their freedom on Saint Lucia in 1795. The 31st Regiment under his command lost 863 men out of 915 (94 percent). "Every description of fever prevailed amongst them, and they fell off so rapidly within a few months" that the handful of survivors had to commandeer a small boat and row to safety on another island. The British, who had claimed Jamaica in the mid-seventeenth century to grow sugar, lost eight thousand soldiers to disease even though no fighting occurred there. And British merchant seamen were not immune. According to the calculations of the historian J. R. McNeill, approximately five thousand British sailors died each year in the West Indies during the 1790s.[53]

By 1798, the British had lost too many soldiers to keep up the fight. One British commander reported, "All of our boasted army has dwindled to nothing." Defeated by slave revolutionaries who were ably assisted by yellow jack, the British evacuated Saint-Domingue.[54]

As news of the mortality rates began spreading to England, the British public accused the government of gross incompetence for not protecting the troops. British officials tried to hide the full extent of the disaster, making it difficult to determine the exact number of deaths. The best estimates are that during the five years of the British invasion, 1793 to 1798, perhaps twenty-five thousand troops served in Saint-Domingue. About fifteen thousand, or nearly two-thirds, died, mostly of yellow fever. Scholars' best guess today is that between fifty and seventy thousand British troops perished in the West Indies during the 1790s.[55] When the prominent conservative politician Edmund Burke discovered the magnitude of the disaster, he voiced his dismay about the "recruits to the West Indian grave" and the futility of fighting to conquer a cemetery in the West Indies. Britain had lost thousands of its countrymen and squandered a huge portion of its national treasury for no obvious advantages.[56]

Britain's attempt to seize Saint-Domingue failed utterly, foiled by the courage and skills of the revolutionary army, assisted by the yellow fever virus. Together they had decimated the invading troops. When the British withdrew in 1798, Toussaint Louverture quickly solidified his power and his independence from his French allies. The new constitution declared him governor for life in 1801, just two years after Napoleon Bonaparte staged a coup d'état and seized power in France. His revolutionary principles earned Louverture the nickname the "Black Napoleon."[57]

Meanwhile, his namesake had decided to renew French claims in the West Indies and carve out a new empire in the immense territory known as Louisiana, which France had recently reacquired from Spain. Bonaparte planned to retake control of Saint-Domingue and reinstate a plantation economy there that would again produce the sugar and coffee that had made it the most valuable colony in the world. The plan included reviving slavery in the French Caribbean. Nonetheless, Bonaparte hoped that black troops could be reconverted to French loyalty, and that France eventually would conquer many of the West Indian islands. At the same time Louisiana would become the breadbasket of the French Empire in North America, supplying food for the slaves on Saint-Domingue and elsewhere. As a bonus, French farms in Louisiana would serve as a buffer to limit the expansion of the United States.

In 1802, Bonaparte entrusted the command of about sixty-five thousand of his best soldiers and sailors, most of them veterans of wars in Europe and Egypt, to his brother-in-law General Charles Leclerc. The troops were ostensibly sent to help protect Saint-Domingue from foreign invaders, but Louverture was not fooled. Along with his lieutenant Dessalines, he retreated to the mountains and organized another guerrilla campaign. The struggle resembled the war they had waged against the British half a dozen years earlier. The rebels set fire to the city of Cap Français, reducing it to a "pile of cinders." They kept the French soldiers confined to the ports and the plains until the fever season could come to their aid.[58]

Both Louverture and Dessalines knew that yellow jack would be on their side if they could stall the French long enough. "Do not forget that while waiting for the rainy season, which will rid us of our enemies," Louverture wrote to his lieutenant, "we have only destruction and fire as our weapons." Dessalines explained the strategy to his troops. "The whites from France cannot hold out against us here in St. Domingue," he declared. "They will fight well at first, but soon they will fall sick and die like flies." And "when the French are reduced to small, small numbers, we will harass them and beat them."

Thanks to yellow jack, events turned out exactly as Louverture and Dessalines anticipated.[59]

The French found it relatively easy to occupy the cities and parts of the plains after their arrival. But with the spring rains, yellow fever broke out among the troops. Leclerc lost about forty men to disease each day in May. That number grew to more than a hundred casualties daily throughout the summer. As the epidemic raged and the guerrilla fighting grew more intense, racial genocide began. Dessalines did not hesitate to slaughter his enemies. Nor did Leclerc, who had advocated killing all black males over twelve years old, or as many as two hundred thousand people, to win the war. Louverture was finally captured in 1802 and deported to France, where he would quickly die in prison, but soon afterword Leclerc was himself cut down by yellow jack. General Rochambeau assumed command of the French, following Leclerc's strategy of torturing and massacring as many black people as possible. The French fought for another year, but their numbers continued to dwindle against the onslaught of both revolutionaries and yellow jack. When Dessalines defeated Rochambeau near Cap Français in November 1803, the French surrendered, and were removed from the island as prisoners of war on warships supplied by Britain, which was again at war with France.[60]

After fifteen years of struggle, the new nation of Haiti was established. With Louverture in a French prison, Dessalines claimed leadership of the new country, and issued Haiti's Declaration of Independence in 1804. Haiti's slave revolution was the only such rebellion to lead to a free and independent nation. Born out of one of the most brutal slave regimes in history, midwifed by yellow fever, it was a spectacular achievement. The slaves of Saint-Domingue had defeated the best troops that European nations could send against them, and it was the Bolama fever, legacy of a failed antislavery colony, that had enabled them to do it.

At the height of the Revolution, in late June 1793, the *Hankey* sailed into Cap Français, where Captain Cox hoped to pick up a cargo of refugees among the white planters and merchants who were desperately trying to arrange passage off the island for themselves and their families. Still searching for a cargo so that he could earn money for the ship's owners, Cox offered his services. In the chaos of the conflict, he probably suspected that no one would ask questions about the *Hankey* and its deadly reputation. In addition, the ship had an empty hold already outfitted for passengers. Cox made a tidy profit by taking on as many refugees as his ship could hold. The *Hankey* anchored in the magnificent harbor only long enough to pick up paying passengers and then sailed north, away from the turmoil of the Revolution.

As the *Hankey* wended its way toward North America, it was part of a wave of approximately fifteen thousand islanders—one-third black slaves and two-thirds white refugees—who were fleeing to seaports in the United States. About a thousand of them, including those on the *Hankey,* sailed to Philadelphia. The *Hankey* arrived at the new nation's capital, its largest, most cosmopolitan city, in July 1793. It anchored, along with another ship, the *Sans Culottes,* off a wharf in the northern reaches of the city. We do not know how the *Hankey*'s passengers fared on the voyage. But we do know that the *Hankey*'s voyage of destruction was far from finished. The United States was about to experience the ferocious power of yellow jack.

CHAPTER 8

Calamity in the United States Capital

ﾝﾍﾞ

The *Hankey* docked in Philadelphia for only a week—long enough to disembark sick refugees from Saint-Domingue, try to find a cargo, and trade empty water casks and jugs for full ones on the piers. Virus-carrying *Aëdes aegypti* and their eggs traveled in or flew alongside the containers. Almost immediately, yellow fever broke out quayside. Other craft from Saint-Domingue and elsewhere in the West Indian islands undoubtedly also contributed infected passengers and mosquitoes, setting loose a disease that burned through the city during the next three months. Yellow jack had not visited Philadelphia for more than thirty years, so residents without immunity furnished tinder aplenty.[1]

Chaos soon followed. People of means fled the city precipitously. Other residents hid in their rooms and houses, refusing to venture outdoors, preferring to go hungry rather than risk contact with someone who might pass along the disease. The civil government disintegrated. The church bells tolled unceasingly for the dead.

Remarkably, however, the city began to revive well before the death toll dropped. After the initial panic, many Philadelphians, as individuals and in groups, dedicated themselves to helping their neighbors. Physicians tried to devise a cure. The free black community nursed the sick and buried the dead. Moved by their conscience and sense of duty, a number of common citizens created or restored civic organizations to help the city. From Saint-Domingue to Philadelphia, the voyage of the *Hankey* did more than spread death; it redrew the map of the United States, reconfiguring the political and geographic landscape of the early American republic.

The pestilence started in late July 1793 in a brothel next to the pier where the *Hankey* had docked. Some contemporary accounts identified it as a legitimate boardinghouse, run by one Richard Denny and his wife. However, its location on Water Street, along the northern wharves in a section of Philadelphia known as Hell Town, combined with its clientele of sailors, prostitutes, and immigrants, strongly suggests that it facilitated not only sleeping but also sexual congress. Two French or West Indian mariners, probably from one of the ships that had arrived recently (perhaps even from the *Hankey*), had rented a room from the Dennys. Attacked by a violent fever that blazed through him quickly, one of the seamen died. An English boarder in the house sickened and perished a few days later. Mrs. Parkinson, an Irish lodger, suffered for a week before she expired. Both managers of the boardinghouse died within another week, as did the second French sailor. At the house next door, two people suffered severe seizures, high temperatures, and black vomiting before dying.[2]

These fatalities drew scant attention except from the inexperienced doctors who served the poor in those areas. Isaac Cathrall—a dedicated young doctor who several years later would eat the black vomit of a yellow fever–infected patient to prove that the disease was not contagious (it worked; he did not get sick)—treated Mrs. Denny, but to no avail. Not for three more weeks, when the virus attacked respectable Philadelphians in the care of esteemed physicians, would news of the disease become public.[3]

Once the information got out, the first step was to identify the disease—not an easy task in eighteenth-century urban centers whose residents frequently suffered from a host of fevers and sicknesses. Authorities and the citizenry initially resisted reports about the contagion because of the looming horror it implied. However, as dying people and dead bodies began to collect in alleys, in tenements, and even in the capitol building housing the Pennsylvania legislature and the U.S. Congress, it was no longer possible to ignore the epidemic.

On Monday, August 19, Dr. Benjamin Rush emerged from his house to see a new patient.[4] The slender, confident signer of the Declaration of Independence, now forty-seven, walked slowly not just because of his chronic cough (for which he bled himself regularly) but perhaps also because he was worried. He had been seeing a number of patients with mysterious fevers lately. One boy, who lived near the wharves on Front Street, suffered from fevers, skin eruptions, nausea, and vomiting, which produced a black substance similar to coffee grounds. The boy had died a few days earlier. Still, disease was far from unusual at this time of year, when a combination of ailments and fevers, popularly referred to as the "summer complaints" and the "fall agues," would regularly sweep through the city. Many wealthier residents retreated to their homes outside the urban center during the summer to escape the heat and contagion. Rush was going to see a patient who lived half a dozen blocks away, near the Delaware River, in the midst of Hell Town.[5]

In a few weeks, the whole of the new nation's political, social, economic, and cultural capital, hailed by many as the "Athens of the Western world," would become a Hell Town. Rush lived in a prosperous, stable neighborhood a few blocks from the city center, near the corner of Walnut and Third Streets, but yellow jack would take up residence even here. The houses of his neighbors—another doctor, a judge, a lawyer, a cabinetmaker, a merchant tailor, a gentlewoman, a barber, several grocers, and two master shoemakers—were predominantly red brick rather than inexpensive wood. Most of the buildings were comfortable and spacious, at least by the standards of the time. The gentlewoman, tailor, and physician each owned three-story brick homes, with a separate kitchen in the back. The barber, his wife, and his two children lived in more modest circumstances, typical of most Philadelphians. They inhabited the ground floor of a wooden structure measuring twelve by twenty-seven feet, while a family of boarders lived on the second floor.[6]

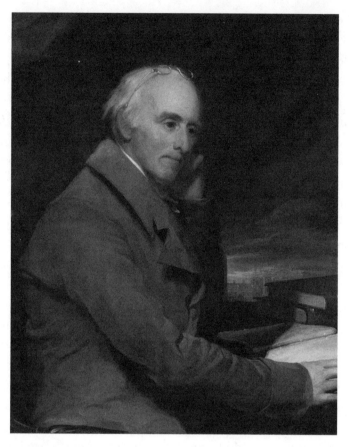

Thomas Sully, *Benjamin Rush,* 1813. Rush was the preeminent doctor in America at the end of the eighteenth century. He was also active politically and was a signer of the Declaration of Independence. Property of Dr. Lockwood Rush. Photo: Smithsonian American Art Museum, Washington, D.C./Art Resource, N.Y.

These houses paled in comparison to many mansions that had recently been constructed in the city. Just a block south of Rush, William Bingham, a merchant, land speculator, and U.S. senator, had built a virtual palace. The huge, three-story brick house with two extended wings contained a library, banquet room, ballroom, card room, and study, all capped off by a white marble staircase. Valuable paintings decorated the interior, while behind the mansion were laid out an English-style garden, a greenhouse with five hundred exotic plants, an orchard, a milk house, an icehouse, and stables. Comparable to the "most luxurious part of Europe," according to one contemporary architect, the house reflected the exorbitant fortunes garnered by some elite Philadelphians. The tall fence setting it off from the street and the public symbolized the wide and growing gap between rich and poor in the city. Class divisions, which had already been significant before the Revolution, had grown even more marked during the subsequent decade.[7]

A gentle breeze greeted Rush as he turned north on Third Street. It carried the pungent bouquet from outhouses (not even the rich had indoor plumbing) and from Dock Creek, a stream running through the heart of the city toward the Delaware River. For decades, tan yards had dumped hides, tanning astringents, and even cow carcasses into the creek; these, along with excrement and other garbage, often rendered it a stagnant sludge that "exhaled the most noxious effluvia," according to one magazine report.[8] Besides irritating the sensibilities of smell and sight, Dock Creek also threatened the health of the city's residents, even if they were unaware of the fact. Since it was also used for drinking water, the stream was the source of some of the dysentery (called the "bloody flux" by contemporaries) endemic in the city.

Clouds of mosquitoes harassed Rush as he walked over the footbridge spanning the creek. It had been a bad year for the pests (or a spectacularly good one when considered from the insect perspective). Heavy spring rains had filled Dock Creek and the Delaware River to overflowing and turned the city's unpaved alleys into muddy quagmires. An unusually hot and dry summer had then dried them up again, leaving the creek a marsh and creating bogs on the banks of the Delaware. The city's rudimentary sewer system likewise dried up, and wells fell below pump level. Residents carted water from the river to fill barrels and cisterns next to their homes, producing an ideal breeding ground for mosquitoes, especially *Aëdes aegypti*. Had they tried, Philadelphians hardly could have created a better environment for the yellow fever–carrying insects. Mosquitoes plagued the city, "constantly lighting on face and hands, stinging everywhere," according to one visitor; many residents kept their windows closed even during the heat of the day to protect themselves from the "myriads of flies and mosquitoes." Nobody at the time, of course, suspected that these tiny, ubiquitous creatures could transmit fatal diseases.[9]

The next several blocks of Third Street through which Rush walked were in the midst of a transformation. Originally attracting businesses that required access to the water in Dock Creek, this neighborhood was becoming the financial center of the nation. In the decade since independence, the Bank of the United States and the federal Department of the Treasury had both established offices in the area; these and other government buildings were beginning to force tan yards and curriers to the outskirts of town. As foul-smelling industries moved out, wealthy citizens moved into the neighborhood, building homes to take advantage of the short walking distance to the wharves and the main marketplace.[10]

Reaching High Street, Rush emerged into the center of the most impressive market in North America. Stretching from Front to Fourth Street, three brick halls, open on the sides and roofed on top, occupied the middle of the street. Slaughtering cattle, pigs, and poultry in the New Shambles Hall, butchers made this market, according to one French visitor, "only second to that of London-hall" in its display of animal flesh. "Besides the customary sorts of meat," a German visitor wrote, "Europeans find in season several dishes new to them, such as raccoons, opossums, fish-otters, bear-bacon, and bear's foot, as well as many indigenous birds and fishes." Calves' heads were a delicacy, and wild pigeons had been particularly numerous this season.[11]

Rush shooed away the flies and stepped over the mounds of garbage, including animal entrails left by butchers from the previous market day. He also avoided the droppings left by animals wandering the streets. Pigs, dogs, and even cows ran wild here, scavenging in the rubbish, while horses pulled carriages and carts. Turning east on High Street, Rush passed Jersey Hall, where farmers from New Jersey brought peas, corn, and other vegetables to sell.[12]

Socializing was almost as important as buying foodstuffs. On the evenings before market days, church bells drew people from both the

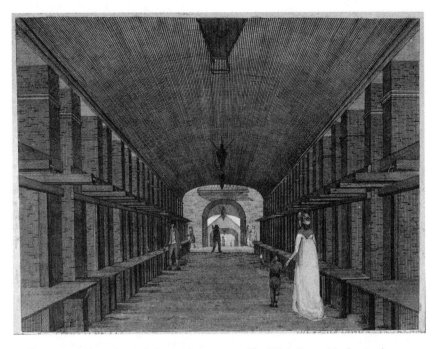

William Russell Birch, *High Street Market,* 1800. The High Street Market in the center of town was rarely empty except during times of epidemic, when people feared catching a disease by venturing onto the street. In William Russell Birch, *The City of Philadelphia, in the State of Pennsylvania North America* (Philadelphia, 1800). Courtesy the Library of Congress, Washington, D.C.

city and the countryside to dances held in the halls. Farmers rumbled into town "in great covered wagons, loaded with all manner of provender, bringing with them rations for themselves and feed for their horses—for they sleep in their wagons." These nights were busy times not only for tavern keepers but also for constables and prostitutes. Streetwalkers congregated at the west end of the market, near the house where Benjamin Franklin had lived. Arrested for "skulking about Country Wagons in High Street at a late Hour of the Night," one prostitute, Margaret Britton, "acknowledged that she wished to have carnal Intercourse with them [farmers] to get money." Although the entertainment was now abolished, just a few years earlier Rush could have watched public whippings and prisoners being exhibited in stocks in the middle of the market. The large crowds that had gathered to see the spectacles, according to one grateful vendor, allowed him to raise the price of eggs and butter considerably.[13]

On Wednesdays and Saturdays, the market attracted one of the most diverse collections of people in the country. The Quaker open-mindedness regarding religious freedom that characterized Philadelphia from its founding had encouraged a varied group of immigrants. Rush consequently heard a medley of tongues—not just different dialects of English but also Dutch, German, French, Spanish, Portuguese, and Gaelic, as well as a host of African and Native American languages. "People swarm to the Market House thicker than Flies to a Hogshead" of sugar, noted one resident. "Everything is full of life," reported an awed visitor, who never tired of watching "this multitude of men and women all moving about and going in every direction."[14]

Crossing Front Street, Rush strolled by the carts where women peddled their husbands' catch of fish and oysters every day. Elizabeth Hill was among the women who gathered here routinely, although she was not there that day since she had just fallen ill with a strange fever. As Rush started down the hill to the Water Street wharves, he saw a lattice of spars and masts on the dozens of vessels docked in the harbor. He also could see and smell a huge mound of putrid coffee on a wharf a block north. The coffee in the hold of the *Amelia,* one of the refugee ships that accompanied the *Hankey* from Saint-Domingue several weeks earlier, had gone bad during the voyage, and the captain had dumped it on a pier and put it up for auction. Given the aroma, no buyers came forward.[15]

To Rush's right was the London Coffee House, a large building where merchants, shopkeepers, and ship captains drank coffee and rum while making business deals, many of which revolved around the ships in the harbor and the maritime trade—the foundation of the city's economy. Philadelphia was an entrepôt, where farmers brought grain and livestock products to be sent abroad, while European manufactured items ranging from textiles to shoes were floated into the port to be sold throughout the Delaware Valley. Fully one-fourth of the nation's export goods at the time passed through the harbor. The

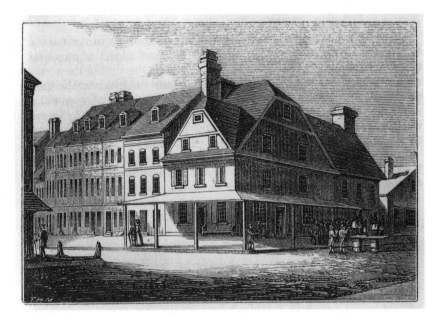

William L. Breton, *The London Coffee House,* c. 1830. The London Coffee House
served as a commercial center, especially for Philadelphia's merchants and ship
captains, and as a social gathering place for wealthier residents in the eighteenth and
early nineteenth centuries. Courtesy the Library of Congress, Washington, D.C.

livelihood of most of the region's citizens depended either directly or
indirectly on trade with merchants scattered throughout the Atlantic
commercial routes, from Native Americans in the backcountry to
farmers and storekeepers in the neighboring countryside, to planters,
manufacturers, and dealers operating from the West Indies, Portugal,
and Britain. Merchants and captains earned money managing the
exchanges, carters and stevedores stowed staples on ships, and coopers
and carpenters fashioned barrels to stow flour and other products
bound for the sea.[16]

The London Coffee House buzzed with talk about foreign affairs,
especially current events in France and Saint-Domingue. Having arrived in Philadelphia ten days earlier, the minister plenipotentiary
from France, Edmond Charles Genêt (known as Citizen Genêt) was
in the process of botching French-American relations. Citizens of the

United States were passionately divided about the recent revolution in France. Some identified it with their own struggle for liberty and equality, while others feared that it had gone too far in its violence and radicalism. Reminding the Americans about the crucial support France had provided during their rebellion against Britain, Genêt actively, if ineptly, courted an American alliance in the current French war against Britain. He illegally commissioned four American privateers to capture British vessels. That one of them, the *Sans Culottes,* bore the sobriquet of the working-class French radicals was thought likely to appeal to American laborers sympathetic to the French Revolution. It had docked in Philadelphia at the same time as the *Hankey,* at a wharf near Rush's destination. The privateer brought a captured sloop, the *Flora.* All the ships carried refugees from Saint-Domingue.[17]

Many Democratic-Republicans—adherents of Thomas Jefferson's emerging political party—cheered the *Sans Culottes* and demanded that the United States join in the war against England. Federalist followers of Alexander Hamilton, like most merchants in the London Coffee House, were outraged because Genêt's actions endangered America's official neutrality, which President Washington had declared four months earlier. Both the city's shipping and prosperity had boomed since the Americans began to carry the trade of both France and Britain under the flag of a nonaligned nation, and ship captains did not want that to end. Genêt would fail in his efforts. When, a year later, the French government recalled him to face the guillotine, Hamilton, in an uncharacteristically generous moment, persuaded Washington to grant Genêt asylum instead.[18]

Descending the hill, Rush entered Hell Town, which comprised three or four blocks along the waterfront. Turning north on Water Street, he found himself on the narrowest, most populous, filthiest street in the city. Abutting the docks, the pathway was nearly always damp, muddy, and pockmarked with stagnant pools of water. "It is," according to one resident, "confined, ill-aired, and, in every respect, a disagreeable street." It was also home to many down-and-out Philadelphians: vagrants, criminals, prostitutes, itinerants, and fugitive slaves and servants, as well as the insane, incapacitated, and homeless. These men, women, and children accounted for one of every ten people in the city, and they often appeared on the dockets of the almshouse, workhouse, prison, and hospital.[19]

The nearby Three Jolly Irishmen epitomized this section of the city. It had earned the reputation as one of the toughest taverns in town, no small feat in a city containing hundreds of licensed and un-licensed drinking establishments. The inns in this district also served as hubs of neighborhood life, where working-class and poor people gathered not only to drink but also to gamble on cards, dice, cock-fights, bull baitings, and boxing matches. Sailors and dockworkers sometimes paid small fees to see exotic animals like leopards, trained pigs, and camels, or to buy narcotics and aphrodisiacs like "Opium and Spanish Flies," as advertised openly in newspapers. The taverns served families as well, especially on holidays like May Day, the Fourth of July, and Christmas, when workers gathered to celebrate with "picnic dinners" and numerous toasts.[20]

In a city filled with transient mariners and poor immigrants, prostitution flourished. Constables often apprehended streetwalkers like Biddy Cummings and Sarah Evans as they plied their trade, charging a dollar—a day's wages for a male laborer—for their ser-vices. When arrested, they faced thirty days in the workhouse. After serving her apprenticeship as a maid in a house a half block east of the Three Jolly Irishmen, Cummings joined a number of "filles de joie," who employed their days in prostitution and petty theft, spending winter months in the Almshouse to make ends meet. Evans, a widow, did not have much luck avoiding night watchmen; she was arrested a dozen times in the early 1790s for vagrancy, keeping bad company, disorderly conduct, and being a drunk and "Lewd Girl." She briefly ran a brothel, apparently without success, since she had to take refuge in the Almshouse several times.[21]

Apprentices, slaves, and servants gravitated to Hell Town for their evening pleasures, often in integrated company, and usually against their masters' wishes. Occasional stories in newspapers cautioned mas-ters about the activities of their bound people:

> At the last city sessions a negro was tried and convicted for keeping a disorderly house; it appeared upon this occasion that the offender kept a place of resort for all the loose and idle characters of the city, whether whites, blacks or mulattoes; and that frequently in the night gentlemen's servants would arrive there, mounted on their master's horses (for which the landlord had provided a stable in the neighborhood) and indulge in riotous mirth and dancing till the dawn, when they posted again to their respective homes. These facts are laid before the public . . . as a hint to masters to watch the conduct of their servants.

Even George Washington's bound people were attracted to the neighborhood. In 1794, he committed a servant and a slave to the workhouse for a week as punishment for sneaking out at night.[22]

On this August Monday, Rush advanced up Water Street until, a few doors past the Dennys' brothel, he reached the home of Peter LeMaigre. A successful merchant-importer who had moved to the city a decade earlier, LeMaigre had spent the previous month seeking contributions for the refugees from Saint-Domingue. When five ships, including the *Hankey,* had landed from that colony at LeMaigre's dock three weeks earlier, he and his wife, Catherine, had extended their compassion to the refugees, inviting some of them, though ill, to stay in their home. Now Catherine lay dying. Her stomach was on fire, her pulse weak, and she could not stop vomiting black bile. Rush met with two other physicians at her bedside to consult about the case. Dr. Hodge, who lived nearby, had just lost his daughter to a disease manifesting similar symptoms. At least half a dozen people had recently died within sight of LeMaigre's pier. Obviously, some horrific pestilence was erupting on Water Street.[23]

The three men could not offer any lifesaving remedy for the patient. But following the conversation with his two colleagues, Rush put the clues together: he announced that the "bilious remitting yellow fever" had come to the city by way of the coffee rotting on the nearby

wharf and polluting the air. Eventually, in the "instant" history written immediately after the epidemic, the author informed Philadelphians (though not all would believe him) that in reality the Bolama
fever had come from the West Indies, having been introduced into
Grenada by the *Hankey*. It did not matter whether he was credible:
within ten days Philadelphia was stricken as never before.[24]

Sickness, rumors, and fear intensified after Rush's pronouncement.
Catherine LeMaigre died on Tuesday, August 20, and half a
dozen other residents of Water Street followed her to graveyards over
the next few days. The fever quickly spread, first to Front Street, then
to alleys and courts a little way from the docks. A few tailors did not
show up at their workbenches, a handful of stevedores failed to appear to unload ships, sailors and prostitutes gossiped fearfully about
illnesses and fatalities in nearby boardinghouses along the wharves.
During a normal August, church bells would chime three or four times
a day to mark funerals. Now they began to toll more often: thirteen
times on Thursday, ten on Friday, and seventeen on Saturday. Philadelphians grew frightened.[25]

On the day after seeing LeMaigre, Rush visited Mayor Matthew
Clarkson to announce the arrival of the new disease. Since it was
"highly contagious," Rush contended (incorrectly), an epidemic was
unavoidable. The only way to limit its destructiveness was to purify
the putrid miasma that emanated from the city's filth. This entailed
cleaning the streets, especially the decaying coffee on the wharf.
Clarkson took immediate action, cautioning inhabitants about "a dangerous, infectious disorder" in the Friday newspapers and ordering
scavengers to scour the city, starting with Water Street. Privately and
publicly, Rush and other doctors advised inhabitants to leave the city
as the only certain way to avoid the disease. In the meantime, the bells
kept tolling.

Clarkson's warning was one of two short pieces about the fever
that appeared in the newspapers on Friday. Over the next few days,
stories about yellow fever supplanted all other domestic and foreign

news, including reports about Citizen Genêt and America's position in the European war. Many notices offered suggestions about how to forestall the "present raging sickness," although medical advice had not changed much since the time of the bubonic plague in London in 1665, when people were advised to sprinkle vinegar and diffuse tobacco smoke in their houses, carry tarred rope in their pockets, and wear bags of camphor around their necks. Chewing garlic and smoking cigars were also thought to ward off the disease. One doctor advocated spreading several inches of dirt in every room, then changing it daily, followed by warm baths containing the "Asiatic remedy of myrrh and black pepper." Rumor had it that fire would clean the air of infection, so some residents began setting bonfires in front of their homes—a dangerous practice in a city still partly built of wood. Fire companies, another letter writer suggested, should use their engines to wash the streets every day.[26]

An anonymous writer who signed only his initials, "A.B.," inadvertently identified the true source of the problem. "The late rains," he noted, "produced a great increase of mosquitoes in the city, distressing to the sick, and troublesome to those who are well." The insects' numbers "may be diminished," he explained, by pouring a little oil in rainwater casks and water barrels. Although most residents ignored his counsel, A.B. had anticipated by a century the efforts of medical pioneers Carlos Finlay and Walter Reed, who helped identify the mosquito vectors that spread yellow fever. (Reed also successfully established a program to eradicate the insects and to end, at least temporarily, the disease in Cuba.)[27]

Fear itself, one newspaper contributor claimed, "creates susceptibility in the body to disease." And the malady began to terrify residents. In a scene foreshadowing chaotic exoduses from New Orleans and other southern cities threatened by hurricanes in our own times, Philadelphians began to flee. The first wave consisted primarily of the wealthy who owned country homes or people who could take refuge with relatives living outside town. On Sunday the 25th, in the midst of a severe rainstorm that turned the roads to mud, several thousand people exited the city by carriage, cart, coach, or horse, often leaving behind their homes, furniture, and personal belongings, as well as their servants to guard them. It is a reflection of eighteenth-century America that the health of the poor was considered less important than the sanctity of private property.[28]

That same day, at the mayor's request, the College of Physicians met to analyze the crisis and suggest an appropriate response. This group of prestigious Fellows disagreed from the outset, mostly because their explanations of the causes (or even existence) of the disease differed so fundamentally. Dr. William Currie, a distinguished former army surgeon during the Revolution and a well-known advocate of smallpox inoculation, led the opposition to Rush. While admitting the existence of widespread sickness, Currie considered the contagion primarily an intensified version of the usual summer complaints and fall agues. Even if a new malignant fever had appeared in the city, according to Currie, attributing it to foul air created by decomposing coffee or putrefying animal flesh was simply nonsense. Miasma might nurture ailments, but it could not initiate an infection. Most new maladies, argued "contagionist" medical theorists like Currie, occurred when migrants brought them into the port. The several thousand recent arrivals from the West Indies, whom everyone in the city had noticed, added strong empirical evidence supporting this hypothesis. The appropriate response was to quarantine the immigrants in a "pest house" on an island in the Delaware. This precaution of isolating sick newcomers before they even reached the city dated back at least half a century.[29]

The difference of opinion greatly disturbed Rush. The climate had changed during the past decade, he believed, making Philadelphia more vulnerable to ailments spread by bad air. Certain that he had correctly identified both the yellow fever and its causes, Rush was confident to the point of arrogance. During the next few weeks, he would also develop a miracle "cure" for the disease, consisting primarily of heavy doses of mercury and the purgative root jalap for catharsis as well as, in his words, "copious bloodletting." This medical breakthrough, he thought, would not only save many lives but also make him more famous. He was partly correct: he subsequently became infamous for bleeding people nearly to death.[30]

Rush won the initial debate in the College of Physicians. He drafted the report submitted to the mayor and published in the newspapers. Few of its recommendations were drastic, most merely commonsensical to Philadelphians at the time. Residents should avoid infected victims of the disease and carry handkerchiefs liberally doused with camphor and vinegar when caring for the sick. Marks or flags were to be set on the doors of all ill persons as a warning. It was important to dress appropriately, avoid fatigue, refrain from standing long in the sun or open air, and limit the consumption of alcohol. Government officials needed to purify the streets, markets, and wharves, and most important, establish a large, well-ventilated hospital for victims of the illness. Although it was a good idea to burn gunpowder or shoot guns to clear the air, people should stop building fires in their houses or on the streets. The dead should be interred privately, carried to graveyards in closed carriages so as not to alarm citizens. Finally, the tolling of church bells for funerals should stop since they only frightened both the sick and the well. Significantly missing from the list of proposals was any plan to quarantine immigrants. Since the disease derived from the city's filth, according to Rush, passengers on arriving ships were not a concern.[31]

These primitive measures were for naught, and scores more people soon fell ill. A few mariners were discovered dying in rented rooms or in doorways of boardinghouses where they had crawled after becoming sick. Bodies began to appear in Pewter Platter Alley, Chancery Lane, and Letitia Court. Passersby were too afraid of catching the disease to assist the sick and the dying. On August 27, by order of the mayor, the bells finally stopped tolling, but the silence, after a week of continual ringing, seemed eerie, almost more terrifying than the bells.[32]

Meanwhile, the government began to disintegrate. Magistrates, councilmen, judges, and aldermen either became sick or fled. Among the several constables and two dozen night watchmen, only about half showed up for their duties. Nobody wanted to perform the dirty work of clearing the city of dangerous garbage, much less carting off the dead. Even some of the Guardians of the Poor, the officials charged with caring for the neediest Philadelphians, began to run away to avoid their responsibilities.

This organization, known officially as the Overseers and Guardians of the Poor, had its origins managing the Bettering House, a large building on the western end of the city, built strategically out of sight of wealthier citizens. Designed to shelter and care for the poor, the combination Almshouse and House of Employment consisted of two buildings intended to serve different functions. The Almshouse east wing provided a refuge for the "deserving poor" who were incapable of working; the House of Employment contained indigents physically capable of laboring for their livelihood. Perhaps the largest building ever constructed in the American colonies, its size reflected the growing problem of urban poverty during the decade before the Revolution. During and after the war, as destitution grew more severe, the overseers and guardians began to assume different duties. Managing the Almshouse, the six overseers transformed the institution into something more like a jail to punish the poor than a refuge to assist them. The overseers funded construction of a tall brick wall around the Bettering House, confined inmates behind locked doors, and took extraordinary steps to reform the "morals" of their charges. The guardians, meanwhile, supervised the needy outside the institution. While charged with providing the poor with such necessities as food, firewood, and medical care, and burying them in potter's field, officials possessed virtually no public financial resources to carry out those duties.[33]

As the number of sick and dead grew, the burdens of the overseers and guardians increased enormously. Rather than risk spreading the disease among the nearly four hundred paupers in the Bettering House, officials initially limited new admissions to the healthy, then forbade entirely any new applicants from entering the poorhouse. The Pennsylvania Hospital for the Sick Poor, one of the many institutions founded by Benjamin Franklin, quickly followed suit, refusing admission to

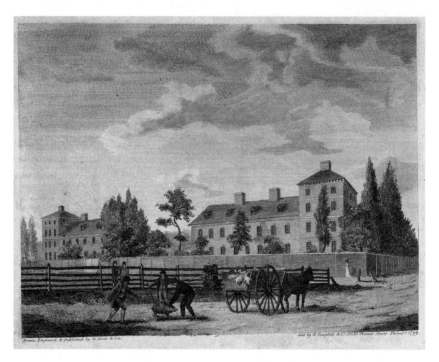

William Russell Birch, *Almshouse in Spruce Street,* 1800. The Almshouse is on the right
and the Workhouse on the left, both surrounded by a high fence to confine inmates
to the grounds. Because it was located in the western part of the city, the Almshouse
largely escaped the epidemic. In William Russell Birch, *The City of Philadelphia, in
the State of Pennsylvania North America* (Philadelphia, 1800). Courtesy the Library of
Congress, Washington, D.C.

new patients suffering from yellow fever. Fear of the supposedly contagious nature of the disease made caring for the noninstitutionalized
poor nearly impossible, since officials could not hire nurses to care for
patients or coach drivers to cart away bodies, or gravediggers to inter
them.[34]

Desperate for a place to send poor victims of the disease, the guardians remembered that Ricketts Amphitheater, at the western end of the
city, was temporarily empty. John Bill Ricketts, an expert equestrian
performer, had funded the recent construction of the building as a
place to entertain the public, including the president, federal officials,
wealthy merchants, and the Guardians of the Poor. Currently, the
circus was on tour in New York City for the season. The guardians

directed seven infected poor patients to the enclosed amphitheater, where they lay on the floor for several nights. Despite offering high wages, officials could not hire anybody to care for their needs. Two of the patients died where they lay, while another crawled into the street before succumbing. When a carter finally was engaged to remove one of the bodies, he was unable to fit it into the coffin by himself. A servant girl in a nearby house bravely helped him complete the gruesome task of wrestling the maggot-ridden corpse into the wooden box, but not before eliciting a promise from the carter not to tell the family with whom she lived; if they knew, they would surely turn her out. (The anonymous girl survived the epidemic.) Terrified by the sight of the body on the street, neighbors of the circus threatened to burn the amphitheater down if it continued to be used as an infirmary.

Half the members of the Guardians of the Poor—one of the few official agencies that continued to operate throughout the epidemic—met with the mayor. They pledged to establish a hospital "in an airy and healthy place" that would be staffed with doctors and nurses. They already had considered Bush Hill, one of the area's oldest mansions, built half a century earlier on a 150-acre farm—about half the size of the entire incorporated city—on the northwest edge of town. But they were hesitant to seize private property, especially from a wealthy man. When they discovered that he was currently living in England, however, they went ahead and confiscated the estate, over the strenuous objections of the tenant living there.

As frightening as August was, September and October would be worse. The temperatures remained warm enough for mosquitoes to spread over the large field of unprotected hosts. Amid the febrile onslaught, the federal government would cease to operate. The increasingly deserted streets would be piled with more and more dead bodies. Yellow jack was in its element.

CHAPTER 9

Journal of the Plague Months

ଽ୯୯

"They are dying on our right hand and on our Left; we have it opposite us, in fact, all around us, great are the number that are called to the grave. To see the hearse go by is now so common that we hardly take notice of it; in fine, we live in the midst of death." So wrote Philadelphian Isaac Heston to his brother on September 19, 1793, at a time when yellow fever claimed the lives of roughly seventy city residents a day. "When I see the Metropolis of the United States depopulated," the twenty-two-year-old moaned, "it is too distressing and affecting a scene for a person young in Life to bear." A mosquito carrying the yellow fever virus stung Heston about the time he wrote the letter; he died ten days later.[1]

After the initial shock of learning that yellow jack was stalking their city, Philadelphians tried to ignore it, hoping that Dr. Benjamin Rush and other physicians had misdiagnosed the disease, or that it wouldn't spread. Soon they were forced to face family and friends with sunken eyes, jaundiced skin, and blood trickling from nose and mouth. Many people panicked and in their haste to escape the contagion left behind infected loved ones who lay ill. Descriptions of people abandoning family and friends during the crisis left a lasting impression on eighteenth- and nineteenth-century Americans.[2]

Because the wealthiest Philadelphians usually took up residence at their country estates in July or August to avoid the various illnesses of the warmer months, many of the wives and children of rich men had already left the city before the fever made its appearance. But beginning in September, residents of other classes began leaving the city in record numbers. As "Death now began," in Daniel Defoe's description of an earlier London plague, "to look into their Houses, and Chambers, and Stare in their Faces," Philadelphians shrank away in horror. As the prominent lawyer and Federalist Alexander Graydon reported, "Those whose property enabled them to do it fled with precipitation."[3]

"So great was the general terror," Mathew Carey observed, "that for some weeks, carts, wagons, coaches, and [sedan] chairs, were almost constantly transporting families and furniture to the country in every direction." Carey, a Philadelphia printer, wrote one of the first instant histories, publishing an account of the epidemic in mid-October, before it had even run its course. "The terror now became universal. The migrations to the country were very great—and about the middle of September, it is supposed that 15,000 of the inhabitants of Philadelphia had deserted the city." The actual number of refugees was even higher: more than a third of the city's 50,000 inhabitants abandoned their homes. By the end of the epidemic, half the original residents had taken flight.[4]

Officials and employees of the federal government joined the refugees. Secretary of State Thomas Jefferson, who lived in a rented country mansion on the Schuylkill River, stopped going to work in downtown Philadelphia. His mansion was a civilized retreat, removed from a world consumed by fear. But this very retreat besmirched his reputation, especially after he left for Monticello, his home in Virginia. His Federalist political opponents were very happy to label Jefferson a coward, just as they had when he fled from the British advance on Philadelphia during the Revolution. Indeed, reactions to the epidemic would become fodder for a great deal of political maneuvering.[5]

Secretary of the Treasury Alexander Hamilton and his wife, Elizabeth, contracted the fever in early September. Having grown up in the West Indies, the secretary had believed that he enjoyed immunity to the ailment. He was wrong. He caught the new strain of yellow fever and almost died. However, even after he grew ill, he let politics shape his decisions. Both Alexander and Elizabeth refused to take Dr. Rush's "republican cure," which involved considerable bloodletting, since Rush was affiliated with the Democratic-Republicans, the party of Thomas Jefferson and James Madison. The Hamiltons instead chose the "French" therapy brought from the Caribbean: bed rest, fluids (especially wine), and light bleeding and purging. When President Washington learned that the Hamiltons had fallen sick, he sent them a bottle of wine (probably delivered by one of his slaves) and best wishes for a speedy recovery.[6]

As we know today, the Hamiltons made the right choice. Basic nursing care, providing patients with water and food, often can save victims of yellow fever. The affluent, such as the secretary of the treasury and his wife, were fortunate to have servants and slaves to care for them. The lack of nurses and regular hydration condemned many sick Philadelphians to almost certain death. After Hamilton and his wife both survived, the Federalists—the party of Hamilton and John Adams—made it their preferred treatment. The culture wars were as intense during the 1790s as in modern America.[7]

Government officials of all political stripes soon were running away from the disaster. During the 1790s, Philadelphia served as capital not only of the nation but also of the state of Pennsylvania. In late August, when the official door attendant of the statehouse was found lying dead at his post, slain by yellow jack, the Pennsylvania Assembly grew unnerved. As members began searching for quick exits from the city, they received a message from Governor Thomas Mifflin requesting a bill authorizing the quarantine of all newly arriving ships and their passengers. The assembly responded immediately, dusting off an old Quarantine Act and voting it into law; the governor affixed his signature the same day. Mifflin now possessed emergency powers to isolate the ill and take necessary steps to protect the state's residents. With that business completed, both houses of the state assembly adjourned, and the members made their getaway. When his head began to throb and his skin started to turn yellow, the governor also turned tail. Through most of the epidemic, he lay a few miles outside town, at his summer retreat near the falls of the Schuylkill.[8]

Deeply disturbed by Hamilton's illness and the spreading death around him, President Washington chose to leave as well. In mid-September, a local newspaper carried the following notice: "This morning, the President of the United States set out from town for Mount Vernon." Washington had made a habit of spending some of the autumn months in Virginia each year, to supervise the slaves on his plantation and enjoy the favorable weather during harvest season. Yet this year's routine trip to Virginia with his family seemed like a bad omen to residents of the city.

Before departing, the president requested that General Henry Knox, the secretary of war, send him weekly reports about the progress of the fever in the city. "I sincerely wish, and pray, that you and yours may escape untouched," he wrote Knox. "When we meet again, may it be under circumstances more pleasing than the present." With that message, Washington escaped the epidemic that was killing Philadelphians with increasing regularity. (Ironically, Washington died six years later, a victim not of yellow fever but of too much bloodletting by his three physicians, who practiced a treatment similar to the republican cure recommended by Benjamin Rush.)[9]

Washington's early exodus intensified the fear in Philadelphia. When Knox fled soon afterward, residents grew gravely concerned. After most of the other prominent politicians ran away, the alarm became panic. As government workers left or became sick, the federal government began to dissolve. Six clerks at the Treasury Department fell ill, followed by seven officials in the Customs Service and three employees at the Post Office. Before long, mail delivery shut down. So did the Office of the Attorney General. A few federal agencies purportedly remained open, but without a staff or people in charge.

From his relatively safe lodging outside of town, Jefferson seized the opportunity to criticize his political enemies in the federal government, especially Hamilton. "He has been miserable several days from a firm persuasion he should catch" yellow fever, Jefferson wrote. "A man as timid as he is on the water, as timid on horseback, as timid in sickness, would be a phenomenon if his courage of which he has the reputation in military occasions were genuine." Jefferson also had scorching words for Henry Knox after his departure.[10]

The city government also collapsed. Every one of the magistrates and roughly half the Guardians of the Poor—central to administering the city—either slipped away in the night or became too ill or too frightened to discharge his duty. By mid-September, Mayor Matthew Clarkson was the only elected administrator remaining in Philadelphia. Admirably, he went to his office each day, serving as a symbol of calm and order in the midst of chaos and death.[11]

Fear moved up and down the East Coast as Philadelphians fled the epidemic. Many people, including doctors, believed that the disease was contagious, and refugees from the epidemic could spread the fever. As a result, escapees from the Quaker City often received rough handling when they attempted to enter other villages or urban centers. Officials in Chestertown, Maryland, decreed that no stagecoaches from the infected region could travel through their town. In Baltimore and Trenton, neither humans nor goods from Philadelphia were to be allowed within city boundaries. The Virginia governor proclaimed a three-week quarantine of all vessels, regardless of their place of origin, arriving in the commonwealth's harbors. As far south as Charleston, officials confined ships that had so much as entered the Delaware Bay, far to the south of Philadelphia. In New York City, the mayor initially declared that any traveler who had passed through Philadelphia needed to be registered. He required physicians to notify his office of new arrivals and confine the ill in the public hospital. A few days later, as fear intensified, he ordered that anyone from Philadelphia be removed from the city; the New York Corporation passed a resolution "to stop all intercourse [with] Philadelphia entirely."[12]

When these measures failed to halt the flow of refugees, officials took even more sweeping steps. They stationed guards at boat landings to send away everyone coming from Philadelphia. Passengers leaving Philadelphia on the stagecoaches to New York did not get near enough to test the new law. "They were refused a passage through New Jersey," according to one newspaper report, and returned exhausted and humiliated to the stagecoach office in Philadelphia. In addition, "the inhabitants of Trenton, Newark, New York, and a great many other towns have behaved most inhumanely," according to one refugee, "stopping well and hearty persons from taking refuge in their towns, and even not permitting them to pass through." Matters grew so heated during a confrontation in Trenton that guards fired at one of the drivers, who "had a very narrow escape with his life [with] the ball passing within a few inches of one of his ears." Even Hamilton's status as secretary of the treasury did him no good. When he left Philadelphia after surviving his bout of yellow fever, soldiers caught and confined him in a makeshift jail north of New York City.[13]

Once the most admired city in America, Philadelphia had become its most feared, the epicenter of death. Yet as hostile as fleeing residents found the outside world, those left behind in the City of Brotherly Love also encountered the numbing, at times savage, effects of the unending scenes of horror. When anyone could be contagious, mercy and compassion were in short supply.

Yellow jack was by no means a stranger to Philadelphia. The disease had periodically devastated the city since its founding in 1682. The worst outbreak occurred in 1699, when more than a third of the residents died. The infection appeared at least five more times during the colonial era, driving the death rates to extraordinary heights each time. By 1793, however, it had not visited the city for more than three decades, leaving most Philadelphians vulnerable to their first attack by the virus.[14]

The sheer lack of knowledge about the causes, spread, and treatment of yellow jack also created extreme unease. Was it contagious, spreading from neighbor to neighbor? Did the miasma, the foul air, in Philadelphia account for the blossoming of the disease? Was it an entirely new disease, imported on ships from the Caribbean or Europe or Africa? Medical men couldn't answer the questions definitively, so rumors and folk cures ran rampant among ordinary people.

Death carts, their drivers crying "bring out your dead," rumbled through the streets every morning, afternoon, and evening. Burials increased daily throughout September. By mid-October, the drivers of the carts and drays were hauling away 120 corpses each day. The epidemic eventually claimed more than 5,000 souls, or one in ten of the city's occupants. Those who could escape enjoyed much better odds of surviving. Among Philadelphians who stayed, the fatality rate was considerably higher: as many as one in five poorer residents perished. The number of deaths was unimaginable in its scope, equivalent in our own times to a million people dying of a disease in New York City or Los Angeles.[15]

Mortality was highest along the northern wharves, where the *Hankey* and other ships carrying refugees from Saint-Domingue had docked. The hardest-hit area was Water Street, which, true to its name, fronted the river. Small pools of water dotted the unpaved street, creating a favorable habitat for mosquitoes. As a result, a staggering two-thirds of the residents there perished.

The worst effects of the fever extended four or five blocks west from the Delaware toward the heart of the city. The infectious *Aëdes aegypti* mosquito typically traveled only about that distance during its lifetime, but it could lay its eggs in the host of water barrels that stood next to almost every house, and its progeny could carry on the destruction. If they avoided going downtown or to the waterfront, people fortunate enough to live on the western, northern, or southern fringes of the city tended to survive.

Yellow jack took an especially heavy toll in the small alleys, courts, and lanes near the water, places largely inhabited by impoverished people. The small red flags that by order of the Board of Health adorned the doors of houses containing people infected by the fever proliferated in these narrow byways. A third of the residents of Moravian Alley, for example, and fully half those in Fetter Lane succumbed to the disease. More than sixty women living in Apple Tree Alley became widows within a few months. Jacob Flake, a tailor residing at the end of Moravian Alley, lost six children to the pestilence, as "whole families," according to Mathew Carey, sank "into

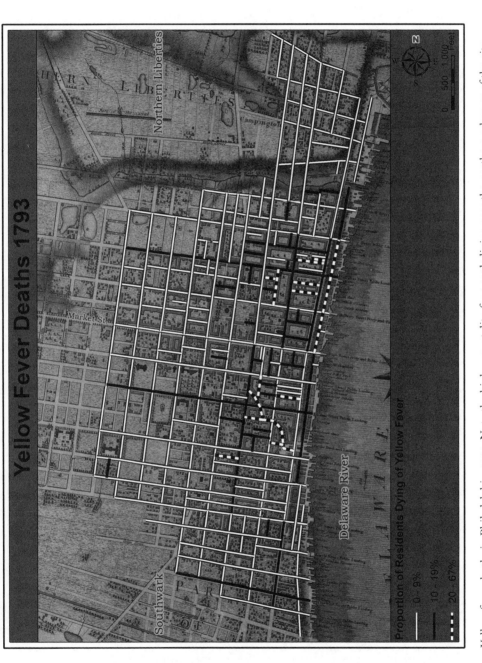

Yellow fever deaths in Philadelphia, 1793. Note the higher mortality for people living near the northern wharves of the city. Residents who lived five blocks from the Delaware River experienced many fewer deaths. Map produced by the GIS Mapping Philadelphia project: Billy G. Smith, Paul Sivitz, Stuart Challender, Alex Schwab, Tara Chesley-Preston, and Alice Hecht.

one silent, undistinguished grave." As one English visitor commented, it was "not at all uncommon for four out of five in a family to die."[16]

The yellow fever virus attacked along class lines, afflicting mainly Philadelphia's "lower sort," as they were labeled by contemporaries. Similar to when Hurricane Katrina hit New Orleans in 2005, poor and black people unable to escape the city bore the brunt of the suffering. The disease was "dreadfully destructive among the poor," Carey noted. "It is very probable that at least seven eights of the number of the dead, was of that class." His observation is confirmed by the preponderance of mariners, laborers, artisans, clothes washers, and prostitutes on the lists of the deceased. Inferior diets, overcrowded housing, and deadly sanitary conditions heightened the vulnerability of the lower classes to any disease. In the case of the yellow fever epidemic, even more important was their inability to leave town or to afford nursing care if they grew ill. As one newspaper essayist pointed out, departing the city was impossible for "the poor who have neither places to remove to or funds for their support, as they depend on their daily labor for daily supplies."[17]

Yellow fever killed Philadelphians selectively in other ways. The disease claimed most of its victims from a cohort of young and middle-aged adults and American-born white males. Once afflicted, children and infants survived in greater numbers because, as is the general pattern, they experienced milder cases of the disease than did adults. Women fared better than men, most likely because they left the city sooner, often sent away by their husbands and fathers. The French residents in the city who had escaped the slave revolution in Saint-Domingue apparently suffered relatively few fatalities, probably because they had gained immunity by exposure to the microbes during their childhood in the West Indies. Black Philadelphians may have experienced slightly lower death rates than whites, since a few of them were migrants from Africa or the West Indies where they too may have been protected by prior exposure. The great majority of black residents of the city, however, were not immune to the disease since they were born in colonial America.[18]

After the vast rush of people leaving the city in early September, a disquieting calm settled over streets usually bustling with life and energy. Terror haunted the avenues, lanes, and alleys. "Dismay and affright were visible in almost every person's countenance," Carey wrote. "Many shut themselves up in their houses and were afraid to walk the streets." By late October, grass grew in many of the roads. When forced to go outdoors to find food or water or medicine, most people shunned the sidewalk. Instead, they walked down the middle of the streets to avoid infection as they passed houses where others had died. Acquaintances and friends kept their distance in the streets, signifying their regard only by a nod. The old custom of shaking hands fell into such general disuse as many shrank back at even the offer of a hand. Everyone shunned people wearing a black cape or other dress suggesting mourning. And many survivors employed hasty maneuvers to put themselves upwind of every person they met. When people summoned up the courage to walk abroad, the sick carts conveying patients to the hospital or the hearses carrying the dead to the grave soon dampened their spirits.[19]

Afraid of catching the fever, captains refused to dock their ships, and farmers and fishermen declined to bring their food into the urban market. "Business," Carey declared, "then became extremely dull." Virtually all the stores closed, as did the coffeehouses, taverns, inns, libraries, and other establishments where the public gathered. Residents who remained in the city, even if they did not contract the fever, began to suffer from unemployment, poverty, and, in many instances, an absence of the necessities of life. Hunger spread at a time when social services organized by the city had ceased completely.[20]

To ward off the disease, Philadelphians used a litany of prophylactic measures, sometimes trying all at the same time. Many of the measures were designed to clean the foul air thought to be responsible for the disease. They fired muskets, chewed garlic, burned bonfires, rang bells, smoked their bedding and houses with tobacco, and carried pieces of tarred rope. Men, women, and children continually puffed on cigars. Most kept handkerchiefs soaked in camphor or small bottles full of red wine and herbs held at their noses. Some tucked garlic and pieces of tarred rope in their shoes and pockets. A few obsessively washed their rooms with vinegar. Even though the mayor forbade bonfires in the street, nobody paid much attention to the decree since there were no constables to enforce the order. A handful of people obtained cannon and shot them down the streets to clear the air of disease. Most of these were home remedies, dating back to plagues of earlier decades, probably all the way back to the Middle Ages.

None of these measures, save perhaps the cigar and bonfire smoke, which chased away the mosquitoes, had much effect. Consequently, cadavers piled up faster than draymen could cart them away, regardless of how often the carriages of death rumbled through the streets. By the end of September, the cemeteries—including potter's field, across the street from the buildings of the federal and state governments—became so heavily used that, as one visitor noted, the "burying grounds are like ploughed fields." During the three months of the epidemic, gravediggers buried more than four thousand bodies there. In early October, the cart men picked up more than a hundred bodies a day. They started burying people in common graves in potter's field. "They drag them away like dead beasts," one Philadelphian moaned to a friend in Virginia, "and put ten or fifteen or more in a hole together." In the chaos, by one British visitor's account, "there are many buried alive." According to a morbid aphorism from the time, the gravediggers "were up to their arse in business and didn't know which way to turn."[21]

Thinking it too dangerous to stand close to potentially infectious bodies, people stopped attending funerals, even for their loved ones. "The corpses of the most respectable citizens, even of those who did not die of the epidemic," Carey noted, "were carried to the grave on the shafts of a [sedan] chair, the horse driven by a Negro, unattended by a friend or relation, and without any sort of ceremony. People hastily shifted their course at the sight of a hearse coming towards them."[22]

The stories of inhumanity during the panic constituted one of the most appalling features of the epidemic. Whether they were literally true, they were passed along as verities: Widow Morris buried her husband, and on her return, her father, fearing contagion, would not allow her back into their home. From then on she slept on the street, in stables, or in the marketplace. One man, learning that his wife was ill, immediately fled their home, abandoning her to a sure death. When he returned several days later with a coffin and a death cart, however, he discovered his wife alive and well. The following day, true to the moral of the story, the man caught the fever and died shortly thereafter. His wife buried him in the coffin purchased for her.[23]

Such anecdotes became morality tales of the epidemic, told repeatedly in newspapers, novels, and accounts of the event. "While affairs were in this deplorable state, and people at the lowest ebb of despair," Carey wrote in his instant history, "we cannot be astonished at the frightful scenes that were acted, which seemed to indicate a total dissolution of the bonds of society in the nearest and dearest connections." The restraints of civilization were loosening. "Who, without horror, can reflect on a husband, married perhaps for twenty years, deserting his wife in the last agony, or a wife unfeelingly abandoning her husband on his death bed, or parents forsaking their only children, or children ungratefully flying from their parents and resigning them to chance, often without an enquiry after their health or safety? Who, I say, can think of these things without horror? Yet they were daily exhibited in every quarter of our city."[24]

Some commentators, like Philip Beaver in Bolama, blamed much of the destruction on the peoples' own terror, especially on the bad character that fear elicited in people under extreme stress. "Children! Mothers! Husbands! Think of the duty which God has prescribed to you," admonished Dr. Jean Devèze, the physician who ran the makeshift hospital at Bush Hill. He censured Philadelphians severely for "abandoning to all the bitterness of disease their nearest relations and dearest friends," to be "neglected and left alone to expire in all the horror of despair." Devèze condemned the newspapers, public officials, and other doctors for advising the frightened residents that the fever was passed from person to person. These warnings, along with placing red flags in front of houses where people had died, accomplished little except to further spread fear. "This was, no doubt," Devèze argued, "one of the principal causes of the rapid destruction, which spread devastation through this unfortunate city." Having treated yellow fever in the West Indies, Devèze was confident that it was not contagious, so there was no reason to abandon family or friends when they fell ill.[25]

Among those who did not flee the epidemic was Mr. Stevens, a saddler who became the last of six in his family to die. After he expired, the African American man driving the death cart discovered the five other bodies in his house. The popular Presbyterian leader Reverend James Sproat, along with his wife and two children, also stayed—and died. The fever claimed David Flickwir and five other family members beneath his roof. For Godfrey Gebler, the family death toll was eleven. The disease orphaned scores of Philadelphia's children. Many were forced to find refuge in stables or the marketplace before the Guardians of the Poor began to function more effectively and helped find them shelters. Even pets suffered. Abandoned when their owners had fled or died, cats and dogs wandered the streets, howling or mewing loudly enough to create a public nuisance.[26]

During the second week of October, J. Henry Helmuth, the parson of one of the Lutheran churches, lost 130 parishioners. In a single block of Appletree Alley, Helmuth counted 40 dead. A few of the survivors had gone temporarily mad from the fever, the associated fear, and grief of having their families and neighbors die around them. None among the three bakers, three laborers, painter, shoemaker, wheelwright, and widow who lived in the alley had the financial means to escape the plague that had descended on them. When word spread that the cemetery at Helmuth's church was among the best places to be buried, with plots still available in a favorable, pleasant location, dozens of people arrived carrying coffins containing their loved ones, though most were neither Lutherans nor had ever set foot in the church's sanctuary. The crowds grew so thick that Parson Helmuth had to leave a boy at the entrance to the cemetery with tickets, so that the gravedigger, Martin Brown, would have some order to follow.[27]

In the midst of wrestling with death, Philadelphians found a modicum of dark humor in a few vignettes. Determined to safeguard himself by using the preventive of tar, one boy wrapped a tarred rope tightly around his neck, and then buttoned his collar over it. During the night, he awoke with a start, coughing, grappling with the rope, half-strangled, having almost killed himself in an attempt to save his own life. An inebriated sailor fell asleep for several hours in one of the streets in the northern suburbs. Too afraid to shake him to see if he were still alive, the neighbors sent to city hall for a dray and coffin. The drayman seized the sailor by the feet and dragged him into the wagon. The seamen woke with a jolt, damning the eyes of the dray-man. Frightened, the man took to his heels.[28]

Not all turned their backs on family and neighbors, despite the panic. The question of whether to desert the city raised serious moral issues for a number of Philadelphians. A few weighed the chances that they might kill residents in nearby towns and villages by person-ally carrying yellow jack to them and decided to stay where they were. Some women, embracing the feminine ideal of caring for their friends and families, refused to leave. Polly Stockton, Benjamin Rush's sister, believed it to be her ethical obligation to remain and nurse the sick. Margaret Peale, the wife of famous portrait painter Charles Willson Peale, refused her husband's proposal that she go to her parents in New York. It was her duty, she said, to take care of her spouse and children.[29]

Samuel Garrigues, a member of the Guardians of the Poor, strug-gled with his conscience when the epidemic broke out. Should he fly to safety or stay and help his friends and neighbors? A successful car-penter and devout Quaker, he turned to his religious faith for the an-swer. He decided to stay. Garrigues walked door to door, especially in poorer neighborhoods, asking how he could help. He nursed the sick, comforted widows, found shelter for orphans, arranged care for aban-doned people, and informed death-cart drivers about the whereabouts of corpses. Garrigues grew ill from exhaustion, and then received a visit from yellow jack. After ten days of struggle, he recovered, then immediately returned to helping his neighbors. When yellow fever revisited the city on a number of occasions over the next decade, Samuel Garrigues continued, in his words, to "wrestle the Pale Faced Messenger" of death. He was but one of many of the city's heroes.[30]

Doctors, too, risked death daily, though their acrimonious debates about the proper treatment of the disease offered little comfort to Philadelphians trying to decide how to protect themselves and help infected relatives. Given the state of medical knowledge, physicians could do nothing to halt the pestilence. Yet they tried valiantly, proposing myriad therapies. On one side was Benjamin Rush, the most respected doctor in the country. His advice carried a great deal of weight with the city's residents. On the other side was the distinguished College of Physicians, supported by several newly arrived French doctors who had escaped the rebellion in the West Indies, where they had previously treated yellow fever. The positions outlined by the two sides helped define the debate that would continue for the following century. In the short term, the highly publicized arguments added greatly to the confusion of ordinary Philadelphians.

Dr. Rush had developed a new theory, announcing several years before the epidemic that there was only one fever in the world: all fevers were merely variants of this single disease. The treatment for all fevers was correspondingly simplified. To deal with the "irregular convulsive action of the blood vessels," physicians should adopt "heroic measures." The core of his therapy consisted of bloodletting and administering large doses of jalap (for purging the bowels) and calomel (which contained mercury and caused salivation). Bleeding with lancets, purging with jalap, and facilitating salivation with mercury would restore balance among the fluids in the body and relieve patients of foul humors.[31]

Rush's thinking followed the traditional medical understanding of the time; most doctors believed that disease came from exposure to adulterated air. This theory harked back many centuries, all the way to Galen, a prominent Roman physician in the second century C.E. Galen believed that when people breathed impure air, their phlegm, bile, feces, and blood became unbalanced; thus, they became ill.

Following this logic, Rush identified the putrefied coffee rotting on the city dock as the culprit that had created the dangerous miasmas. Other physicians ridiculed the idea, arguing that ships had imported the disease from abroad. They all agreed, however, that miasmas were deadly.

Rush initially tried out his treatment on several poor patients whom he expected to die anyway. Instead, they apparently survived, although the records are sketchy. Shortly thereafter, he began to experiment on other patients as well. "Four of five," he noted, improved from the new therapy, and a handful were "perfectly cured." In a few short days, Rush got the chance to try the cure on himself.[32]

On the evening of September 14, Rush cut open the veins on a patient's arm and let nearly ten ounces of blood drip out. (At other times, he used leeches.) As he rode back to his house at Walnut and Third, he succumbed to illness. He had been feeling unwell for a couple of days, shivering in his bed during the few hours of sleep he allowed himself each night. Yet he had pushed on despite his chills and profound bodily weakness. After being bled (either by one of his students or a black volunteer), Rush spent the next morning attending to fifty new cases around the city. However, his fever became debilitating in the early afternoon, forcing him to retreat to his home. He drank weak tea and currant jelly mixed with water. The following morning, still feverish, he bathed in cold water, but was unable to leave his house. Later that day, Rush asked his assistant to drain him of another ten ounces of blood and administer a tincture of mercury and jalap. It seemed to help. On September 16, he slept through the night with little more than chills. "Thus you see that I have proved upon my own body," he wrote, "that the yellow fever when treated in the new way, is not more than the common cold."[33]

He was spectacularly wrong, as would eventually become apparent to nearly everyone but Rush. He had always enjoyed a strong ego, and he grew too enthusiastic in his conviction that he had discovered a cure for yellow fever, administering it throughout the city during the ensuing weeks. At one point, having severely miscalculated the amount of blood in human beings, Rush prescribed draining out of sick people more blood than their bodies contained. Rush trumpeted that he routinely "drew from many persons seventy or eighty ounces of blood in five days"—perhaps half the quantity present in his patients. The other elements of his "cure," jalap and mercury, can be extremely harmful if taken in excessive quantities. Mercury, also commonly used at the time to treat venereal disease, caused patients' teeth and hair to fall out. It also burned holes in their stomach linings. But some of Rush's patients survived in spite of his cure, convincing him that it was efficacious.[34]

Like most doctors at the time, Rush did not keep careful records of his patients, simply cataloguing what worked and what didn't, especially during the chaos of the epidemic, when he often tended more than a hundred patients every day. Moreover, while he was a man of the Enlightenment, he also deeply believed in God's will. He sometimes dismissed medical evidence that contradicted his views. "Reason produces, it is true, great and popular truths," Rush acknowledged, but "it seems to be reserved to Christianity alone to produce universal, moral, political, and physical happiness."[35]

When the epidemic began, Rush searched within himself, then "resolved to perish with my fellow citizens rather than dishonor my profession or religion by abandoning the city." He cannot be faulted for his bravery or commitment to helping thousands of sick people. His ignorance was also partially defensible: the mosquito vector that spread yellow fever was not discovered for another century.[36] His belief that he had found a cure for yellow fever, however, and his insistence on using it despite the experts arrayed against it, was another question entirely.

A number of Philadelphians, both laypeople and doctors alike, disputed his cure. It became so controversial that even his own mother would not take it when she grew ill. She survived. When Rush claimed that virtually all his patients lived if given his treatment early enough, William Cobbett, a prominent printer, publicly challenged him to prove it. Cobbett performed a statistical study of the city's Bills of Mortality. Since the death rate had increased enormously at the same time Rush was treating hundreds of patients in the city, Cobbett concluded that Rush was killing people rather than saving them. Although crude, it was one of the first statistical analyses of the effectiveness of therapies, an approach to recordkeeping by doctors and hospitals that would grow enormously during the next century and become a crucial contribution to the improvement of medical practice. An irate Rush sued Cobbett for libel, ultimately winning a judgment of five hundred British pounds, a substantial amount at the time.[37]

The city's renowned College of Physicians also disputed Rush's contention. The college advocated that doctors follow a more traditional, much milder treatment of the disease. We have seen that William Currie, a distinguished member of the college, prescribed an emetic to his patients to produce a mild purging. However, reasoning that victims of yellow fever were already debilitated from the disease, he rarely bled them. The French doctors from the West Indies agreed. Jean Devèze tried to provide his patients with gentle remedies and pleasant surroundings, including comfortable beds and plenty of wine, lemonade, and cold water. His cure was much closer to the recommended treatment today—bed rest and plenty of fluids.[38]

Besides disagreements about treatment, the city's physicians also sharply divided over both the origin of yellow fever and whether it was contagious. The debate quickly grew politicized, for this was the nation's capital, and two new political parties were just beginning to emerge and compete with one another. The Federalists declared that immigrants had imported the disease, an argument that fit with their desire to limit the arrival of the Irish and French, who tended to vote against the party of Alexander Hamilton. Quarantining new arrivals on ships and curtailing immigration would prevent outbreaks of yellow fever, they believed. The Democratic-Republicans, including Rush, were certain that yellow fever had domestic origins, erupting out of filthy conditions in the city. Quarantining incoming ships would accomplish little except hamstringing the commercial economy. Instead, Philadelphians needed to clean and purify their town, to provide residents with fresh drinking water, and to renew their commitment to their community. During the next decade, solutions proposed by both political parties would be adopted.[39]

A few brave physicians ran bold, if distasteful, experiments on themselves to determine whether the fever was communicated from one person to another. As the medical student John Coxe recalled, "Experiments were made by swallowing the black vomit or by inoculating with it with perfect impunity." Contrary to his mentor, Rush, Coxe reached the correct conclusion: "Not a single instance could be adduced in favor of contagion." Most Philadelphia doctors, except those associated with Rush, agreed that the disease was not contagious. Moreover, heroic measures like excessive bleeding and strong purgatives were inappropriate since the illness was all but incurable, they claimed. A decade later, even Rush would finally admit that the disease did not pass from person to person, and that it was imported from Bolama. Still, the issue of contagion remained hotly debated for the next century, as governments and physicians squabbled about whether to quarantine ships arriving from infected areas.[40]

Philip Freneau expressed the city's and the nation's exasperation in verse. Nicknamed the poet of the American Revolution, he summed up the situation in "Pestilence":

> Hot, dry winds forever blowing,
> Dead men to the grave-yards going:
> Constant hearses,
> Funeral verses;
> Oh! what plagues—there is no knowing!
> Doctors raving and disputing,
> Death's pale army still recruiting—
> What a pother
> One with t'other!
> Some a-writing, some a-shooting.[41]

Being a physician was a dangerous profession at any time in the eighteenth century, but especially during an epidemic. At least ten of the city's medical men died during the first five weeks. "Scarcely one of the practicing doctors who remained in the city escaped sickness," Mathew Carey claimed. "Some were three, four, and five times confined." Rush survived his bout with his own brutal therapy and lived for another two decades, his reputation a bit besmirched by his mistaken enthusiasm for his "cure" for yellow jack. However, Rush paid the ultimate price for his erroneous theories: he died when he ordered his assistants to bleed him after he caught typhus. His physicians advised strongly against Rush's "favorite system of depletion," but could not change his mind. Ironically, Rush succumbed to his own therapy.[42]

More than any other group except doctors, African Americans risked their lives to help save their community. As federal, state, and local governments ceased to function, Mayor Clarkson grew desperate. He decided to appeal directly to the ordinary citizens of Philadelphia for assistance. The most pressing needs were nurses to care for the sick, cart men to carry away bodies, and gravediggers to bury them. But these duties were considered too dangerous since they brought the workers into contact with sources of the infection. Nobody wanted to perform these jobs.

A large cohort of black Philadelphians stepped into the breach. At a banquet celebrating the opening of the first free black church in North America, members of the congregation learned about the mayor's plea for help. Benjamin Rush, himself an abolitionist and a supporter of the free black community, also pleaded for their assistance. Mistakenly believing that yellow fever "passes by [misses] persons of your color," Rush argued that black people's supposed immunity placed them "under an obligation to offer your services to attend the sick." Doing so would be "pleasing to God."[43]

During the church banquet, the worshipers solemnly resolved that "it was our duty to do all the good we could to our suffering fellow mortals." In conjunction with the Free African Society—an organization founded in 1787 that emphasized helping one another—they volunteered their service. Since most black people could not afford to travel to the countryside, several thousand remained in the city. Their assistance would make an important difference for people's survival in the City of Brotherly Love.

Two clergymen, Absalom Jones and Richard Allen, co-founders of the African Methodist Episcopal Church, took the lead. When they visited City Hall, the mayor responded enthusiastically and without hesitation, despite the racism that permeated even Philadelphia's comparatively liberal society. He even agreed to free black prisoners—most confined for running away from bondage—in the Walnut Street Jail so that they could help.

Jones and Allen, along with William Grey, a leader of the Free African Society, placed ads in those newspapers still publishing, announcing that black Philadelphians stood willing to care for the sick and to collect and bury the dead. Even in this generous offer of aid, they couched the announcement in the deferential terms demanded of them by white society. "As it is a time of great distress in this city, many people of the black color, under a grateful remembrance of the favors received from the white inhabitants, have agreed to assist them." Members of the church and the Free African Society "set out to see where we could be useful." In groups of two, they walked the streets every day, stopping to make house calls to see where their services were needed.[44]

For one of the first times, a black community wielded enormous public authority in America. African Americans cared for the stricken, carted away the ill to the hospital and the dead to the cemetery, and organized workers to dig graves and bury the dead. They also patrolled the streets, kept watch on temporarily abandoned properties, apprehended looters, and tried to maintain order, performing the jobs of constables as well as nurses.[45]

Benjamin Rush was ecstatic about the involvement of the black community, since he could use them as foot soldiers to administer his miracle cure. Rush taught his black helpers how to bleed and purge patients with jalap and mercury. Jones, Allen, and Grey worked tenaciously themselves and supervised a large group of others willing to help. For good or for ill, they applied the treatment to more than

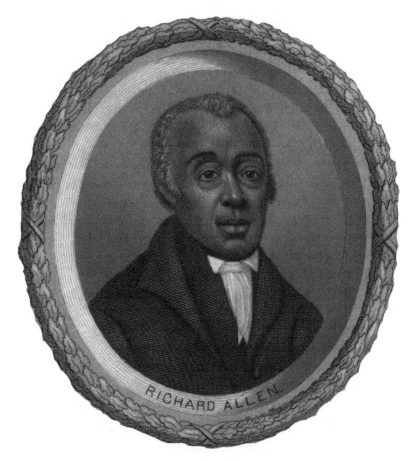

Richard Allen (1760–1831) organized his first church in Philadelphia in 1794 and subsequently became the founder of the African Methodist Episcopal Church. Born into slavery, he purchased his freedom in 1780. Allen organized free blacks to care for the sick during Philadelphia's 1793 yellow fever epidemic. Courtesy the Library of Congress, Washington, D.C.

eight hundred patients during the epidemic. They followed up after Rush visited his patients, and even cared for Rush and his family during their illnesses. In a letter to his wife, Rush praised the activities of the black helpers: "You will see by this day's paper what my African brethren have done for the city. They are extremely useful in attending the sick. Billy Grey and Absalom Jones have been very active in procuring nurses."[46]

Black volunteers likewise had a significant impact in transforming the house in Bush Hill from a mansion to a hospital. When authorities first assumed control of the building, it served primarily as a warehouse for sick people on their way to the grave. Lacking beds, medical supplies, food, blankets, doctors, and nurses, it quickly became known as a house of death. Many sick people refused to go to the hospital during the early weeks of the epidemic, preferring to take their chances at home.[47]

As black laborers and draymen steadily carted supplies and water to Bush Hill, Anne Saville, a member of the Free African Society, took over the nursing responsibilities, not only caring for individual patients but also organizing the staff, both blacks and whites. The institution changed within weeks under her direction, from "a great human slaughterhouse" to a place where most patients survived the disease. Saville was an extremely "valuable woman," according to the French doctor who oversaw Bush Hill. She "deserves the gratitude of the public for the manner in which she acquitted herself."[48]

Volunteers encountered horrifying incidents of the epidemic in the course of their duties. They discovered hundreds of corpses alone in homes, reported Jones and Allen, "many of whose friends and relations had left them, [who] died unseen, and unassisted." Some lay "on the floor, without any appearance of their having had even a drink of water for their relief; others were lying on a bed with their clothes on, as if they had come in fatigued, and lain down to rest; some appeared, as if they had fallen dead on the floor, from the positions we found them in."[49]

The encounters with orphans were particularly heartrending. "We found a parent dead and none but little innocent babes to be seen, whose ignorance led them to think their parent was asleep. On account of their situation, and their little prattle, we have been so wounded and our feelings so hurt, that we almost concluded to withdraw from our undertaking." Fear of catching the disease kept next-door neighbors and kin from offering help, giving them the "appearance of barbarity." When possible, the humanitarian patrols "picked up little children that were wandering they knew not where, and took them to the orphan house."[50]

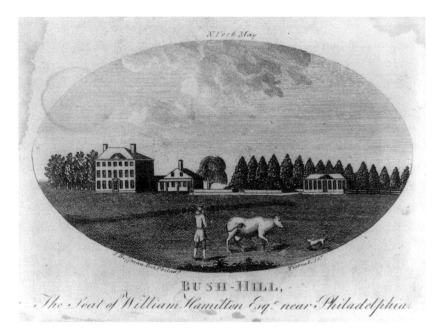

Bush Hill Hospital. William Hamilton's mansion on Bush Hill served as a hospital during the 1793 epidemic. Vice President John Adams had lived there for several years previously. Courtesy the Library of Congress, Washington, D.C.

A number of African Americans began to sicken and die as they exposed themselves to yellow jack by going into homes around the city, especially near the Delaware. Despite popular belief, most black residents possessed no biological immunity to yellow fever. Allen and Jones cited the increase in burials to draw attention to the sacrifice of the African American community. "In 1792, there were 67 of our color buried, and in 1793 it amounted to 305; thus the burials among us have increased more than fourfold." They concluded that just "as many colored people died in proportion as others." They weren't far off the mark.[51]

After the epidemic, many whites praised black people for their invaluable service to the city. The mayor and Benjamin Rush both commended African Americans for their work. Other white citizens agreed. Before his premature death, Isaac Heston noted gratefully, "I don't know what the people would do if it was not for the Negroes,

as they are the Principal nurses." Black volunteers had been responsible for saving countless lives.[52]

However, racism would devise its own interpretation. African
Americans drew criticism in an account that was widely read in the
United States and Britain. In his instant history of epidemic, which
quickly went through four editions, the author and printer Mathew
Carey accused black nurses and gravediggers of extorting money
for their services. Caretakers had come under attack for ineptitude,
thievery, and neglect of their patients in virtually all epidemics for
the previous century. Yet this attack was different, focusing as much
on the race of the alleged miscreants as on their actions. Black leaders
were appalled. Their community was being excoriated at one of its
finest hours. If this was the reaction to their dangerous, even deadly
work in helping save the city during the epidemic, then what hope
did African Americans have of gaining acceptance and some measure
of equality from the larger white community?[53]

Outraged, Allen and Jones responded forcefully to Carey's censure, publishing a remarkable pamphlet in rebuttal, *A Narrative of the
Proceedings of the Black People, During the Late Awful Calamity in Philadelphia in the Year 1793*. The document provides an extraordinary eyewit-
ness report of the conduct of one of the earliest free black communities.
Even more important, it also publicly articulated the anger many black
people felt toward Carey specifically and the institution of slavery in
general. The expression of these feelings had rarely found its way into
print in early America.

Carey had actually praised Jones and Allen by name in his account, so the two ministers had no personal motive for replying to
his attacks. Their heated response indicates that they identified deeply
with their tightly knit community, believed they needed to defend its
reputation, and desired to establish an African American voice independent of the control of whites. Carey's accusations also required a
response because they undermined any claim that might be made
that the behavior of blacks during the epidemic demonstrated that
they had a right to equality and full citizenship. Regarded in prag-
matic economic terms, African Americans likewise had to counter

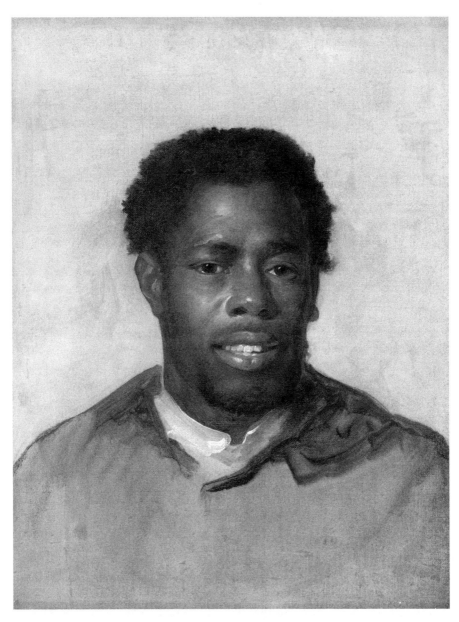

John Singleton Copley, *Head of a Negro,* c. 1777–78, oil on canvas. This painting, done by an American-born artist who moved to Britain shortly before the Revolution, is one of the relatively few eighteenth-century portraits that depicted an African American in a dignified fashion. Detroit Institute of the Arts/The Bridgeman Art Library.

accusations that they had engaged in profiteering and theft simply because many would depend on whites for employment after the epidemic.[54]

Jones and Allen were partially successful in setting the record straight. In later editions of his book, Carey deleted some of his criticism of the black community. He also added a note indicating that some white nurses had acted improperly. In addition, a number of prominent white citizens, including the mayor, came to the defense of black volunteers.

In a striking correlation with the motives that had spurred the colonization of Bolama, the epidemic that the *Hankey* had spread became one of the first platforms for black Americans to denounce slavery in a public forum. Jones and Allen pointed out that slaves were not content with their lot, contrary to what many whites believed. Were they "to attempt to plead with [their] masters, it would be deemed insolence," the authors explained. "We do not wish to make you angry, but excite your attention to consider, how hateful slavery is in the sight of that God, who hath destroyed kings and princes, for their oppression of the poor slaves." Jones and Allen also warned whites of the danger inherent in keeping people in bondage. American slaves might be driven to rebel, like their counterparts in Saint-Domingue, whose revolution made "our hearts sorrowful for the late bloodshed of the oppressors, as well as the oppressed."[55]

Jones and Allen addressed other African Americans as well. As Christian ministers, the authors exhorted slaves to take solace in religion and to love their masters regardless of their misdeeds. Individual slaves should try to convince their owners to grant them an opportunity to gain their freedom. The two ministers, along with thousands of other slaves, had achieved their liberty through self-purchase or individual manumission in the previous decade. They advocated the same avenue for others.[56]

The laudable behavior of Philadelphia's black population during the 1793 epidemic helped soften the racial attitudes of white Philadelphians during the 1790s despite Carey's criticisms. "We have been beholden to the poor; to the despised blacks, for nurses to attend the sick," read the report of the Committee to Alleviate Suffering, "as if Providence were determined to convince us that they are equally the objects of His care, with ourselves."[57]

Still, the wider American society ultimately refused to embrace free black Americans as either citizens or equals. Carey's attack, coupled with the clear findings that blacks did *not* enjoy a special immunity to yellow fever, discouraged many African Americans from attending to the sick in subsequent epidemics. One result was that the mortality rate for white Philadelphians increased in some of the later outbreaks.[58]

Finally, after three months of misery and death, the weather accomplished what no selfless individual had been able to do. It lessened the grip of yellow jack. The nights grew cold. White blankets of frost began to cover the ground. New instances of the fever declined dramatically. On Wednesday, October 23, a bitter wind blew hard out of the north; even in the peak heat of the day, the thermometer climbed only as high as 50 degrees. That day, only fifty-four people died, compared to the average of nearly a hundred a day at the height of the epidemic. The number of internments fell in pace with the temperatures. Although relieved, Philadelphians were not entirely surprised, since cold weather usually ended the mysterious fall agues. What they did not realize was the explanation for this particular diminution of disease. The lower temperatures killed the insects that carried the fever.

"The whole of the disorder, from its first appearance to its final close," wrote Mathew Carey, "has set human wisdom and calculation at defiance." As the threat of death receded, the refugees who had fearfully left the city began to return. There was one last, slight uptick in the number of afflicted, probably caused by infectious mosquitoes who had found shelter from the cold in abandoned houses.[59]

Dr. Benjamin Rush carefully watched the fever's dominance dissipate. On October 24, he saw just six new patients. Two days later, not a single person sought his assistance, and yellow jack had disappeared from his own immediate neighborhood. He checked with physicians in other parts of the city and declared that "the disease visibly and universally declines." Thanks to the number of physicians who had adopted his protocol of bleeding and purging, Rush proclaimed, he had saved the city. He was enormously popular among many Philadelphians, though others were not so sure. During future epidemics Rush's cure would become increasingly discredited.[60]

Rush made plans for his wife, Julia, and the rest of his family to return home. His servants washed his house at Walnut and Third Streets with vinegar, both inside and out. "Our little back parlor has resembled for two months the cabin of a ship," he wrote his wife. "It has been shop, library, council chamber, dining room, and at night a bed chamber for one of the servants." He also reminisced about the difficulties of the past hundred days. "Sometimes seated in your easy chair by the fire," he wrote to Julia, "I lose myself in looking back upon the ocean which I have passed, and now and then find myself surprised by a tear in reflecting upon the friends I have lost, and the scenes of distress I have witnessed." He quoted an appropriate verse from the Song of Solomon: "The winter is gone. The flowers appear upon the earth, the time of the singing of birds is come, and the voice of the turtle is again heard in our land."[61]

The siege of yellow jack ended in early November—at least for that year. Tench Coxe, the U.S. commissioner of revenue, notified Vice President John Adams that Philadelphia was returning to normal. The city's markets and shops began to open, and people once again found work when ships docked in the harbor. President Washington and his Cabinet made their way back to their offices. The city and state governments were reconstituted, and the temporary committees slowly handed management of the institutions back to the appropriate civil departments. Even the Guardians of the Poor found a new footing. There remained talk of restricting trade with ships and wagons from other cities and ports, not to mention managing the size of Philadelphia in order to minimize the threat of future outbreaks, but trade was slowly settling back into its normal routines.

Governor Thomas Mifflin celebrated the end of the first major urban epidemic in the new nation by declaring December 12 a day of thanksgiving and prayer. All Pennsylvanians, he advised, using the fashionable deist terminology, should confess "with contrite hearts, their manifold sins and transgressions—in acknowledging, with thankful adoration, the mercy and goodness of the Supreme Ruler of the universe" for having saved Philadelphia from the infection.[62]

In the weeks and months to follow, conservative Christian preachers often interpreted the epidemic as God's punishment for the myriad sins of the people of Philadelphia, ranging from not attending church to allowing a theater to operate, from engaging in excessive swearing on Sundays to the spread of deism and atheism among the city's inhabitants. "It is a judgment on the inhabitants for their sins," reported one Quaker. The city had grown too wealthy, too secular, too evil—and God had punished it. A group of nineteen Philadelphia ministers enjoined their brothers and sisters, "When His judgments are in the land, the inhabitants should learn righteousness."[63]

Others strongly disagreed. Living in the primary center of the American Enlightenment, a considerable number of Philadelphians understood the tragedy in secular terms, as a health issue that doctors and natural philosophers (scientists) needed to address. Yellow fever had stricken the city because of natural rather than supernatural reasons. Regardless of whether the city's residents behaved morally, preventive measures, like cleaning the city and quarantining ships with sick passengers, were necessary to prevent future epidemics.

The official ineptitude in Philadelphia had outraged many Americans. In the wake of the epidemic, municipalities strengthened the power of boards of health, granting them new powers to quarantine ships and detain infected people in their homes. They developed public policies to protect the well-being of citizens, including bringing cleaner drinking water to cities. Not everyone agreed with increasing the authority of officials. After rancorous political debates, some Philadelphians rioted in the early nineteenth century to protest the new restrictions imposed on individual freedom.[64]

The 1793 epidemic also affected the location of the nation's capital, helping to finalize the decision that made Washington rather than Philadelphia the political center of the country. Early in the 1790s,

Alexander Hamilton and Thomas Jefferson and their two political parties struck a deal to construct a new capital city located between Maryland and Virginia—in part as an acknowledgment of the power of the southern states. Many Philadelphians wanted their city to remain the capital, and politically powerful northerners like John Adams agreed. The continual outbreaks of yellow fever in Philadelphia, however, destroyed those hopes. (Ironically, city planners built Washington, D.C., on a series of swamps that contained swarms of infectious insects. Malaria, also spread by mosquitoes, became endemic to the nation's new capital. While the Bolama fever did not break out in epidemic proportions near the capitol building, it did plague nearby Baltimore early in the nineteenth century and Alexandria in 1803.)[65]

Meanwhile, physicians, government officials, sailors, and residents of Philadelphia began to identify individual ships—such as the *Hankey*—as the primary culprits diffusing the black vomit. Among the first physicians to recognize the damage wrought by the ship, Colin Chisholm presented his conclusions in 1795 in his long but aptly named *Essay on the Malignant Pestilential Fever Introduced into the West Indian Islands from Boullam, on the Coast of Guinea, as It Appeared in 1793 and 1794.* The *Hankey,* he claimed, caused all the havoc. (Chisholm likewise would implicate the *Zephyr* as the vessel that introduced yellow fever to New York from Saint-Domingue in 1795.)[66] And in fact, the *Hankey*'s legacy was far from over.

The summer after the Philadelphia epidemic, the Bolama fever began waging relentless war on North American port cities that would last for the next fifteen years. In 1794, the virus shifted to Charleston, South Carolina. The *Aëdes aegypti* found spectacular breeding grounds in that hot, humid city interlaced with marshes. Moreover, Charleston's lively commerce with the tropics meant that infected mosquitoes continued to arrive in ships. The city suffered yellow fever epidemics annually until the close of the century.[67]

At the same time, the mosquitoes and fevers drifted north from Philadelphia to New York, Boston, Providence, Portsmouth, New Haven, and New London, as well as south to Baltimore, Wilmington, Norfolk, and Savannah. Yellow jack afflicted most of those cities repeatedly. In a particularly brutal outbreak of the disease, six thousand people died in both Philadelphia and New York during the summer and fall of 1798, surpassing the five thousand who perished in 1793. Epidemics recurred in Philadelphia at least seven times over the next fifteen years, threatening its survival as an urban center.[68]

The numerous, severe epidemics tempered the passionate optimism felt by many citizens when the Constitution was ratified just a few years earlier. The inhabitants of the new country began denouncing the cities. "The American plague generates in our cities," the minister William Marshall announced, adding, "It is the wickedness of our cities [that] is the moral cause of our plagues." Suspicions of urban corruption deepened among Americans.[69]

Thomas Jefferson expressed the view of many politicians that "yellow fever will discourage the growth of great cities in our nation." He went further: "The yellow fever epidemics spelled the doom of large cities." This certainly buttressed Jefferson's opposition to the Hamiltonians, who advocated greater government funding for manufacturing and other programs that would lend assistance to municipalities. When state and federal leaders had to flee yellow fever epidemics on an almost annual basis, they grew disenchanted with the idea that the nation's future lay in encouraging the expansion of its urban centers.[70]

Jefferson had always envisioned a rural nation, different from and better than the more urbanized Europe. Yellow jack strongly reinforced his and others' philosophical commitment to a yeoman republic of small farmers. For the next half century, many Americans embraced the rural countryside and disdained cosmopolitan areas. Rather than focus on constructing large cities, they spread westward into the land bought by the United States in the Louisiana Purchase—an acquisition the Bolama fever helped facilitate.[71]

In 1803, Thomas Jefferson received the greatest boon the infant nation had ever known. Having grown disillusioned with dreams of an empire in North America, the young dictator of France offered a vast swath of the Great Plains to the United States. Napoleon Bonaparte had witnessed the widespread slaughter of his proud French troops in Saint-Domingue—not only by an army of rebellious slaves and free black people but also by an unseen pestilence that had struck soldiers when they were lying in their tents. He decided to turn his back on the whole filthy business and offered the United States the Louisiana Territory.

The importance of the Louisiana Purchase to westward expansion in the United States can hardly be exaggerated. Americans had long been coveting the right to navigate the Mississippi and control the river's mouth at New Orleans. More than a third of the nation's products, all coming from the interior of the country between the Allegheny Mountains and the Mississippi River, flowed through New Orleans—but only if Spain or, later, France permitted it.

Both the Republican and Federalist Parties engaged in intense political jockeying over New Orleans during the early nineteenth century. After discovering that Napoleon had forced Spain to cede the Louisiana Territory to France in the Treaty of San Ildefonso in 1801, President Jefferson at once sent a representative to France with an offer to buy New Orleans. Jefferson favored diplomacy and peaceful relations with France, but he still feared that if Napoleon would not make compromises, people in the United States would be forced to "marry ourselves to the British fleet and nation."[72]

As was his wont, Hamilton, still influential in politics even if out of office, was considerably more energetic in proposing the use of an American army to resolve the problem. American "independence and liberty" depended on dislodging Napoleon from New Orleans, he wrote. The French presence "threatens the early dismemberment of a larger portion of the country, more immediately, the safety of all the Southern States, and remotely, the independence of the whole Union." Moreover, Napoleon's was a "most flagitious, despotic, and vindictive government," which was undertaking "hasty and colossal strides to universal empire." The U.S. response, Hamilton believed, should be to construct a navy, raise an army, invade New Orleans and Florida, and then negotiate from a position of strength. If Jefferson followed his advice, he might "save the country and secure a permanent fame." Hamilton held out little hope: "For this, alas! Jefferson is not destined."[73]

Hamilton was wrong. He did not foresee that the conclusion of the Haitian Revolution would be the factor that determined the ownership of New Orleans. As the revolution in Saint-Domingue moved ineluctably toward its conclusion—Toussaint Louverture issued a constitution and called for sovereignty in 1801—Napoleon made one more attempt to create an empire in the Western hemisphere, sending his army to overthrow the victorious rebels and retake the island for France. General Leclerc, at the head of the French forces, soon arrested Louverture and sent him back to France, where he died in prison. However, the military tactics of Jean-Jacques Dessalines and his insurgents, coupled with the decimation of French troops by yellow fever, made the French imperial effort hopeless.

At that historical juncture, Napoleon made a bold decision.[74] For Napoleon, the money for his planned invasion of Britain was of more value than regaining Saint-Domingue. Once the rich sugar island was lost, he saw little use in owning New Orleans, let alone the 828,000 square miles of the territory stretching north and west of the port. It had originally been seen as the breadbasket of France's West Indian empire, but there were no more French slaves in Saint-Domingue, so crops to feed them were no longer needed. In addition, New Orleans was nearly indefensible from attacks by the powerful British navy or even the weaker United States, where Federalists like Hamilton had been advocating a preemptive invasion.

Napoleon decided to sell not just New Orleans but the entire Louisiana Territory to the United States, in order to keep Louisiana from falling into the hands of his main enemy, Britain. His offer to sell the vast territory to the United States for $15 million (approximately $220 million today) stunned the U.S. emissaries, whom Jefferson had authorized only to bargain for New Orleans, with a top price of $10 million. At about three or four cents an acre, it was an offer that they couldn't refuse. Even though it exceeded their authority, the representatives grabbed the deal and signed the Louisiana Purchase Treaty in Paris on April 30, 1803, an act that transformed the history of America. As one of the treaty signers, James Livingston presciently noted, "We have lived long, but this is the noblest work of our whole lives. From this day the United States take their place among the powers of the first rank."[75]

As Americans poured into the Mississippi River valley and moved westward during the nineteenth century, they expanded what Jefferson called the "empire of liberty." Vast new social and economic opportunities opened up, especially for white males, many of whom could now claim land and a farm for the first time in their lives. Acquiring the Louisiana Territory likewise changed how Americans thought about themselves as a nation. They now looked west for empire and toward a future as a great continental power. It was, as the slogan became, "manifest destiny" that the United States would dominate the continent and perhaps even the world.

For other people, the expansion brought tragedy. For Native Americans, the national move westward meant dispossession of their property, forced transformation of their cultures, and even death. By the time of the purchase, President Jefferson was already setting the foundation of a policy of "removal" of Native Americans from their lands between the Allegheny Mountains and the Mississippi River. Andrew Jackson implemented that policy vigorously, resulting in the heartbreaking Trail of Tears, the forcible movement of southeastern Native American peoples to Oklahoma. The government would adopt a similar but even more fatal policy toward Indians in the lands encompassed by the Louisiana Territory.[76]

The Louisiana Purchase also solidified slavery in the new nation by enabling its expansion westward. Masters moved or sold several million bound people into the new territories, ranging from the sugarcane fields of Louisiana to the farms on the plains of Kansas and Nebraska. African Americans experienced it as one more forced migration, this time within the continent rather than across the ocean. They once again endured the painful breakup of families and communities they had struggled successfully to create while in bondage, especially in the older states of Virginia, Maryland, and the Carolinas. However, the expansion of slavery also greatly exacerbated the political tensions between the North and South over the issue of slavery or freedom in the West, eventually culminating in a civil war that would finally settle the conflict over racial bondage in the United States.[77]

History sometimes works in circuitous, interrelated ways, in this instance on a journey around the Atlantic Ocean. The well-intentioned but disastrous Bolama expedition organized by Britons inadvertently helped the Haitian revolutionaries cast off the shackles of their French oppressors, contributing to Napoleon's decision to divest France of the Louisiana Territory. Taking advantage of Napoleon's problems, the United States then purchased the region, laying claim to a large swath of land in the middle of North America. The immediate fates of Native Americans and African slaves in the land rush that followed made an ironic counterpoint to the intentions underlying the voyage of the *Hankey*.

Epilogue
The Living and the Dead

෬෬

I n July 1793, after docking for a few days in Philadelphia, where he unloaded sick refugees and infectious mosquitoes, Captain Cox needed to sail the *Hankey* south to join the convoy of British merchant vessels from the West Indies to London. Britain and France were at war, and French flying squadrons threatened to seize lightly armed commercial vessels as prizes. Cox was eager to have the protection that the Royal Navy afforded the convoy on the last leg of the voyage home. The *Hankey* joined the fleet as it was massing in Golden Rock harbor at Saint Kitts in the Caribbean. There it encountered HMS *Charon* and HMS *Scorpion,* the two ships that several months earlier had loaned seamen to the *Hankey* at Cape Verde, and whose captains had organized the convoy. Cox was probably happier to see the ships than their commanders were to see him. The British naval officers surely remembered that yellow fever had killed a number of their own mariners after their previous encounter with the *Hankey.*[1]

On July 28, the ship of death raised its sails alongside the merchant and warships bound for London. Warnings about the ship's infestation, probably issued by the governor of Grenada, were finally beginning to catch up with the *Hankey.* Because of its growing reputation, no other commander wanted to cruise too close, and it kept falling behind the flotilla during the Atlantic crossing. (For once, the problem was not due to Captain Cox's incompetence.) The other commanders' fears of contagion were justified: two new sailors aboard the *Hankey* died during the voyage.[2]

While the *Hankey* was sailing across the ocean, its reputation was traveling even faster. Rumors and newspaper reports abounded on both sides of the Atlantic about the ship and the deadly cargo it had carried from Africa to the Americas. Interest was particularly keen on London's wharves, where fear inflated the rumors. Britons who worked on the docks dreaded catching the African disease from this mysterious death ship. (Officials subsequently estimated that as many as a hundred thousand residents of Britain's capital, one of the most populous cities in the world, might have died if a yellow fever epidemic as severe as the one in Philadelphia had broken out there.)[3]

Before the *Hankey* sailed up the Thames, the British Privy Council issued an order to sink the vessel, along with its cargo and even its passengers, if necessary. Although there is no direct surviving evidence, it would not be surprising if Henry Dundas, who had opposed the Bolama expedition from the beginning, had had a hand in writing the order. However, word of the extreme measure came too late to stop the vessel from reaching Britain. In an era before easy communication at sea, officials had a hard time contacting ships, so the *Hankey* continued under sail as part of the fleet.

The *Hankey* finally dropped anchor on October 2, 1793. Heeding the order of the Privy Council, officials immediately commanded Captain Cox and the ship into quarantine at Stangate Creek near Chatham well before it reached London docks. As the *Times* cautioned, "A very dangerous distemper has for some time raged on board the Ship *Hankey,* now performing quarantine. It is thought that she will be ordered to be burnt." The *Evening Post* subsequently published a similar account, claiming that the *Hankey* had been "so thoroughly impregnated with the contagion of yellow fever that no means were sufficient to render it healthy and safe. Nothing but scuttling at last would answer."[4]

A fortnight of quarantine passed. Bureaucrats cautiously went aboard to inspect the cargo, while a doctor examined the passengers.

Because of the war with France, the Royal Navy, desperate for sailors, immediately impressed the entire crew, save for Captain Cox, into His Majesty's service. Reportedly, all the impressed men died shortly thereafter; if so, the causes of their deaths are unknown. After serving their time in quarantine, the few surviving passengers carried their personal belongings onto launches bound for London. Meanwhile, tales began to spread that some sailors had contracted fevers just from being near the *Hankey*.[5]

Officials at last set the *Hankey* on fire. Its own timbers became its funeral pyre as the ship burned to the waterline. The waters eventually snuffed out the flames; what remained of the hull slipped beneath the confluence of waves near where the brown and turbid Thames meets the cold Atlantic of the English Channel. The *Hankey* was gone, but its devastating legacy of disease and death would live on.[6]

Only a handful of survivors from the Bolama expedition returned to England on the *Hankey*. On board was Elizabeth Rowe, the widow of John, the physician of the colony, who had escaped the colony but died in Bissau. It was Elizabeth who informed Philip Beaver when they met in England about the secret plot hatched by the slaver Captain Moore to kill him and enslave the grumettas. Her account clarified why James Johnson and other grumettas had rebelled against Beaver's authority: Beaver had welcomed to the colony a man who threatened their freedom.[7]

Another original passenger, John Paiba, survived the Bolama expedition. He accompanied his parents to the colony, but his father and stepmother took the first opportunity to return home on the *Calypso*. The younger John Paiba stayed on the island, hoping to claim land and to become financially successful, but he finally acknowledged defeat after his wife and child died and left on the *Hankey*. After the ship docked in England, he became a key source of information for doctors, government officials, and newspaper printers, relating the events on Bolama and the ship of death.[8]

Thomas Blake, described in the records as a "boy," probably in his late teens, had journeyed to Bolama as a personal servant to John

Munden. Blake had been in trouble with authorities in London since at least 1788, when a judge condemned him to a whipping for stealing a pair of boots. His legal problems probably encouraged him to sign on as a servant. When his master died during the homecoming voyage of the *Hankey,* Blake may have been relieved to be released from his contract. He still had the burden of locating new employment in England, however. Possibly, he was the same Thomas Blake found guilty of stealing a petticoat, parasol, and satin cloak in 1801 and sentenced to deportation. If so, he probably regaled his shipmates with tales of his adventures as they sailed past Bolama on the way to the penal colony of Australia.[9]

Joseph Glover enjoyed moderate success after returning to London. He had traveled to Bolama as a cabin boy on the *Beggar's Benison,* working for John Birkhead, the cutter's master. Both left Bolama on the *Hankey,* although Birkhead died in Bissau, before they ever left Africa. Later in life, Glover became a coach smith, in partnership with his brother or father. It was not a bad career and surely a success story for someone who had started as a cabin boy.[10]

Among the original council members, John Curwood had worked energetically to organize the expedition. Having stayed on Bolama after the *Calypso* left, Curwood spent months trying to convince Beaver and the others that they should abandon the colony. Disease claimed his wife and two children, but he survived to reach England on the *Hankey,* though probably in an emotionally devastated state. What had started so promisingly for the family had turned into a catastrophe.[11]

Captain John Cox disappeared from the historical record after returning to Britain. His poor seamanship throughout the disastrous journey had exacerbated the colonists' problems. His professional experience had been limited before the voyage—probably a reason that the Bolama Association could hire him so cheaply—and his reputation was ruined by the time he returned to England. Apparently, he never sailed out of England again as a ship captain.[12]

Among those who left on the *Calypso,* the tailor's widow, Ann Baker, and her three daughters also made it back to England alive.

Ann and her husband had decided to try their luck in Bolama, hoping
to provide a financial future for their daughters, but their decision
had led to a tragic end. Aaron Baker was among the first colonists to
die, a victim of the initial attack by Bijago combatants, who also
dragged off Susan and Julia Baker. They apparently recovered from
the ordeal after being ransomed, and they had returned to the colonists unharmed physically. Ann and her daughters left on the *Calypso,*
along with most of the European women who had traveled to Bolama. Without a male head of household to earn a livable wage, the
four Baker women found their financial circumstances in England
extremely difficult. They moved in with the families of the two married daughters who had not gone to Bolama. All the women struggled hard to scrape out a living by needlework, but they could never
find sufficient employment. After a few years, authorities imprisoned
the husband of the eldest daughter for debt. He languished in a damp
cellar in Fleet Prison, crowded in with other debtors, where after ten
weeks he died of tuberculosis. Constables then arrested the husband
of the other daughter, who had acted as security for his brother-in-
law, and who now had to pay the debt or take his place in prison.
Shortly thereafter, Ann herself landed in jail for stealing food, a
measure of the desperation of their lives. The court sentenced her to
transportation to Australia, and the family disappeared from the historical record.[13]

One of the best-known survivors of the Bolama expedition did
not sail home on the *Hankey.* Philip Beaver had parted ways with the
handful of remaining colonists when they reached Sierra Leone. He
caught a ride on a ship sailing up the coasts of West Africa and Europe, ultimately returning six months after the arrival in England of
the *Hankey* itself. The Bolama Association awarded Beaver a gold
medal when he reached London in recognition of his vigorous efforts
to make the colony succeed amid so many trials. Shortly afterward,
the Bolama Association disbanded, its funds exhausted. The investors
had lost almost all of their money. A few people associated with the
venture continued for another decade to advocate a second attempt to
colonize Africa, but the talk came to nothing. Many decades later,

the British government would engage in the scramble for colonies in Africa, although Bolama itself became part of the Portuguese rather than the British territorial booty.[14]

Returning to the Royal Navy as a lieutenant after his two years in Bolama, Beaver saw a fair amount of military action and rose quickly through the ranks. In 1795, he participated in Britain's capture of the Cape of Good Hope, which had until then been controlled by the Dutch. Four years later, he became commander of HMS *Dolphin,* ironically the name of the ship (perhaps the same vessel) that had carried yellow fever from Philadelphia to Spain a few years earlier. His last battle action came in 1810, when he helped land troops on the Isle de France (Mauritius), which the British had recently conquered. Afterward, he cruised around the Indian Ocean as captain of HMS *Nisus.*

On Beaver's death at age forty-seven in 1813, the London *Times* ran an obituary lauding his naval career, which had lasted through thirty-six years of active service. The death notice did not mention his participation in the attempt to colonize Bolama, but Beaver summarized his dreams for the colony in his own account: "I hope that the day is not far distant, when some enlarged and liberal plan will be adopted to cultivate the western coast of Africa, without interfering with the freedoms of its natives. Such a plan, pursued with a wise policy, is the surest way of introducing civilization, and at the same time of abolishing slavery."[15]

In 1805, when Beaver's *African Memoranda* appeared, Britain was in the midst of a spirited debate about the Atlantic slave trade. Even though Parliament would end the nation's involvement in the trade two years later, the outcome was still uncertain. The history of the colony on Bolama became part of that dispute.

Beaver denied the existence of the disease known as the Bolama fever, and he minimized the sickness and death on the island, calling it, with what even he must have recognized as hyperbole, the "healthiest spot on the coast." Bolama was a bountiful place for Europeans, he claimed; he laid the blame for the deaths of the colonists primarily on their own behavior. The British would never establish an antislavery

colony in Africa, Beaver feared, if the widely circulated stories about
the high mortality rate held sway. He also contended that the Bolama
colony had succeeded in its major goal by demonstrating that Europeans could hire Africans more efficiently and cheaply than enslaving
them. Half a century later, abolitionists in the U.S. Congress cited
the Bolama expedition as evidence of exactly that point.[16]

Meanwhile, proponents of the slave trade cited the Bolama disaster in support of their own cause. Since Britons could not survive on
African soil, the failure of the enterprise demonstrated that colonizing Africa and hiring local peoples to grow sugarcane and other cash
crops was not feasible. Slave-trade enthusiasts also trumpeted news of
the Bolama fever that had killed so many on both sides of the Atlantic. This misbegotten adventure, according to proslavery advocates,
had resulted in countless deaths rather than in bettering the condition
of slaves and Africans. Moreover, the arguments went, resistance to
yellow fever and other tropical diseases enjoyed by Africans made
them biologically more capable of working in tropical climates.[17]

The campaign to convince the British, other Europeans, and the
Americans to end the slave trade was far from easily won, in part because of the durability of the economic, social, and ideological forces
arrayed in support of slavery. Racial bondage had been an accepted
part of life for most white people, and it had made a good many of
them rich. It was another seventy years before the Atlantic slave trade
finally ended. Even though Denmark banned the trade in 1803, Britain in 1807, and the United States in 1808, the number of people forcibly transported across the Atlantic actually increased during the early
decades of the nineteenth century. Not until 1850, when officials from
Brazil began to seize the human cargo on slave ships, did the volume
of traffic decline significantly. The last recorded transatlantic voyage
carrying African slaves, from the Congo River area to Cuba, occurred
in 1867.[18]

While the *Hankey* was spreading the yellow fever virus, affairs
on Bolama Island largely reverted to the way they had been
before the short-lived attempt at British colonization. The Bijago

quickly reclaimed the land, cultivating rice and cashews in the more than fifty acres of forests cleared and prepared by the grumettas and colonists. They put the blockhouse to use for shelter and storage. Both the British and the Portuguese attempted to invade the island in 1814, but the Bijago successfully defended their territory. There is no record of whether Jalorem and Bellchore, the elderly Bijago leaders when the British settlers arrived, had died by then or whether they were alive to lead their villages in resisting the invasions. Unfortunately, we know almost nothing about the fate of men like James Johnson and other grumettas who worked on Bolama.[19]

The British and Portuguese squabbled for decades over ownership of the island of Bolama. Officials in Great Britain, who had wanted nothing to do with the colony, later held that Philip Beaver had purchased it legitimately from not one but *two* of the local groups who had claimed ownership in 1792. Officials in Portugal insisted that Bolama belonged to their own colonial holdings in "Portuguese Guinea," claimed more than three centuries earlier. The Canabac leaders believed that Beaver had merely rented, not purchased, Bolama, but their opinion was sought by neither European nation. Finally, in 1870, Ulysses S. Grant, president of the United States, chaired an international commission to arbitrate the dispute. The commission, which had no representatives from the people who lived on the islands, officially awarded the Bijago Archipelago, including Bolama, to Portugal. The Bijago living on Bolama did not give up easily; they fought the Portuguese just as they had resisted the British.[20]

In 1879, Portugal renewed its colonial claim on Portuguese Guinea, making Bolama its first capital. It was a poor choice. Over the next half century, the Bijago rebelled against the Portuguese colonists on seven different occasions. In 1936, the exhausted Portuguese tacitly relinquished autonomy to the Bijago, granting them self-rule. Five years later, the Portuguese transferred their colonial capital to Bissau, much closer to the mainland, after which Bolama declined in importance and population. Portuguese Guinea became a province of Portugal in 1952. It remained in Portuguese hands until a nationalist guerrilla war, joined by Bijago, won Guinea-Bissau independence in

1974. More recently, Guinea-Bissau society has become chaotic. Cap-
italizing on the increased European demand for cocaine, the country
currently is an important narco-state, serving as a major conduit for
drugs shipped from South America to Europe.[21]

The Bijago still govern their islands. At present, they number approximately thirty thousand people, a third of whom reside on the
island of Bolama. They engage primarily in rice production and subsistence fishing, while still cultivating cashew nuts as a commercial
crop. They are among the most impoverished people in the world.[22]

The voyage of the *Hankey* created a pandemic that reshaped, to
varying degrees, the histories of West Africa, the West Indies,
North America, and Europe. Carrying its deadly cargo of mosquitoes, it inadvertently threaded together isolated pockets of illness
among peoples in discrete coastal locations into a deadly necklace,
disfiguring commercial relationships, societies, and nations. The epidemic launched by the *Hankey* would not be matched until 1918,
when the Spanish flu killed an estimated fifty to a hundred million
people worldwide.

The *Hankey* had help taking yellow jack to Europe: before the
ship reached London, the virus had made landfall via other contaminated vessels. These ships had been exposed to the *Hankey*'s Bolama
fever in North America and the West Indies and carried the infectious mosquitoes back across the Atlantic. Outbreaks of the disease in
Spain and southern Europe occurred during the summer of 1793. On
August 8, the *Dolphin,* a commercial ship flying the flag of the United
States, brought the scourge to Cádiz. Its passengers and crew had
probably picked up both the virus and infectious mosquitoes when
the ship made a brief stop in Charleston, South Carolina, to purchase
provisions and hire three new sailors. All the new mariners died during the ocean voyage to Spain. As soon as the ship made port, the
surviving passengers and sailors fled, unrestrained by officials who
should have ordered them quarantined. Yellow jack subsequently
found many new victims in Cádiz. For the remainder of the decade,
epidemics broke out from Gibraltar to Jerez, Seville to Valencia. At

least eighty thousand people perished of the fever in Spain before 1800, and another hundred thousand, roughly 1 percent of the nation's entire population, died during the first four years of the nineteenth century.[23]

Epidemics threatened the Mediterranean coasts of France and Italy and continued to rage through southern Spain early in the nineteenth century. Gibraltar lost more than five thousand people to yellow jack in 1804, becoming, according to Dr. William Pym, a "scene of horror beyond all description," much like Philadelphia and other cities in which a severe eruption of the Bolama fever had appeared. Although the figure is probably an exaggeration, Pym claimed that out of fourteen thousand civilians, only twenty-eight successfully escaped the disease, and a dozen of these had contracted the fever previously in Philadelphia, the West Indies, or Spain. Of forty-two hundred soldiers stationed at Gibraltar, Pym estimated that three thousand caught the ailment. The final tally: about a third of the population perished. Gibraltar continued to suffer severe yellow fever epidemics in 1810, 1812, and 1814.[24]

Wars among major European powers facilitated the spread of microbes throughout the Atlantic world. Those conflicts provided thousands of new victims in the form of military personnel and civilian refugees who were not immune to the disease. Yellow jack even made brief forays into other areas of Europe: Italy, Hungary, Saxony, Prussia, Austria, and the Netherlands.[25]

Patterns of trade across the Atlantic Ocean during the 1790s and early nineteenth century also helped transport yellow fever. The United States, officially neutral in the wars, became active in what was termed the "carrying trade." To gain the status of a neutral carrier, a ship had to drop supplies at a U.S. port and then reload them onto its own or another vessel. Ship entrances and clearances boomed in eastern ports—the places that harbored the yellow fever virus. Whenever infected mosquitoes were loaded on board along with water casks, the departing ships became vectors for the disease.[26]

The number of deaths in Bolama and on the *Hankey,* though heartbreaking, pales in comparison to the hundreds of thousands of

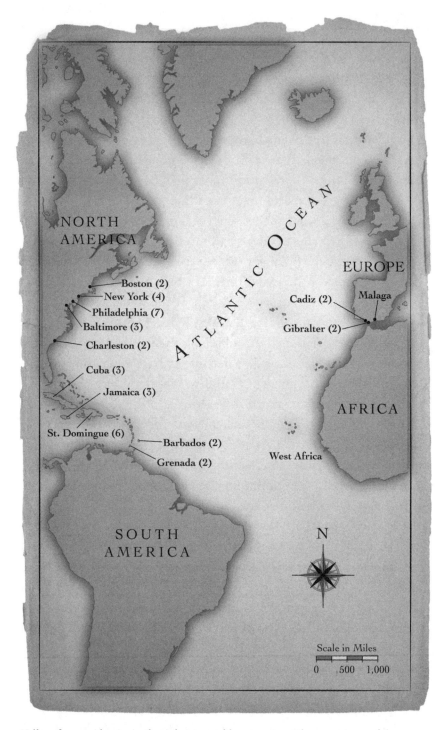

Yellow fever epidemics in the Atlantic world, 1793–1805. These are some of the known epidemics of yellow fever that broke out in the dozen years after the *Hankey* sailed. Only a handful of epidemics occurred during the thirty years before 1793. The numbers in parentheses indicate the annual outbreaks of yellow fever in each area. Map drawn by Michele Angel.

deaths that trailed behind the ship as it plied the trade lanes of the Atlantic. For a dozen years after the voyage of the *Hankey,* the commercial web of ships cruising the Atlantic Ocean spawned virulent new waves of the ailment. But starting in 1807, yellow fever epidemics mysteriously declined for a decade along the Atlantic rim. Perhaps the virus took on a new, less virulent form for a brief while, as sometimes happens with these types of diseases. After the Napoleonic Wars ended in 1815, yellow fever again found a foothold in U.S. port cities along the Atlantic coast. The mosquitoes and virus discovered an especially favorable environment in New Orleans and cities on the Gulf Coast, which the fever would plague for the next century. The heat and humidity, with some similarity to West African coastal regions, made New Orleans a particularly welcoming environment for mosquito vectors of the disease.

Modern chaos theory posits that tiny, seemingly insignificant events, like the beating of the wings of a butterfly (or a mosquito), can have enormous consequences half a globe away. The so-called butterfly effect surely characterized the voyage of the *Hankey,* presenting local peoples throughout the Atlantic world with common dilemmas. Pestilence, one of the Four Horsemen of the Apocalypse, remains at large in our own times. In 1793, Pestilence took the form of a sailor on a ship rather than a rider on a horse. Newer plagues, perhaps similar to Marburg, Ebola, or HIV, will probably emerge from humans invading the preserve of animals like monkeys and apes. Or viruses like swine flu and bird flu, originating on domestic pig farms in the United States or in poultry operations in Asia, may sweep the planet. The next pandemic could be carried by a passenger on an airplane, on the wings of a wild bird, or even in the hold of a ship, and could have consequences as dire as those brought by the *Hankey.*

The Legacy of the *Hankey*

ဘာ

The tale of the *Hankey* and its passengers—both human and insect—brings together peoples who lived thousands of miles apart who discovered, perhaps to their surprise, that far-distant events could have impacts, sometimes fatal, on their own lives. The close-up view from the ship's deck allows us to see in greater detail, and sometimes for the first time, clusters of ordinary men and women who built the societies on the perimeter of the ocean. Whether they lived in Britain, West Africa, the Caribbean, or Philadelphia, their lives were interconnected; sometimes they shared similar quests to shape their communities and their lives, at others they came into conflict with one another when their interests diverged.

An observation from the *Hankey*'s topmast provides a wider perspective. Virtually all the peoples bordering the Atlantic wrestled with the larger forces of the Atlantic world: slavery and the slave trade, the aggressive expansion of western Europe and North America, the extension of commercial capitalism, rising social inequality, and the spread of deadly diseases. Some of these forces bear remarkable similarities to our own times of intensified globalization.

Of all these larger forces, slavery and the traffic in human beings lay at the heart of the Atlantic world, shaping it in virtually every aspect. Free, unfettered trade allowed ship captains and merchants to earn staggering profits by forcibly moving millions of people across the ocean. When the English colonists migrated to Bolama, many hoped to change the world by challenging the slave trade and, ultimately, racial bondage itself. In the process, they set in motion a series of events that changed societies, for good or ill, on both sides of the Atlantic.

The voyage of the *Hankey* became legendary in the decades following the ship's destruction. The threat of the "Bolama fever" brought terror to port cities throughout the West Indies, the United States, Spain, and France. Doctors and laypeople passionately debated its causes and effects in newspapers and magazines, while politicians and officials created new policy in its wake.

But the saga of the *Hankey* was recast in the early nineteenth century to meet new imperial agendas. The history of global expansion by Europeans and North Americans for decades was narrated in those continents through the escapades of explorers seeking out exotic parts of the globe. Even scholars frequently focused on imperial ventures and political and intellectual forces that spread from England, France, Holland, Portugal, and Spain to their colonies, writing from the perspective of the aggressors. Western expansion has been portrayed as the story of struggling colonists and brave ship captains, with barely a mention of the people whose land was being invaded or colonized.

The story of Captain Philip Beaver and the colony of Bolama was no exception: Beaver's narrative of the disaster (though he would have rejected that label) became immensely popular as an adventure story, the kind that enthralled British boys during the early years of the British imperial century. Conveniently omitted was any mention of the yellow fever pandemic sparked by the *Hankey*.

In the new version the stalwart British pioneers sailed three thousand miles to a remote island off the coast of West Africa motivated purely by philanthropy: the desire to challenge the slave trade and "civilize" the "savages" in West Africa. Beaver's narrative contained plenty of excitement: cannibals, witches, exotic animals. Even though the outpost lasted only a short time and failed miserably in its goals, Beaver labeled it a success and urged his readers to carry on the good work, both on Bolama itself and around the world. The echo in our own times is hard to miss. When one people assumes the superiority of its own culture and tries, sometimes forcibly, to change the behavior and values of other peoples, the results can be disastrous for both parties involved. We can see this in today's world as in Beaver's, when politicians and "nation-builders" deny failure and claim success in restructuring other nations.

The saga of Bolama and the *Hankey* is a much broader and more vital story than the adventure tale recounted by Beaver and his contemporaries. The only way to understand a more balanced, accurate narrative of the Bolama colonists and their legacy is through multiple perspectives: the colonized as well as the colonizers, free blacks as well as free whites, slave revolutionaries as well as famous physicians. This richer story contains important lessons for our own times of rapid globalization, lessons that are also part of the *Hankey*'s bequest to the modern world.

ᘛᐧᘚ

Notes

Chapter 1: The *Hankey*

1. Descriptions of the *Hankey* are taken from the *Independent Gazetteer* (Philadelphia), June 27, 1784; and *Lloyd's Register of Shipping,* volumes 1784 to 1792, National Maritime Museum, Greenwich, England.

2. This chapter draws heavily on four personal accounts as well as official records. Members of the expedition wrote the first two reports, and subscribers with access to the papers of the Bolama Association published two additional accounts. The quotations in this paragraph are from Philip Beaver's detailed, five-hundred-page account of the Bolama expedition, *African Memoranda: Relative to an Attempt to Establish a British Settlement on the Island of Bulama, on the Western Coast of Africa, in the Year 1792 . . . and the Introduction of Letters and Religion to Its Inhabitants but More Particularly as the Means of Gradually Abolishing African Slavery* (London: Baldwin, 1805; repr. Westport, Conn.: Negro Universities Press, 1970), 14. Joshua Montefiore wrote the pamphlet *An Authentic Account of the Expedition to Bulam, on the Coast of Africa, and the Settlement of Sierra Leone* (London: J. Johnson, 1794). Subscriber C. B. Wadstrom published *An Essay on Colonization, Particularly Applied to the Western Coast of Africa, with Some Free Thoughts on Cultivation and Commerce; Also Brief Descriptions of the Colonies Already Formed, or Attempted, in Africa, Including Those of Sierra Leona and Bulama* (London: Darton and Harvey, 1794; repr. New York: Kelley, 1968). Andrew Johansen's *Account of the Island of Bulama, with Observations on Its Climate, Productions, etc. and an Account of the Formation and Progress of the Bulam Association, and of the Colony Itself . . .* (London: Martin and Bain, 1794) is, like the other three narratives, available at the Library Company of Philadelphia. Interactions between the Bolama expedition and the British government are in the Records of the Colonial Office, 267/9 and 267/10, British National Archives, Kew, England. Among the relatively few historians who have noted the Bolama mission are Deidre Coleman, in *Romantic Colonization and British Anti-Slavery* (Cambridge: Cambridge University Press, 2005) and "Bulama and Sierra Leone: Utopian Islands and

Visionary Interiors," in *Islands in History and Representations,* ed. Rod Edmond and Vanessa Smith (London: Routledge, 2003), 63–80; and Philip D. Curtin, *The Image of Africa: British Ideas and Action, 1780–1850* (Madison: University of Wisconsin Press, 1964).

3. Wadstrom, *Essay on Colonization,* 270. The lands bordering the Atlantic Ocean and making up the Atlantic world have attracted a great deal of scholarly attention during the past few decades. In this book, the term "Atlantic" references the shared history of those regions. Among the numerous recent studies are Thomas Benjamin, *The Atlantic: Europeans, Africans, Indians and Their Shared History, 1400–1900* (Cambridge: Cambridge University Press, 2009); Douglas R. Egerton, Alison Games, Jane G. Landers, Kris Lane, and Donald R. Wright, *The Atlantic: A History, 1400–1888* (Wheeling, Ill.: Harlan Davidson, 2007); Jack P. Greene and Philip D. Morgan, eds., *Atlantic History: A Critical Appraisal* (New York: Oxford University Press, 2008); David Armitage and Michael J. Braddick, eds., *The British Atlantic, 1500–1800,* 2nd ed. (Houndmills, U.K.: Palgrave Macmillan, 2009); and Peter Linebaugh and Marcus Rediker, *The Many-Headed Hydra: Sailors, Slaves, Commoners, and the Hidden History of the Revolutionary Atlantic* (Boston: Beacon, 2000).

4. Manchester abolitionist, quoted in Amanda Vickery, *The Gentleman's Daughter: Women's Lives in Georgian England* (New Haven: Yale University Press, 2003), 293; Wadstrom, *Essay on Colonization,* 340. See also Deidre Coleman, "Conspicuous Consumption: White Abolitionism and English Women's Protest Writings," *English Literary Review* 61, no. 2 (Summer 1994): 341–62.

5. The description appears in Blake's *Milton: A Poem.*

6. Beaver, *African Memoranda,* 3. (For ease of reading, the spelling, punctuation, and grammar of eighteenth-century quotations have occasionally been slightly and silently modernized.) "The resemblance of Mr. Beaver's situation to that of Columbus," wrote Wadstrom, "is too striking to escape the notice of intelligent readers" (*Essay on Colonization,* 165).

7. The old saying about Benin is quoted in Marcus Rediker, *Between the Devil and the Deep Blue Sea: Merchant Seamen, Pirates, and the Anglo-American Maritime World, 1700–1750* (Cambridge: Cambridge University Press, 1989), 47.

8. The colony's constitution and the questions posed by officials are located in the Records of the Colonial Office, 267/9, British National Archives, Kew. Dava Sobel discusses clock setting in *Longitude: The True Story of a Lone Genius Who Solved the Greatest Scientific Problem of His Time* (New York: Walker, 2003).

9. Beaver, *African Memoranda,* 12, 15; Johansen, *Account of the Island of Bulama,* 6.

10. Emma Christopher, *A Merciless Place: The Fate of Britain's Convicts After the American Revolution* (Oxford: Oxford University Press, 2010), 83–84; see also James Walvin, *Britain's Slave Empire* (Gloucestershire, U.K.: Tempus, 2007). The British economist Malachy Postlethwayt was an exceptionally strong proponent of the colonization of Africa.

11. J. H. Elliott, *Empires of the Atlantic: Britain and Spain in America, 1492–1830* (New Haven: Yale University Press, 2006).

12. The intensity of interest in trade is apparent in the correspondence between the African Committee of Merchants and Secretary Dundas found in Records of the Colonial Office, 267/10, British National Archives, Kew.

13. Paine was writing *The Age of Reason* while Wollstonecraft was finishing *A Vindication of the Rights of Woman.*

14. Beaver, *African Memoranda,* 367. I have substituted modern spellings of place names throughout. In the eighteenth and nineteenth centuries, for example, Britons and Americans commonly used variants of Bulama, Bulam, and Bullom for Bolama. To his credit, Beaver, unlike most other European imperialists, at least tried to use local names and "native pronunciation" for places; see *African Memoranda,* 21.

15. Ibid., 16.

16. Ibid.

17. Ibid.

18. A list of the subscribers is included in Wadstrom, *Essay on Colonization,* 359–61.

19. Beaver, *African Memoranda,* 17.

20. Ibid., 16–17. The *Hankey's* sailing appears in *Lloyd's Register of Shipping,* vol. 1792, National Maritime Museum, Greenwich. A copper-sheathed 300-ton ship, the *Hankey* contained a single wooden deck built over beams.

21. The captains of the *Hankey* are recorded in *Lloyd's Register of Shipping,* volumes 1784 to 1792, National Maritime Museum, Greenwich.

22. On Beaver, see William Henry Smyth, *The Life and Services of Captain Philip Beaver* (London: John Murray, 1829); *London Gazette,* June 24, 1800, May 30, 1809, and January 21, 1812; J. K. Laughton and Andrew Lambert, "Beaver, Philip," *Oxford Dictionary of National Biography,* available at http://www.oxforddnb.com/public/index -content.html. On rebels in Britain, see Michael T. Davis, " 'That Odious Class of Men Called Democrats': Daniel Isaac Eaton and the Romantics, 1794–1795," *History* 84, no. 273 (January 1999): 74–92.

23. James Boswell, *The Life of Samuel Johnson . . .* (Boston: Carter, Hendee, 1832), 1:151.

24. On John Paiba and his family, see the *Times* (London), April 4, 6, and 10, 1788; and Beaver, *African Memoranda,* 446–50.

25. Information about Ann and Aaron Baker and their children is in Wadstrom, *Essay on Colonization,* 174; and in various computer-searchable criminal cases in the *Proceedings of the Old Bailey,* London, 1674 to 1834, January 10, 1787, and June 4, 1794, http://www.oldbaileyonline.org.

26. Information about James Watson is from Beaver, *African Memoranda,* 173–76, 193, 212–14, 237, 241–46, 264, 269, 274, 282, 436, 438.

27. The *Hankey's* earlier voyages transporting indentured servants began soon after the American Revolution, as recorded in the *Independent Gazetteer* (Philadelphia), June 2, 1784.

28. Conditions for passengers aboard ships are discussed in Marianne S. Wokeck, *Trade in Strangers: The Beginnings of Mass Migration to North America* (University Park: Pennsylvania State University Press, 1999), chap. 4. The *Hankey's* numerous previous

voyages are recorded in *Lloyd's Register of Shipping,* volumes 1784 to 1792, National Maritime Museum, Greenwich. They also appear in ship entrances and clearances in dozens of issues of the London *Times* in the 1780s and early 1790s.

29. In the eleven volumes of logbooks that Beaver kept of subsequent voyages as a navy officer, he was routinely mentioned issuing limes, sauerkraut, and mustard to the crew to combat scurvy, as well as ensuring that there was sufficient water on board; Logbooks of Captain Philip Beaver, February, 28, 1795, to April 1813, National Maritime Museum, Greenwich.

30. Rediker, *Devil and the Deep Blue Sea;* Lt. Philip Beaver, H.M.S. *Stately,* "Log from Europe to India," 1:1795–96, National Maritime Museum, Greenwich.

31. On heavy alcohol consumption, see W. J. Rorabaugh, *The Alcoholic Republic: An American Tradition* (New York: Oxford University Press, 1981). On drinking breaks during the workday, see Alfred F. Young, *Liberty Tree: Ordinary People and the American Revolution* (New York: New York University Press, 2006), 42.

32. Beaver, *African Memoranda,* 24.

33. On the Barbary pirates, see Linda Colley, *Captives: The Story of Britain's Pursuit of Empire and How Its Soldiers and Civilians Were Held Captive by the Dream of Global Supremacy, 1600–1850* (New York: Pantheon, 2002), chap. 2. Contemporary advances in measuring longitude are considered in Sobel, *Longitude.*

34. My discussion of the Canary Islands draws on Alfred W. Crosby, *Ecological Imperialism: The Biological Expansion of Europe, 900–1900,* 2nd ed. (Cambridge: Cambridge University Press, 2004), chap. 4; Elliott, *Empires of the Atlantic,* 18–32; Felibe Fernández-Armesto, *The Canary Islands After Conquest: The Making of a Colonial Society in the Early Sixteenth Century* (Oxford: Oxford University Press, 1982); John Mercer, *The Canary Islands: Their Prehistory, Conquest and Survival* (London: Rex Collings, 1980); and Roberto Nodal, "Black Presence in the Canary Islands (Spain)," *Journal of Black Studies* 12, no. 1 (September 1981): 83–90.

35. The quote from Pliny is cited by Alice Carter Cook, "The Aborigines of the Canary Islands," *American Anthropologist* 2, no. 3 (July–September 1900): 452.

36. Cook, "Aborigines of the Canary Islands"; Ronald Ley, "From the Caves of Tenerife to the Stores of the Peabody Museum," *Anthropological Quarterly* 52, no. 3 (July 1997): 159–164.

37. Beaver, *African Memoranda,* 33.

38. Philip Beaver relates the story of Hayles in *African Memoranda,* 159, 164–65, 169, 173, 229–30, 250, 261–65, 279–80, 445, 450, although Beaver did not discover his true identity until a year after Hayles joined the expedition. On ships resupplying at Santa Cruz, see William Henry Portlock, *A New, Complete, and Universal Collection of Authentic and Entertaining Voyages and Travels to All the Various Parts of the World* (London: Alexander Hogg, 1794), 223. On "worth his salt," see the Phrase Finder, http://www.phrases.org.uk/meanings/worth-ones-salt.html.

39. Beaver, *African Memoranda,* 43.

40. Ibid., 44.

41. Mark Twain, *Following the Equator* (1895; Washington, D.C.: National Geographic, 2005).

Chapter 2: The British Colonists

1. Information about the *Zong* in this and succeeding paragraphs is from James Walvin, *The Zong: A Massacre, the Law and the End of Slavery* (New Haven: Yale University Press, 2011). There were gradations among antislavery supporters and abolitionists at the time. A contingent of antislavery advocates was against the horrendous international slave trade but did not oppose slavery itself. Other antislavery supporters believed that by ending the trade in humans, the institution of racial bondage would gradually fade away as slaves became less available. Abolitionists promoted ending the slave trade as well as slavery itself, either gradually or immediately. For ease of language, *antislavery* and *abolitionist* are used interchangeably in the text.

2. Letter from Granville Sharp to William Baker about the *Zong* incident, May 23, 1783, D3549 13/1/B1, British National Archives, Gloucestershire, England.

3. Steven M. Wise, *Though the Heavens May Fall: The Landmark Trial That Led to the End of Human Slavery* (Cambridge, Mass.: Da Capo, 2005).

4. Jerome Nadelhaft, "The Somersett Case and Slavery: Myth, Reality, and Repercussions," *Journal of Negro History* 51, no. 3 (July 1966): 193–208; Mark S. Weiner, "New Biographical Evidence on Somerset's Case," *Slavery and Abolition* 23, no. 1 (April 2002): 121–36.

5. Statistics about the slave trade are available at the Trans-Atlantic Slave Trade Database, www.slavevoyages.org. For spectacular maps of the slave trade, see David Eltis and David Richardson, *Atlas of the Transatlantic Slave Trade* (New Haven: Yale University Press, 2010).

6. On the British abolitionist movement, see the excellent account by Adam Hochschild, *Bury the Chains: Prophets and Rebels in the Fight to Free an Empire's Slaves* (New York: Mariner, 2006); and Linda Colley, *Britons: Forging the Nation, 1707–1837*, rev. ed. (New Haven: Yale University Press, 2009), 250–56.

7. Hochschild, *Bury the Chains*.

8. Colley, *Britons*, 365–70; C. A. Bayly, *The Birth of the Modern World, 1780–1914: Global Connections and Comparisons* (Malden, Mass.: Blackwell, 2004), 186–88.

9. All three men appear in criminal cases in the *Proceedings of the Old Bailey, 1674–1913*, at www.oldbaileyonline.org (cited hereafter as *Old Bailey*): Frasier t17891028-35; Griffiths t17840915-73; and Blake t17880402-51. The comment by Johnson is from James Boswell, *The Life of Samuel Johnson, LLD* (London: Routledge, 1865), 1:199. On debtors going to Bolama, see C. B. Wadstrom, *An Essay on Colonization, Particularly Applied to the Western Coast of Africa, with Some Free Thoughts on Cultivation and Commerce; Also Brief Descriptions of the Colonies Already Formed, or Attempted, in Africa, Including Those of Sierra Leona and Bulama* (London: Darton and Harvey, 1794; repr. New York: Kelley, 1968), 235.

10. For an account of British criminals transported to West Africa, see Emma Christopher, *A Merciless Place: The Fate of Britain's Convicts After the American Revolution* (Oxford: Oxford University Press, 2010), 82.

11. The classic history of workers in early factories is Edward P. Thompson, *The Making of the English Working Class* (New York: Vintage, 1966).

12. Bell appears in numerous court cases during the 1780s at the *Old Bailey*, including t17860426-16, t17860222-87, t17860222-19, and t17861025-18.

13. Quotes from the trial of Bates in *Old Bailey,* t17851214-86; Wadstrom, *Essay on Colonization,* 228.

14. An outstanding account of escaped slaves where the scholar dug deeply into the historical record to find the runaways is Cassandra Pybus's *Epic Journeys of Freedom: Runaway Slaves of the American Revolution and Their Global Quest for Liberty* (Boston: Beacon, 2007). See also Monday B. Abasiattai, "The Search for Independence: New World Blacks in Sierra Leone and Liberia, 1787–1847," *Journal of Black Studies* 23, no. 1 (September 1992): 107–16. On the Loyalists, see Ellen Gibson Willson, *The Loyal Blacks* (New York: Capricorn, 1976); Maya Jasanoff, *Liberty's Exiles: American Loyalists in the Revolutionary World* (New York: Knopf, 2011).

15. Susan E. Klepp, *Revolutionary Conceptions: Women, Fertility, and Family Limitation in America, 1760–1820* (Chapel Hill: University of North Carolina Press, 2009).

16. Information about Ann and Aaron Baker is in Wadstrom, *Essay on Colonization,* 174; and in *Old Bailey,* t17870110-31, t17940604-19, and t17911207-38.

17. Philip Beaver, *African Memoranda: Relative to an Attempt to Establish a British Settlement on the Island of Bulama, on the Western Coast of Africa, in the Year 1792 . . . and the Introduction of Letters and Religion to Its Inhabitants but More Particularly as the Means of Gradually Abolishing African Slavery* (London: Baldwin, 1805; repr. Westport, Conn.: Negro Universities Press, 1970), 446.

18. Ibid., 443, 470–71; information about Bates is in *Old Bailey,* t17920215-31 and s17920215-1.

19. Beaver, *African Memoranda,* 16, 19, 20, 205, 441.

20. Ibid., 449.

21. Scholars have long debated the complex motivations of the antislavery and abolitionist movement of the late eighteenth century. See, for example, Eric Williams, *Capitalism and Slavery* (1944; Chapel Hill: University of North Carolina Press, 1994); David Brion Davis, "Reflections on Abolitionism and Ideological Hegemony," *American Historical Review* 92, no. 4 (October 1987): 797–812; Davis, *The Problem of Slavery in the Age of Revolution, 1770–1823* (Ithaca: Cornell University Press, 1975); Davis, *Inhuman Bondage: The Rise and Fall of Slavery in the New World* (New York: Oxford University Press, 2006); Seymour Drescher, "Whose Abolition? Popular Pressure and the Ending of the British Slave Trade," *Past and Present* 143, no. 1 (1994): 136–66; Drescher, *Mighty Experiment: Free Labor Versus Slavery in British Emancipation* (New York: Oxford University Press, 2002); Michael J. Turner, "The Limits of Abolition: Government, Saints and the 'African Question,' c. 1780–1820," *English Historical Review* 112, no. 447 (April 1997): 319–57; Steven A. Diouf, ed., *Fighting the Slave Trade* (Athens: Ohio University Press, 2003); Philip D. Curtin, *The Image of Africa: British Ideas and Action, 1780–1850* (Madison: University of Wisconsin Press, 1964); Deirdre Coleman, *Romantic Colonization and British Anti-Slavery* (Cambridge: Cambridge University Press, 2005); Christopher Leslie Brown, *Moral Capital: Foundations of British Abolitionism* (Chapel Hill: University of North Carolina Press, 2007).

22. Quotations from this and the following paragraphs are from Dalrymple's testimony, *Abridgment of the Minutes of Evidence, Taken Before a Committee of the Whole House,*

to Whom It Was Referred to Consider of the Slave-Trade, vol. 3 (London, 1790), 291–325. The questions posed by the parliamentary examiners are in *Questions to Be Proposed to Such Gentlemen as Have Been Resident on the Coast of Africa . . .* (London, 1788). On Dalrymple, also see Curtin, *Image of Africa,* 106–7; Simon Shoma, *Rough Crossings: The Slaves, the British, and the American Revolution* (New York: Harper Collins, 2007), 297; and Coleman, *Romantic Colonization,* 81–89.

23. Dalrymple testimony, *Abridgment of the Minutes of the Evidence . . . ,* 118.

24. Ibid., 119–21.

25. For a firsthand account of the terrors of slave life in the West Indies, see Angelo Costanzo, ed., *The Interesting Narrative of the Life of Olaudah Equiano* (New York: Broadview, 2001), 120–28. On slavery in the British Caribbean, see, for example, Richard S. Dunn, *Sugar and Slaves: The Rise of the Planter Class in the English West Indies, 1624–1713* (1972; Chapel Hill: University of North Carolina Press, 2000).

26. Dalrymple, *Abridgment of the Minutes of the Evidence . . . ,* 119.

27. Wadstrom, *Essay on Colonization,* 3.

28. The opposition to a military colony by black Londoners is noted in Committee Minutes of the Black Poor in London, August 4, 1786, T 1/634, British National Archives, Kew, England. See also A. P. Kup, "John Clarkson and the Sierra Leone Company," *International Journal of African Historical Studies* 5, no. 2 (1972): 203–20; Coleman, *Romantic Colonization;* Stephen J. Braidwood, *Black Poor and White Philanthropists: London's Blacks and the Foundation of the Sierra Leone Settlement, 1786–1791* (Liverpool: Liverpool University Press, 1994).

29. Details about the Old Slaughter's Coffeehouse are from D. G. C. Allan, "Shipley, William," *Oxford Dictionary of National Biography,* available at http://www.oxforddnb .com/view/article/25412. Quotation from Bolama's constitution, Colonial Office Series, 267/9, British National Archives, Kew.

30. Details about Philip Beaver's life in this and the next few paragraphs are from William Henry Smyth, *The Life and Services of Captain Philip Beaver* (London: John Murray, 1829); "Biographical Memoir of Philip Beaver, Esquire," *Belfast Monthly Magazine,* February 28, 1814, 117–28.

31. "Biographical Memoir of Philip Beaver," 118; on Montesquieu, see Davis, *Inhuman Bondage,* 74–75.

32. Beaver, *African Memoranda,* xiii.

33. Todd M. Endelman, "The Checkered Career of 'Jew' King: A Study in Anglo-Jewish Social History," *Association of Jewish Studies* 7 (1982–1983): 69–100; Todd M. Endelman, "King, John," *Oxford Dictionary of National Biography,* available at http:// www.oup.com/oxforddnb/info/online/.

34. Maud Maxwell Vesey, "Benjamin Marston, Loyalist," *New England Quarterly* 15, no. 4 (December 1942): 622–51; Violet Mary-Ann Showers, "The Price of Loyalty: The Case of Benjamin Marston" (master's thesis, University of New Brunswick, 1982); Benjamin Marston Diary, http://www.lib.unb.ca/Texts/marston/index.html.

35. James Stark, *Loyalists of Massachusetts, and the Other Side of the American Revolution* (Boston: W. B. Clark, 1910), 222.

36. Beaver, *African Memoranda,* 115.

37. Marston to Elizabeth Watson, London, March 9, 1792, Benjamin Marston Diary.

38. Ibid.

39. Ibid.

40. Ibid.

41. Information about Le Mesurier is from "Le Mesurier, Paul," *Oxford Dictionary of National Biography;* Obituary, *Gentlemen's Monthly Magazine* (London), 1806, 571–73; Coleman, *Romantic Colonization,* 82. On criminals, see Gwenda Morgan and Peter Rushton, eds., *Eighteenth-Century Criminal Transportation* (Houndmills, U.K.: Palgrave Macmillan, 2004). Also see the criminal cases at *Old Bailey.*

42. Equiano's *Interesting Narrative* (London, 1789) was reprinted several times before the *Hankey* set sail; see also Vincent Carretta, *Equiano, the African: Biography of a Self-Made Man* (Athens: University of Georgia Press, 2005).

43. Le Mesurier's bond is in the Records of the Colonial Office, 267/9, British National Archives, Kew.

44. Gary B. Nash and Jean R. Soderlund, *Freedom by Degrees: Emancipation in Pennsylvania and Its Aftermath* (New York: Oxford University Press, 1991); Gary B. Nash, *The Unknown American Revolution: The Unruly Birth of Democracy and the Struggle to Create America* (New York: Penguin, 2006).

45. Laurent Dubois, *Avengers of the New World: The Story of the Haitian Revolution* (Cambridge, Mass.: Belknap, 2004).

46. Quotations from the London Corresponding Society appeared in the *London Chronicle,* November 12, 1792.

47. Robert M. Maniquis, "Filling up and Emptying out the Sublime: Terror in British Radical Culture," *Huntington Library Quarterly* 63, no. 3 (2000): 369–405; Clive Emsley, "The London 'Insurrection' of December 1792: Fact, Fiction, or Fantasy?" *Journal of British Studies* 17, no. 2 (Spring 1978): 66–86; Emsley, "Repression, 'Terror' and the Rule of Law in England During the Decade of the French Revolution," *English Historical Review* 100, no. 397 (October, 1985): 801–25.

48. On the desire by many Britons to extend their ideas of liberty abroad, see Jasanoff, *Liberty's Exiles,* and Ralph A. Austen and Woodruff D. Smith, "Images of Africa and British Slave-Trade Abolition: The Transition to an Imperialist Ideology, 1787–1807," *African Historical Studies* 2, no. 1 (1969): 69–83.

Chapter 3: West Africa

1. Joshua Montefiore, who sailed to Bolama on the *Calypso,* wrote the most detailed account of its voyage to and arrival in Africa in *An Authentic Account of the Expedition to Bulam, on the Coast of Africa, and the Settlement of Sierra Leone* (London: J. Johnson, 1794). This chapter also relies on Philip Beaver, *African Memoranda: Relative to an Attempt to Establish a British Settlement on the Island of Bulama, on the Western Coast of Africa, in the Year 1792 . . . and the Introduction of Letters and Religion to Its Inhabitants but More Particularly as the Means of Gradually Abolishing African Slavery* (London: Baldwin, 1805; repr. Westport, Conn.: Negro Universities Press, 1970); and C. B. Wadstrom, *An Essay on*

Colonization, Particularly Applied to the Western Coast of Africa, with Some Free Thoughts on Cultivation and Commerce; Also Brief Descriptions of the Colonies Already Formed, or Attempted, in Africa, Including Those of Sierra Leona and Bulama (London: Darton and Harvey, 1794; repr. New York: Kelley, 1968).

2. On Dalrymple, see Deirdre Coleman, *Romantic Colonization and British Anti-Slavery* (Cambridge: Cambridge University Press, 2005), 81–89; and Ellen Gibson Wilson, *The Loyal Blacks* (New York: Putnam, 1976), 191–93. Dalrymple's lengthy testimony about slavery and the slave trade before the House of Commons is also revealing about his own life. See *Abridgment of the Minutes of the Evidence, Taken Before a Committee of the Whole House, to Whom It Was Referred to Consider of the Slave-Trade,* vol. 3 (London, 1790), 116–29; and Thomas Clarkson, *The History of the Rise, Progress and Accomplishment of the Abolition of the African Slave Trade by the British Parliament* (London: Longman, 1808).

3. Abdoulaye Camara and Joseph Roger de Benoïst, *Histoire de Gorée* (Paris: Maisonneuve et Larose, 2003).

4. Walter Rodney, *A History of the Upper Guinea Coast, 1545 to 1800* (New York: Monthly Review Press, 1970).

5. Quotations in this and the following paragraph are from Montefiore, *Account of the Expedition to Bulam,* 9–10.

6. There are multiple problems involved in determining how to call ethnic and national groups by names of their own choosing. Over the past six centuries, the Britons and Americans used various terms to identify indigenous peoples in Africa. During the eighteenth century, at the time of the sailing of the *Hankey,* the names were wildly inconsistent and sometimes simply made up. The common pejorative connotations of the labels served, in part, as a linguistic method to enable Britons and Americans to separate themselves from Africans, supposedly inferior peoples. This book attempts to treat categories of Africans, like Bijago, with similar linguistic imprecision shared by terms like Americans or Britons, using the article "the" before the names whenever appropriate. Arthur Hawthorne discusses the complexity of these naming issues in *From Africa to Brazil: Culture, Identity, and an Atlantic Slave Trade, 1600–1830* (Cambridge: Cambridge University Press, 2010), 6–20.

7. Beaver notes the oversights in equipment in a letter in the Records of the Colonial Office, 267/10, British National Archives, Kew, England. See also Wadstrom, *Essay on Colonization,* 306.

8. Beaver, *African Memoranda,* 48.

9. Montefiore, *Account of the Expedition to Bulam;* Beaver, *African Memoranda;* and Wadstrom, *Essay on Colonization* all contain information about Canabacs and the Bijago. The accounts require reading with a critical eye because of the biases of their authors. Modern scholars who discuss Canabacs include Philip D. Curtin, *The Image of Africa: British Ideas and Action, 1780–1850* (Madison: University of Wisconsin Press, 1973); Boubacar Barry, *Senegambia and the Atlantic Slave Trade* (Cambridge: Cambridge University Press, 2002); Rodney, *History of the Upper Guinea Coast;* and Christine Henry, *Les îles où dansent les enfants défunts: age, sexe et pouvoir chez les Bijago de Guinée-Bissau* (Paris: CNRS Editions, 1994).

10. Montefiore, *Account of the Expedition to Bulam,* 11–12.

11. Ibid., 14–15.

12. Beaver, *African Memoranda,* 198, 356. Andrew Spielman and Michael D'Antonio, *Mosquito: A Natural History of Our Most Persistent and Deadly Foe* (New York: Hyperion, 2001); Christopher Wills, *Yellow Fever—Black Goddess: The Coevolution of People and Plagues* (Reading, Pa.: Addison-Wesley, 1996).

13. Montefiore, *Account of the Expedition to Bulam,* 15–16.

14. One example of many mistaken contemporary rumors about Bijagos being cannibals is in Elihu Hubbard Smith, "On the Origin of the Pestilential Fever, Which Prevailed in the Island of Grenada, in the Years 1793 and 1794," *Medical Repository* 1, no. 4 (1798): 472.

15. Montefiore, *Account of the Expedition to Bulam,* 25.

16. Beaver, *African Memoranda,* 55.

17. Ibid., 54.

Chapter 4: Cross-Cultural Negotiations

1. Joseph E. Harris, *Africans and Their History,* 2nd rev. ed. (New York: Plume, 1998); Kevin Shillington, *History of Africa,* rev. 2nd ed. (Houndmills, U.K.: Palgrave Macmillan, 2005).

2. This and the next paragraph draw on Paul E. Lovejoy, *Transformations in Slavery: A History of Slavery in Africa* (New York: Cambridge University Press, 2000); John Thornton, *Africa and Africans in the Making of the Atlantic World, 1400–1800* (Cambridge: Cambridge University Press, 1998).

3. David Eltis and David Richardson, *Atlas of the Transatlantic Slave Trade* (New Haven: Yale University Press, 2010), 90–97; David Eltis, Trans-Atlantic Slave Trade Database, http://www.slavevoyages.org/tast/assessment/estimates.faces.

4. Sylvain Meinrad Xavier de Golbéry, *Travels in Africa Performed During the Years 1785, 1786, and 1787 . . . ,* trans. Francis Blagdon (London: Ridgway, 1802), 1:183; Philip Beaver, *African Memoranda: Relative to an Attempt to Establish a British Settlement on the Island of Bulama, on the Western Coast of Africa, in the Year 1792 . . . and the Introduction of Letters and Religion to Its Inhabitants but More Particularly as the Means of Gradually Abolishing African Slavery* (London: Baldwin, 1805; repr. Westport, Conn.: Negro Universities Press, 1970), 320–22.

5. Walter Hawthorne, *Planting Rice and Harvesting Slaves: Transformations Along the Guinea-Bissau Coast, 1400–1900* (Portsmouth, N.H.: Heinemann, 2003); Peter Mark, *"Portuguese" Style and Luso-African Identity: Precolonial Senegambia, Sixteenth–Nineteenth Centuries* (Bloomington: Indiana University Press, 2003); Roberto Nodal, "Black Presence in the Canary Islands (Spain)," *Journal of Black Studies* 12, no. 1 (September 1981): 83–90. Scholars have proposed calling the group of mixed ancestry by various names, including "Eurafricans" and "Luso-Africans," though I do not do so here.

6. K. David Patterson, "Epidemics, Famines, and Population in the Cape Verde Islands, 1580–1900," *International Journal of African Historical Studies* 21, no. 2 (1988): 291–313.

7. Philip D. Curtin, *Economic Change in Precolonial Africa: Senegambia in the Era of Slave Trade* (Madison: University of Wisconsin Press, 1975); Arthur Hawthorne, *From Africa to Brazil: Culture, Identity, and an Atlantic Slave Trade, 1600–1830* (Cambridge: Cambridge University Press, 2010), 93–95.

8. P. E. H. Hair, "'Elephants for Want of Towns': The Interethnic and International History of Bulama Island, 1456–1870," *History in Africa* 24 (1997): 177–93.

9. For firsthand accounts of the militarization of the West African coast, see Thomas Winterbottom, *An Account of the Native Africans in the Neighbourhood of Sierra Leone* (London: C. Whittingham, 1803), 159–60; and Angelo Costanzo, ed., *The Interesting Narrative of the Life of Olaudah Equiano* (New York: Broadview, 2001).

10. Beaver, *African Memoranda,* 335.

11. On the impressive size of the Bijago canoes, see Randy J. Sparks, *The Two Prices of Calabar: An Eighteenth-Century Atlantic Odyssey* (Cambridge: Harvard University Press, 2004), 49.

12. Hawthorne, *From Africa to Brazil,* 93–95. Beaver initially believed that the island had never been inhabited; see *African Memoranda,* 66.

13. Winterbottom, *An Account of the Native Africans,* 174–75.

14. Beaver, *African Memoranda,* 296–97.

15. Joseph Corry, *Observations upon the Windward Coast of Africa . . . 1805 and 1806* (London: G. and W. Nicol, 1807), 56.

16. Ibid.

17. Emma Christopher, *A Merciless Place: The Fate of Britain's Convicts After the American Revolution* (Oxford: Oxford University Press, 2010), 180–83.

18. Alexander Falconbridge noted how speedily information of a slave ship's arrival spread along this part of the African coast and how, in response, Africans would raise the prices of their slaves; *An Account of the Slave Trade on the Coast of Africa* (London: Phillips, 1788), 17–18.

19. Beaver, *African Memoranda,* 56–57.

20. Ibid., 56. The Iroquois in North America, for example, were masters at the strategy of pitting the French against the British; see Daniel Richter, *Facing East from Indian Country: A Native History of North America* (Cambridge: Harvard University Press, 2003).

21. Beaver, *African Memoranda,* 57.

22. The English word "grumetta" is derived from the word *grumete* from the Portuguese/Creole language popular among this Guinea-Bissau part of the African coast. Beaver understood a grumetta to be "the meanest sort of sailor," probably unskilled, perhaps like a cabin boy. Among coastal peoples and European traders, the meaning was expanded to include all "natives who trade for [are paid by] Europeans in canoes, but [it] is generally applicable to all those who labor for others for wages" (*African Memoranda,* 143, 322). Simply put, most grumettas were working people, hired temporarily, not unlike many of the colonists who had migrated to Bolama. A ship captain defined the term as "free black people"; Corry, *Windward Coast of Africa,* 4.

23. Beaver, *African Memoranda,* 58.

24. Ibid., 61.

25. Ibid., 61; Joshua Montefiore, *Account of the Expedition to Bulam, on the Coast of Africa, and the Settlement of Sierra Leone* (London: J. Johnson, 1794), 32.

26. Beaver, *African Memoranda,* 71–73.

27. Ibid., 62.

28. On the early Bijago, see Boubacar Barry, *Senegambia and the Atlantic Slave Trade* (Cambridge: Cambridge University Press, 2002), 42–43, 65, 117; Walter Rodney, *History of the Upper Guinea Coast, 1545 to 1800* (New York: Monthly Review Press, 1970), 110; Rodney, "Upper Guinea and the Significance of the Origins of Africans Enslaved in the New World," *Journal of Negro History* 54, no. 4 (October 1969): 327–45; and Hawthorne, *Planting Rice and Harvesting Slaves.*

29. Beaver, *African Memoranda,* 336.

30. This and the quotations in the following three pages are from Beaver, *African Memoranda,* 64–70, 337–38.

31. Ibid., 70; another European, quoted in C. B. Wadstrom, *An Essay on Colonization, Particularly Applied to the Western Coast of Africa, with Some Free Thoughts on Cultivation and Commerce; Also Brief Descriptions of the Colonies Already Formed, or Attempted, in Africa, Including Those of Sierra Leona and Bulama* (London: Darton and Harvey, 1794; repr. New York: Kelley, 1968), 243; also see John Leyden, *A Historical & Philosophical Sketch of the Discovers & Settlements of the Europeans . . .* (Edinburgh: J. Moir, 1799), 243.

32. Christine Henry, *Les îles où dansent les enfants défunts: age, sexe et pouvoir chez les Bijago de Guinée-Bissau* (Paris: CNRS Editions, 1994); Christine Henry, "Grandeur et decadence des Marins Bijogo," *Cahiers d'études africaines* 29, no. 114 (1989): 193–207. On rice growing in the Americas, see Judith A. Carney, *Black Rice: The African Origins of Rice Cultivation in the Americas* (Cambridge: Harvard University Press, 2002); and the review of Carney's book by Philip D. Morgan, "Carolina Rice: African Origins, New World Crop," *William and Mary Quarterly,* 3rd ser., 59 (July 2002): 739–42.

33. On Native Americans, see Richter, *Facing East.* Gender among West Africans is noted, for example, in the testimony of James Frazer (ship captain) in *Abridgment of the Minutes of the Evidence, Taken Before a Committee of the Whole House, to Whom It Was Referred to Consider of the Slave-Trade,* vol. 3 (London, 1790), 225. See also Winterbottom, *An Account of the Native Africans,* 159–60.

34. Winthrop D. Jordan, *White over Black: American Attitudes Toward the Negro, 1550–1812* (Chapel Hill: University of North Carolina Press, 1968); Dorothy Hammond and Alta Jablow, *The Africa That Never Was: Four Centuries of British Writing About Africa* (Prospect Heights, Ill.: Waveland, 1992), esp. 22–23.

35. Beaver, *African Memoranda,* 68–70.

36. Ibid., 327, 339. Crafting his tale as an adventure story, Beaver wrote his book not only to support the antislave-trade cause but also to appeal to a British public eager for tales of African exploration, like the account of the Scottish traveler Mungo Park, *Travels in the Interior Districts of Africa* (London: Bulmer, 1799).

37. Beaver, *African Memoranda,* 338.

38. Ibid., 72–73. The 473 bars of goods equaled approximately 79 British pounds, according to Beaver. This was about twice the annual salary of a sailor or day laborer in

Philadelphia or London at the time; see Billy G. Smith, *The "Lower Sort": Philadelphia's Laboring People, 1750–1800* (Ithaca: Cornell University Press, 1990), 233.

39. Knox testimony (ship captain), in *Abridgment of the Minutes of the Evidence . . .* , 23.

40. Beaver, *African Memoranda,* 72.

41. Ibid., 74.

42. Ibid., 75–76.

43. Ibid., 75–83.

44. Two of the many reports of cannibalism in this part of Africa are Colin Chisholm, "An History of the Rise and Progress of the Malignant Pestilential Fever," *Newburyport* (Massachusetts) *Herald,* June 14, 1799; and "Extract of a Letter from a Gentleman on Board the Ship *Boris,* Capt. Mount, Africa," *Gazette of the United States* (Philadelphia), August 8, 1800; both are available at the Philadelphia Free Library.

45. Beaver, *African Memoranda,* 79.

46. Ibid., 82.

47. P. E. H. Hair, "Africanism: The Freetown Contribution," *Journal of Modern African Studies* 5, no. 4 (December 1967): 521–39; Jean Baptiste Léonard Durand, *Voyage to Senegal* (London, 1806), 83–86.

48. "The Calypso arrived at London on the 14th of November, 1792, with between eighty and ninety colonists"; Elihu Hubbard Smith, "On the Origin of the Pestilential Fever, Which Prevailed in the Island of Grenada, in the Years 1793 and 1794," *Medical Repository* 1, no. 4 (1798): 496. The *Calypso* appears as a slave ship in 1797 in the Trans-Atlantic Slave Trade Database, http://www.slavevoyages.org/tast/database /search.faces.

Chapter 5: Death in Bolama

1. On John Smith and the Jamestown colony, see Karen Ordahl Kupperman, *The Jamestown Project* (Cambridge: Harvard University Press, 2007).

2. Philip Beaver, *African Memoranda: Relative to an Attempt to Establish a British Settlement on the Island of Bulama, on the Western Coast of Africa, in the Year 1792 . . . and the Introduction of Letters and Religion to Its Inhabitants but More Particularly as the Means of Gradually Abolishing African Slavery* (London: Baldwin, 1805; repr. Westport, Conn.: Negro Universities Press, 1970), 80, 82.

3. Ibid., 90–91.

4. Ibid., 91–93.

5. Ibid., 91–93, 110.

6. Ibid., 96–97. On the Biafada, see Joshua B. Forrest, *Lineages of State Fragility: Rural Civil Society in Guinea-Bissau* (Athens: Ohio University Press, 2003); P. E. H. Hair, "Ethnolinguistic Continuity on the Guinea Coast," *Journal of African History* 8, no. 2 (1967): 247–68.

7. Beaver, *African Memoranda,* 99.

8. Ibid., 101, 103. The Biafada had a long and contentious history with Canabacs, since the latter had often attacked them and sold prisoners as slaves; see Boubacar Barry,

Senegambia and the Atlantic Slave Trade (Cambridge: Cambridge University Press, 2002), 42–43.

9. Beaver, *African Memoranda,* 104–5, 108.

10. Ibid., 106, 108. On the sophistication of African traders and their ability to control much of the trade with Europeans, see Arthur Hawthorne, *From Africa to Brazil: Culture, Identity, and an Atlantic Slave Trade, 1600–1830* (Cambridge: Cambridge University Press, 2010); and John Thornton, *Africa and Africans in the Making of the Atlantic World, 1400–1800* (Cambridge: Cambridge University Press, 1998). Also see comments by Dr. Thomas Winterbottom in *An Account of the Native Africans in the Neighbourhood of Sierra Leone* (London: C. Whittingham, 1803), 172–73; and by Captain Joseph Corry in *Observations upon the Windward Coast of Africa . . . 1805 and 1806* (London: G. and W. Nicol, 1807), 56.

11. Beaver, *African Memoranda,* 111–12.

12. Ibid., 112.

13. Information for this and the following paragraph, ibid., 113–14, 217, 234.

14. Joshua Montefiore, *An Account of the Expedition to Bulam, on the Coast of Africa, and the Settlement of Sierra Leone* (London: J. Johnson, 1794), 25.

15. Beaver, *African Memoranda,* 114.

16. Ibid., 115.

17. Ibid., 79.

18. Ibid., 117, 120.

19. Ibid., 120.

20. Ibid., 121–22.

21. Ibid., 131.

22. On the process whereby mosquitoes become infectious and, in turn, pass fevers to humans, see Andrew Spielman and Michael D'Antonio, *Mosquito: A Natural History of Our Most Persistent and Deadly Foe* (New York: Hyperion, 2001); and J. R. McNeill, *Mosquito Empires: Ecology and War in the Greater Caribbean, 1620–1914* (Cambridge: Cambridge University Press, 2010).

23. Spielman and D'Antonio, *Mosquito;* Christopher Wills, *Yellow Fever—Black Goddess: The Coevolution of People and Plagues* (Reading, Pa.: Addison-Wesley, 1996); James C. Riley, "Mortality on Long-Distance Voyages in the Eighteenth Century," *Journal of Economic History* 41, no. 3 (September 1981): 651–56; Donald B. Cooper and Kenneth F. Kiple, "Yellow Fever," in *Cambridge Historical Dictionary of Disease,* ed. Kenneth F. Kiple (Cambridge: Cambridge University Press, 1993), 365–69.

24. On the technicalities of the yellow fever virus and how it spreads among monkeys and humans via a mosquito vector, see the reports of the World Health Organization, http://www.who.int/csr/disease/yellowfev/en/, and the Centers for Disease Control, http://www.cdc.gov/ncidod/dvbid/yellowfever/ (accessed July 2, 2011). For more on *Aëdes aegypti* and its role in spreading the eighteenth-century pandemic, see Chapter 7, below.

25. Godwin R. A. Okogun, Bethran E. B. Nwoke, Anthony N. Okere, Jude C. Anosike, and Anegbe C. Esekhegbe, "Epidemiological Implications of Preferences of Breeding Sites of Mosquito Species in Midwestern Nigeria," *Annals of Agricultural and*

Environmental Medicine 10 (2003): 217–22. Various theories about the source of the HIV virus in humans are discussed in Jacques Pepin, *The Origins of AIDS* (Cambridge: Cambridge University Press, 2011).

26. Beaver, *African Memoranda*, 125.

27. Ibid., 126.

28. Ibid.

29. Ibid., 127.

30. Ibid.

31. Ibid., 132; Kupperman, *The Jamestown Project*.

32. Beaver, *African Memoranda*, 134–35.

33. *Proceedings of the Old Bailey, 1674–1913,* at www.oldbaileyonline.org, March 29, 1792, John Rowe, t17920329-15.

34. Beaver, *African Memoranda*, 136.

35. Ibid., 141.

36. Ibid.

37. Ibid., 144–45.

38. Ibid., 146, vii.

39. Quoted ibid., 148–49.

40. Ibid., 149.

41. Ibid., 175.

42. Montefiore, *Account of the Expedition to Bulam*, 35.

43. Beaver, *African Memoranda*, 150–53.

44. Ibid., 153–55.

45. Ibid., 155.

46. Ibid., 78.

47. Ibid., 163.

Chapter 6: Grumettas and the Final Days of the "Canabacs' Chickens"

1. The material concerning the end of the colony in this chapter depends primarily on the accounts by Philip Beaver, *African Memoranda: Relative to an Attempt to Establish a British Settlement on the Island of Bulama, on the Western Coast of Africa, in the Year 1792 . . . and the Introduction of Letters and Religion to Its Inhabitants but More Particularly as the Means of Gradually Abolishing African Slavery* (London: Baldwin, 1805; repr. Westport, Conn.: Negro Universities Press, 1970), 45–411; and C. B. Wadstrom, *An Essay on Colonization, Particularly Applied to the Western Coast of Africa, with Some Free Thoughts on Cultivation and Commerce; Also Brief Descriptions of the Colonies Already Formed, or Attempted, in Africa, Including Those of Sierra Leona and Bulama* (London: Darton and Harvey, 1794; repr. New York: Kelley, 1968).

2. Information about James Watson is from Beaver, *African Memoranda*, 194, 237, 264, 269, 274, 282, 448.

3. David Dabydeen, John Gilmore, and Cecily Jones, eds., *The Oxford Companion to Black British History* (New York: Oxford University Press, 2010).

4. Gretchen Gerzina, *Black London: Life Before Emancipation* (New Brunswick, N.J.: Rutgers University Press, 1995), 3–8.

5. Beaver, *African Memoranda,* 164–65, 229–30, 250, 261–62, 279–80, 445, 450.

6. Marcus Rediker, *Between the Devil and the Deep Blue Sea: Merchant Seamen, Pirates, and the Anglo-American Maritime World, 1700–1750* (Cambridge: Cambridge University Press, 1989).

7. James Johnson's story is pieced together from information in Beaver, *African Memoranda,* 162–78, 193–95, 213–15, 229–30, 240, 279–81, 490; and Committee Minutes of the Black Poor in London, August 4, 1786, T 1/634, British National Archives, Kew, England.

8. See John N. Grant, "Black Immigrants into Nova Scotia, 1776–1815," *Journal of Negro History* 58, no. 3 (July 1973): 253–70; Mary Beth Norton, "The Fate of Some Black Loyalists of the American Revolution," *Journal of Negro History* 58, no. 4 (October 1973): 402–26; Neil Mackinnon, *This Unfriendly Soil: The Loyalist Experience in Nova Scotia, 1783–1791* (Kingston, Ont.: McGill-Queen's University Press, 1986).

9. On this enterprise, see the letter from Granville Sharp to Thomas Clark, October 13, 1788, CN 147, the Huntington Library, San Marino, California. Also see the following accounts: Christopher Fyfe, *A Short History of Sierra Leone* (London: Longmans, 1962); Fyfe, "1787–1887–1987: Reflections on a Sierra Leone Bicentenary," *Africa: Journal of the International African Institute* 57, no. 4 (1987): 411–21; Fyfe, "Thomas Peters: History and Legend," *Sierra Leone Studies* 1 (1953): 4–13; Deidre Coleman, *Romantic Colonization and British Anti-Slavery* (Cambridge: Cambridge University Press, 2005); Coleman, "Bulama and Sierra Leone: Utopian Islands and Visionary Interiors," in *Islands in History and Representations,* ed. Rod Edmond and Vanessa Smith (London: Routledge, 2003), 63–80.

10. Johnson appears in the Committee Minutes of the Black Poor in London, August 4, 1786, T 1/634, while Equiano's complaints about corruption are in T 1/643, no. 681, f. 87, British National Archives, Kew. Granville Sharp's comments on black migrants and the difficulties of the voyage can be found in his letter to Thomas Clark, CN 147, the Huntington Library, San Marino, California.

11. Johnson and Jones are recorded among the list of passengers for February 16, 1787, in Committee Minutes of the Black Poor in London, T 1/643, and in T 1/638, no. 249. See also Coleman, *Romantic Colonization;* Stephen J. Braidwood, *Black Poor and White Philanthropists: London's Blacks and the Foundation of the Sierra Leone Settlement, 1786–1791* (Liverpool: Liverpool University Press, 1994).

12. Ira Berlin, "From Creole to African: Atlantic Creoles and the Origins of African-American Society in Mainland North America," *William and Mary Quarterly,* 3rd ser., 53, no. 2 (April 1996): 251–88; Berlin, *Generations of Captivity: A History of African-American Slaves* (Cambridge, Mass.: Belknap Press, 2003), 23–25; Simon Schama, *Rough Crossings: Britain, the Slaves and the American Revolution* (New York: Harper Collins, 2006).

13. Beaver, *African Memoranda,* 320. Beaver never learned any local languages.

14. Ibid., 299.

15. Ibid., 168–69.

16. Ibid., 189; Wadstrom, *Essay on Colonization,* 149–55.

17. Beaver, *African Memoranda,* 162, 203, 210, 216.

18. Ibid., 490–94.

19. Ibid., 237–39, 249, 251–56, 263, 266, 273, 492.

20. Ibid., 170–71.

21. Quoted in Wadstrom, *Essay on Colonization,* 304.

22. Beaver, *African Memoranda,* 311.

23. Ibid., 170–72.

24. Ibid., 177–78.

25. Arthur Hawthorne, *From Africa to Brazil: Culture, Identity, and an Atlantic Slave Trade, 1600–1830* (Cambridge: Cambridge University Press, 2010), 82–85.

26. Beaver, *African Memoranda,* 395.

27. The conversation in this and the following paragraph is recorded ibid., 178–79.

28. Bellchore echoed the refrain, supposedly saying that "all white man witch"; Beaver, *African Memoranda,* 207. See also Hawthorne, *From Africa to Brazil,* 82–88.

29. Beaver, *African Memoranda,* 198; Wadstrom, *Essay on Colonization,* 302.

30. Beaver, *African Memoranda,* 182.

31. Ibid., 200.

32. Quoted ibid. The material in the next few paragraphs is from Beaver, *African Memoranda,* 194–96, 279–81, 296; Wadstrom, *Essay on Colonization,* 155–57.

33. The *Nancy* is recorded in the Trans-Atlantic Slave Trade Database, www.slave-voyages.org.

34. Beaver, *African Memoranda,* 220–21. Some examples of the memory loss can be found on pages 258–59.

35. Ibid., 230, 490.

36. Ibid., 230.

37. Ibid., 241–42.

38. Ibid., 241.

39. Beaver, quoted in Wadstrom, *Essay on Colonization,* 305.

40. Ibid.

41. Ibid., 244–53, 493. Many grumettas gave "Lopez" as their last name.

42. Ibid., 244–50; Jill Lepore, *The Name of War: King Philip's War and the Origins of American Identity* (New York: Vintage, 1999).

43. Beaver, *African Memoranda,* 244.

44. Ibid., 253, 249. On the moral understanding and behavior of slaves in the United States, see Berlin, *Generations of Captivity,* chap. 4.

45. Ibid., 243.

46. Beaver, quoted in Wadstrom, *Essay on Colonization,* 304.

47. Beaver, *African Memoranda,* 254.

48. Ibid., 176, 255.

49. Ibid., 252–53.

50. Ibid., 261–63.

51. Ibid., 263.

52. Ibid., 265.

53. Ibid., 253, 264.

54. The account of the demise of the colony appears ibid., 268–79.

55. Ibid., 277.

56. Emma Christopher, *A Merciless Place: The Fate of Britain's Convicts After the American Revolution* (Oxford: Oxford University Press, 2010), 85–86; Philip D. Curtin, "The End of the White Man's Grave? Nineteenth-Century Mortality in West Africa," *Journal of Interdisciplinary History* 2, no. 1 (1990): 63–88. The Atlantic world has drawn a great deal of attention from historians during the past few decades. See, for example, Alison Games, *The Web of Empire: English Cosmopolitans in an Age of Expansion, 1560–1660* (New York: Oxford University Press, 2009); Douglas R. Egerton, Alison Games, Jane G. Landers, Kris Lane, and Donald R. Wright, *The Atlantic World: A History, 1400–1888* (New York: Wiley, 2007); Jack P. Greene and Philip D. Morgan, *Atlantic History: A Critical Appraisal* (New York: Oxford University Press, 2008); Simon P. Newman, *A New World of Labor: The Development of Plantation Slavery in the British Atlantic* (Philadelphia: University of Pennsylvania Press, 2013).

57. In this imperial spirit in the early nineteenth century, Captain W. H. Smyth wrote a hagiography of Beaver, *The Life and Services of Captain Philip Beaver* (London: John Murray, 1829). Also see "Biographical Memoir of Philip Beaver, Esquire," *Belfast Monthly Magazine*, February 28, 1814, 117–28; and John Stuart Mill, *The Autobiography of John Stuart Mill* (Sioux Falls, S.D.: NuVision Publications, 2007).

58. Beaver, *African Memoranda*, 203, 210, 216.

Chapter 7: Yellow Jack Comes to the Caribbean

1. My reconstruction in the next few pages of the *Hankey*'s voyage from Africa to the West Indies is based on C. B. Wadstrom, *An Essay on Colonization, Particularly Applied to the Western Coast of Africa, with Some Free Thoughts on Cultivation and Commerce; Also Brief Descriptions of the Colonies Already Formed, or Attempted, in Africa, Including Those of Sierra Leona and Bulama* (London: Darton and Harvey, 1794; repr. New York: Kelley, 1968), 148–60; Elihu Hubbard Smith, "On the Origin of the Pestilential Fever, Which Prevailed in the Island of Grenada, in the Years 1793 and 1794," *Medical Repository* 1, no. 4 (1798): 472–80; "Extract from the Log of the *Hankey*," reproduced in Philip Beaver, *African Memoranda: Relative to an Attempt to Establish a British Settlement on the Island of Bulama, on the Western Coast of Africa, in the Year 1792 . . . and the Introduction of Letters and Religion to Its Inhabitants but More Particularly as the Means of Gradually Abolishing African Slavery* (London: Baldwin, 1805; repr. Westport, Conn.: Negro Universities Press, 1970), 192, 470–71; Colin Chisholm, *An Essay on the Malignant Pestilential Fever Introduced into the West Indian Islands from Boullam, on the Coast of Guinea, as It Appeared in 1793 and 1794* (London: J. Mawman, 1795); and several newspaper reports, including an account in the *Gazette of the United States* (Philadelphia), October 7, 1797.

2. Abdoulaye Camara and Joseph Roger de Benoïst, *Histoire de Gorée* (Paris: Maisonneuve et Larose, 2003).

3. Obituary of John Gandell, *European Magazine and London Review*, 1793, 25:85.

4. Charles Darwin, *The Voyage of the Beagle,* entry for January 17, 1832, available at http://www.thebeaglevoyage.com/1832/01/st-jago.html (accessed July 1, 2011).

5. The Bolama Association had asked the British navy to check on the colony, and the *Scorpion* visited the island for a few days in early January 1793. Captain Ferris informed Beaver that the association was sending out additional colonists and provisions, but they never sailed; see Beaver, *African Memoranda,* 184–89. Contemporaries debated the extent to which the *Charon* and the *Scorpion* suffered ill effects from their contact with the *Hankey.* For example, Colin Chisholm, M.D., surgeon to His Majesty's Ordnance in Grenada, was certain that the deaths occurred; see his *Essay on the Malignant Pestilential Fever.* Numerous reports confirm Chisholm's contentions, as reported in *Columbian Centinel,* June 6, 1799. However, Elihu Hubbard Smith claims that yellow fever was never passed to the *Charon* or the *Scorpion;* see "On the Origin of the Pestilential Fever." The preponderance of evidence supports Chisholm.

6. Perhaps the most famous ghost ship was the *Flying Dutchman,* whose tale first appeared in print in 1795, a few years after the voyage of the *Hankey.* A man-of-war from Holland, the ship became lost while trying to round the Cape of Good Hope against strong winds. By some accounts, a series of lurid murders left the *Dutchman* without a crew. Emitting an eerie glow of light, the phantom ship could never make port, doomed to sail forever. Any vessel encountering the *Dutchman* was destined for disaster, usually within the day. Although not directly connected with yellow fever, the tale of the *Flying Dutchman* was part of the lore that the plague generated. Seamen reported seeing this and other ghost ships well into the nineteenth century. George Barrington first recorded the *Flying Dutchman* myth in *Voyage to Botany Bay* (1795; Sydney: Sydney University Press, 2004), 30.

7. William H. McNeill, *Plagues and Peoples* (New York: Anchor, 1976), 222.

8. On the technicalities of yellow fever as well as the disease today, see "Yellow Fever," Media Centre fact sheet 100, January 2011, World Health Organization, at http://www.who.int/mediacentre/factsheets/fs100/en/ (accessed April 13, 2013); "What Is Yellow Fever? What Causes Yellow Fever," *Medical News Today,* December 17, 2009, at http://www.medicalnewstoday.com/articles/174372.php; Mayo Clinic Staff, "Yellow Fever: Causes," August 27, 2011, Mayo Clinic, at http://www.mayoclinic.com/health/yellow-fever/DS01011/DSECTION=causes.

9. Juliet E. Bryant, Edward C. Holmes, and Alan D. T. Barrett, "Out of Africa: A Molecular Perspective on the Introduction of Yellow Fever Virus into the Americas," *PLoS Pathogens* 3, no. 5 (May 2007), available at doi:10.1371/journal.ppat.0030075; Amadou A. Sall, Ousmane Faye, Mawlouth Diallo, Cadhla Firth, Andrew Kitchen, and Edward C. Holmes, "Yellow Fever Virus Exhibits Slower Evolutionary Dynamics than Dengue Virus," *Journal of Virology* 84, no. 2 (January 2010): 765–72.

10. On the transatlantic pandemic, see J. R. McNeill, *Mosquito Empires: Ecology and War in the Greater Caribbean, 1620–1914* (Cambridge: Cambridge University Press, 2010), 265–67.

11. On how altering the environment enhanced the spread of yellow fever, see ibid. On the different species of mosquitoes, see Christopher Wills, *Yellow Fever—Black Goddess: The Coevolution of People and Plagues* (Reading, Pa.: Addison-Wesley, 1996); Sir

Rickard Christophers, *Aëdes Aegypti (L.) The Yellow Fever Mosquito: Its Life History, Bionomics and Structure* (Cambridge: Cambridge University Press, 2009).

12. Information in this and the next paragraph from Christophers, *Aëdes Aegypti;* Wills, *Yellow Fever—Black Goddess.*

13. On the methods of obtaining water and transporting it on ships, see Edward Nathaniel Bancroft, M.D., *An Essay on the Disease Called Yellow Fever . . .* (London: T. Cadell and W. Davies, 1811), 206–7, 225–26; John Hunter, *Observations on the Diseases of the Army in Jamaica and on the Best Means of Preserving the Health of Europeans in the Climate,* 3rd ed. (London: T. Payne, 1808), 122–23; and the Knox testimony (ship captain) in *Abridgment of the Minutes of the Evidence, Taken Before a Committee of the Whole House, to Whom It Was Referred to Consider of the Slave-Trade,* vol. 3 (London, 1790), 22.

14. Michael H. Glantz, *Currents of Change: Impacts of El Niño and La Niña on Climate and Society,* 2nd ed. (Cambridge: Cambridge University Press, 2001), 187; Paul Reiter, "Climate Change and Mosquito-Borne Disease," *Environmental Health Perspectives* 109, no. 1 (March 2001): 141–61.

15. The computerized index of the London *Times* records the *Hankey* as having sailed to Grenada at least a dozen times in the 1780s and early 1790s.

16. Chisholm, *Essay on the Malignant Pestilential Fever.* Also see William Pym, *Observations upon the Bulam Fever, Which Has of Late Years Prevailed in the West Indies, on the Coast of America, at Gibraltar, Cadiz, and Other Parts of Spain: With a Collection of Facts Proving It to Be a Highly Contagious Disease* (London: Callow, Medical Bookseller, 1815), 109; Joseph Gilpin, "Copy of a Letter from Joseph D. A. Gilpin, MD, Inspector of Military Hospital at Gibraltar, to Colin Chisholm," *Edinburgh Medical Surgical Journal* 10 (1814): 41. On Dr. Chisholm, see Gordon Goodwin, "Chisholm, Colin," *Oxford Dictionary of National Biography,* available at http://www.oxforddnb.com/view/article/5322.

17. Chisholm, *Essay on the Malignant Pestilential Fever,* 89.

18. Chisholm, *Essay on the Malignant Pestilential Fever;* Benjamin Spector, ed., *Noah Webster: Letters on Yellow Fever Addressed to Dr. William Currie* (Baltimore: Johns Hopkins University Press, 1947); William Currie, *A Sketch of the Rise and Progress of Yellow Fever* (Philadelphia: Budd and Bartram, 1800); Smith, "On the Origin of the Pestiential Fever."

19. Although Philip Beaver was among those who denied the culpability of the *Hankey* in spreading yellow fever, his transcription of the ship's log clearly identifies the arrival date in Saint George as February 19; see *African Memoranda,* 470–71. Adding to his credibility concerning the date, Beaver kept very detailed logs of his subsequent journeys, eleven volumes of which are located in the National Maritime Museum, Greenwich, England. On the contemporary dispute about the arrival date of the *Hankey,* see James Clark, *A Treatise on the Yellow Fever as It Appeared in the Island of Dominica, in the Years 1793–4–5–6: To Which Are Added, Observations on the Bilious Remittent Fever . . .* (London: Murray and Highley, 1797), 406–7.

20. *Times* (London), October 1, 1793.

21. In 1879, for instance, the term Bullam Fever was still being used in official documents; *Public Health Reports and Papers, Volume 5, Presented at the Meetings of the American Public Health Association in the Year 1879* (Boston: Houghton, Mifflin, 1880), 187.

Bullam Fever continued to be used in the early twentieth century by Dr. W. A. Newman Dorland in the *American Illustrated Medical Dictionary* (Philadelphia: Saunders, 1907), 135. Even Dr. Benjamin Rush, the most famous advocate of locating the origin of yellow fever in the United States, eventually recognized that the disease was imported from Bolama: Rush, *Medical Inquiries and Observations* (Philadelphia: Carey, 1809).

22. Chisholm, *Essay on the Malignant Pestilential Fever,* 123. Dr. Stuart, who treated Captain Remington, confirms Chisholm's account in *New York Gazette,* December 5, 1805.

23. Joseph Mackrill, M.D., *The History of the Yellow Fever, with the Most Successful Method of Treatment* (Baltimore: Hayes, 1796), 9.

24. Chisholm, *Essay on the Malignant Pestilential Fever,* 123.

25. Ibid.

26. Thomas Clarkson, *The Substance of the Evidence of Sundry Persons on the Slave-Trade . . .* (London: J. Phillips, 1789), 92; *Gazette of the United States* (Philadelphia), September 5, 1795, and October 7, 1797.

27. Chisholm, *Essay on the Malignant Pestilential Fever,* 486; *Commercial Advertiser,* October 18 and November 15, 1797.

28. Ibid., 131.

29. McNeill, *Mosquito Empires.*

30. Kenneth F. Kiple, ed., *The African Exchange: Toward a Biological History of Black People* (Durham, N.C.: Duke University Press, 1987).

31. Chisholm, *Essay on the Malignant Pestilential Fever,* 111.

32. James Clark, *Treatise on the Yellow Fever,* 2–5; *New-York Gazette,* December 5, 1805.

33. Clark, *Treatise on the Yellow Fever,* 3; *South-Carolina State-Gazette,* June 20, 1794.

34. *South-Carolina State-Gazette,* June 20, 1794; Kiple, *The African Exchange.*

35. *New-York Evening Post,* September 1, 1803; *Columbian Centinel,* June 6, 1799; Chisholm, *Essay on the Malignant Pestilential Fever,* 145–50; Clark, *Treatise on the Yellow Fever,* 403–4.

36. Medicus Londinensis, "The Yellow Fever at Philadelphia," *Gentleman's Magazine* 64, no. 1 (1794); Clark, *Treatise on the Yellow Fever,* 404; Beaver, *African Memoranda,* 305–6; Chisholm, *Essay on the Malignant Pestilential Fever.*

37. Clark, *Treatise on the Yellow Fever,* 404–6; Chisholm, *Essay on the Malignant Pestilential Fever.*

38. Laurent Dubois, *Avengers of the New World: The Story of the Haitian Revolution* (Cambridge, Mass.: Belknap, 2004), 21–24 (nickname on 22, quotation from Moreau de St. Mery on 24); Dubois, *A Colony of Citizens: Revolution and Slave Emancipation in the French Caribbean, 1787–1804* (Chapel Hill: University of North Carolina Press, 2004), 155–56. See also Stewart R. King, *Blue Coat or Powdered Wig: Free People of Color in Pre-revolutionary Saint Domingue* (Athens: University of Georgia Press, 2007), 122–24.

39. Franklin W. Knight, "The Haitian Revolution," *American Historical Review* 105, no. 1 (February 2000): 103–15. For the marvelously descriptive term *pigmentocracy,* see Deborah Jensen, "Jean-Jacques Dessalines and the African Character of the Haitian Revolution," *William and Mary Quarterly,* 3rd ser., 69, no. 3 (July 2012): 618.

40. McNeill, *Mosquito Empires*.

41. On both the violence and the negotiations inherent in slave societies, see Ira Berlin, *Generations of Captivity: A History of African-American Slaves* (Cambridge, Mass.: Belknap, 2003), prologue.

42. Francis Alexander Stanislaus, *A Voyage to Saint Domingo, in the Years 1788, 1789, and 1790,* trans. J. Wright (London: T. Cadell and W. Davies, 1791), 98, 228.

43. Quoted in Robert Debs Heinl, Michael Heinl, and Nancy Gordon Heinl, *Written in Blood: The Story of the Haitian People, 1492–1995* (Lanham, Md.: University Press of America, 2005), 3.

44. See the articles in "Forum: Jean-Jacques Dessalines and the Haitian Revolution," *William and Mary Quarterly,* 3rd ser., 69, no. 3 (July 2012): 541–638.

45. McNeill, *Mosquito Empires,* 249–51; J. R. McNeill, "Ecology, Epidemics and Empires: Environmental Change and the Geopolitics of Tropical America, 1600–1825," *Environment and History* 5 (1999): 175–84.

46. David Geggus, "The British Government and the Saint Domingue Slave Revolt, 1791–1793," *English Historical Review* 96, no. 379 (April 1981): 285–305; Geggus, "The Cost of Pitt's Caribbean Campaigns, 1793–1798," *Historical Journal* 26, no. 3 (September 1983): 699–706; James D. Goodyear, "The Sugar Connection: A New Perspective on the History of Yellow Fever," *Bulletin of the History of Medicine* 52 (1978): 5–21; Kenneth F. Kiple and Kriemhild Coneé Ornleas, "Race, War and Tropical Medicine in the Eighteenth-Century Caribbean," *Clio Medica: Acta Academia Internationalis Historiae Medicinae* 35 (1996): 65–79.

47. Pym, *Observations upon the Bulam Fever,* 12–14, 236–37.

48. Roger N. Buckley, ed., *The Haitian Journal of Lieutenant Howard, York Hussars, 1796–1798* (Knoxville: University of Tennessee Press, 1985), 43, 49–50. See especially the excellent accounts in McNeill, *Mosquito Empires,* 244–48; and Dubois, *Avengers of the New World,* 215–19.

49. Dubois, *Avengers of the New World,* 215–16.

50. Buckley, *Haitian Journal,* 43, 49–50; McNeill, *Mosquito Empires,* 244–48; Dubois, *Avengers of the New World,* 215–19.

51. Buckley, *Haitian Journal,* 49–50.

52. Ibid.; McNeill, *Mosquito Empires,* 244–48.

53. Henry Hegart Breen, *St. Lucia: Historical, Statistical, and Descriptive* (1844; London: General Books, 2010), 103–4; McNeill, *Mosquito Empires,* 265.

54. Lt. Col. Thomas Maitland, quoted in McNeill, *Mosquito Empires,* 246.

55. Ibid., 248.

56. McNeill, *Mosquito Empires,* 236–49; Dubois, *Avengers of the New World,* 215–25; Geggus, "Cost of Pitt's Caribbean Campaigns"; quoted in David Brion Davis, *Inhuman Bondage: The Rise and Fall of Slavery in the New World* (New York: Oxford University Press, 2006), 166.

57. This and the following paragraphs draw on McNeill, *Mosquito Empires,* 249–60; Dubois, *Avengers of the New World,* 251–79; and Jim Tomson, "The Haitian Revolution and the Forging of America," *History Teacher* 34, no. 1 (November 2000): 76–94.

58. McNeill, *Mosquito Empires,* 273.

59. Louverture quoted ibid., 253; Dessalines quoted in Dubois, *Avengers of the New World,* 273. The memory of the person who later reported the prediction by Dessalines may, of course, been shaped by subsequent events in the Revolution.

60. McNeill, *Mosquito Empires,* 252–65; Dubois, *Avengers of the New World,* 280–301.

Chapter 8: Calamity in the United States Capital

1. Contemporaries debated the importance of the *Hankey* in spreading yellow fever to the continent of North America. See John Bordley, *Yellow Fever* (Philadelphia: Cist, 1794); Andrew Duncan, *Medical Commentaries for the Year 1795* (Philadelphia: Dobson, 1797); James Hardie, *An Account of the Malignant Fever* (New York: Southwick and Hardcastle, 1805); William Currie, *A Sketch of the Rise and Progress of Yellow Fever* (Philadelphia: Budd and Bartram, 1800); Joseph Mackrill, M.D., *History of the Yellow Fever, with the Most Successful Method of Treatment* (Baltimore: Hayes, 1796); James Clark, *A Treatise on the Yellow Fever as It Appeared in the Island of Dominica, in the Years 1793–4–5–6: To Which Are Added, Observations on the Bilious Remittent Fever . . .* (London: Murray and Highley, 1797), 3, 212; Nathaniel Bancroft, M.D., *An Essay on the Disease Called Yellow Fever* (London: T. Cadell and W. Davies, 1811), 212. A host of newspapers in the United States, Britain, and the West Indies excerpted parts of the debates during the 1790s and early nineteenth century.

2. Contemporaries agreed on the neighborhood where the epidemic began, even as they disagreed about its cause; see the city's official report, *An Account of the Rise, Progress, and Termination of the Malignant Fever Lately Prevalent in Philadelphia* (Philadelphia, 1794). Dr. William Currie identified sailors on the *Sans Culottes* as the lodgers at the Dennys' (*Gazette of the United States,* October 5, 1797). The captain of that ship, as was usual in these situations, denied having any sick passengers on board. This chapter draws on both primary documents and secondary sources, including Mathew Carey, *A Short Account of the Malignant Fever, Lately Prevalent in Philadelphia* (Philadelphia, 1794); Billy G. Smith, *The "Lower Sort": Philadelphia's Laboring People, 1750–1800* (Ithaca: Cornell University Press, 1990); J. Worth Estes and Billy G. Smith, eds., *A Melancholy Scene of Devastation: The Public Response to the 1793 Philadelphia Yellow Fever Epidemic* (Philadelphia: Science History Publications, 1997); Anita DeClue, "Living in Fear of the Pale Faced Messenger: The Private and Public Responses to Yellow Fever in Philadelphia, 1793–1799" (master's thesis, Montana State University, 2001); and Bob Arneback, *Destroying Angel: Benjamin Rush, Yellow Fever and the Birth of Modern Medicine* (1999), online book, available at http://bobarnebeck.com/fever1793.html. An excellent account, if frustrating for scholars because it does not identify many specific sources, is J. M. Powell, *Bring Out Your Dead: The Great Plague of Yellow Fever in Philadelphia in 1793* (Philadelphia: University of Pennsylvania Press, 1949).

3. Isaac Cathrall, *Memoir on the Analysis of the Black Vomit, Ejected in the Last Stage of the Yellow Fever* (Philadelphia: R. Folwell, 1800), 19.

4. Although Rush's exact route that day is unknown, the details about his life, vignettes about people, and descriptions of the streets and neighborhoods are factual. To avoid burdensome prose, I have intentionally used assertive rather than conditional

language to describe Rush's activities. David Rittenhouse recorded details about the weather every day for years, and his observations are available in Meteorological Observations, 1784–1805, at the American Philosophical Society, Philadelphia.

5. Benjamin Rush, *An Account of the Bilious Remitting Yellow Fever, as It Appeared in the City of Philadelphia, in the Year 1793* (Philadelphia: Dobson, 1794), 8–11. The boy, the son of Solomon McNair, lived at 5 Front Street, according to Clement Biddle, *The Philadelphia Directory 1791* (Philadelphia, 1791).

6. Many contemporaries referred to Philadelphia as the "Athens of America," including the architect Benjamin Latrobe; John C. Van Horne, *The Correspondence and Miscellaneous Papers of Benjamin Henry Latrobe* (New Haven: Yale University Press, 1988), 3:76. I reconstructed the makeup of Rush's neighborhood from various city directories, the First Census of the United States (1790), the 1789 Provincial Tax List (Philadelphia City Archives), and the U.S. Direct Tax of 1798 (National Archives).

7. Richard G. Miller describes Bingham's mansion in "The Federal City, 1783–1800," in Russell F. Weigley, ed., *Philadelphia: A 300-Year History* (New York: Norton, 1982). The contemporary architect, Charles Bullfinch, is quoted in Joseph J. Kelley, Jr., *Life and Times in Colonial Philadelphia* (Harrisburg, Pa.: Stackpole, 1973), 160–61.

8. *Philadelphia Monthly Magazine,* August 1798, 69.

9. Quotations are in Kenneth Roberts and Anna M. Roberts, *Moreau de St. Mery's American Journey* (New York: Doubleday, 1947), 324; and Charles William Janson, *The Stranger in America, 1793–1806,* ed. Carl S. Driver (New York: Press of the Pioneers, 1971).

10. Elizabeth Gray Kogen Spera, "Building for Business: The Impact of Commerce on the City Plan and Architecture of the City of Philadelphia, 1750–1800" (Ph.D. diss., University of Pennsylvania, 1980), 68, 105–19.

11. Quotations are in Roberts and Roberts, *St. Mery's American Journey,* 316, and Johann David Schoepf, *Travels in the Confederation* [1783–1784], ed. and trans. Alfred J. Morrison (New York: Bergman, 1968), 112.

12. James Mease, *The Picture of Philadelphia: Giving an Account of its Origin, Increase and Improvements in Arts, Sciences, Manufactures, Commerce and Revenue* (Philadelphia: Kite, 1811), 117–19.

13. Roberts and Roberts, *St. Mery's American Journey,* 112; Vagrancy Docket, January 16, 1794, Philadelphia City Archives. Public punishments are noted in Negley K. Teeters, *The Cradle of the Penitentiary: The Walnut Street Jail at Philadelphia* (Philadelphia: n.p., 1955).

14. Harrold E. Gillingham, ed., "Dr. Solomon Drowne," *Pennsylvania Magazine of History and Biography* 48 (1924), 236; Schoepf, *Travels in the Confederation,* 112.

15. Powell, *Bring Out Your Dead,* 12.

16. Smith, *The "Lower Sort,"* chap. 3.

17. Accounts of the *Sans Culottes* and the *Hankey* appeared in the *South Carolina State Gazette* (Charleston), July 24, 1794, and the *Gazette of the United States* (Philadelphia), September 5, 1795.

18. Newspaper stories about the controversial Genêt are in the *Pennsylvania Gazette* (Philadelphia), August 14 and 17, 1793, while the docking of the ships is recorded in the

July 24 edition. See also John Ferling, *Adams vs. Jefferson: The Tumultuous Election of 1800* (New York: Oxford University Press, 2005).

19. Resident, quoted in Powell, *Bring Out Your Dead,* 10; Smith, *The "Lower Sort,"* chap. 1.

20. Kelley, *Life and Times in Colonial Philadelphia,* 16–61; Sharon V. Salinger, *Taverns and Drinking in Early America* (Baltimore: Johns Hopkins University Press, 2002); W. J. Rorabaugh, *The Alcoholic Republic: An American Tradition* (New York: Oxford University Press, 1981), 7–10.

21. "Filles de joie" mentioned in Carey, *Short Account of the Malignant Fever,* 66; Sarah Evans appears in the Vagrancy Docket, April 23, 1794, Philadelphia City Archives; Evans appears thirteen more times in the docket.

Seemingly from firsthand experience, Moreau de St. Mery explicitly described prostitutes and their activities in Roberts and Roberts, *St. Mery's American Journey,* 311–25.

22. Newspaper story in the *Pennsylvania Gazette* (Philadelphia), August 8, 1787. Washington's servant and slave appear in the Vagrancy Docket, July 2 and August 6, 1794, Philadelphia City Archives.

23. Rush, *Account of the Bilious Remitting Yellow Fever,* 12–13; Powell, *Bring Out Your Dead,* 11–12; William Currie, Letter, *Gazette of the United States* (Philadelphia), October 5, 1797.

24. Rush, *Account of the Bilious Remitting Yellow Fever,* 12–13; Powell, *Bring Out Your Dead,* 11–12; "Bullam fever" origins described in Colin Chisholm, *An Essay on the Malignant Pestilential Fever Introduced into the West Indian Islands from Boullam, on the Coast of Guinea, as It Appeared in 1793 and 1794* (London: J. Mawman, 1795); and Carey, *Short Account of the Malignant Fever,* 44.

25. For material in this and the next paragraph, see Carey, *Short Account of the Malignant Fever,* 12–15, and Powell, *Bring Out Your Dead,* 45.

26. Quotations and anecdotes from the following Philadelphia newspapers (all 1793): *Philadelphia Aurora,* August 23 and 25; *Dunlap's American Daily Advertiser,* August 24, 26, and 27; *Gazette of the United States,* August 28; *Philadelphia Gazette,* August 28.

27. *Independent Gazetteer and Agricultural Repository,* August 31, 1793. Reed usually receives primary credit for the discovery of the mosquito vector, although Finlay, a Cuban-born doctor, had proposed it several decades earlier; see John R. Pierce and James V. Writer, *Yellow Jack: How Yellow Fever Ravaged America and Walter Reed Discovered Its Deadly Secrets* (Hoboken, N.J.: John Wiley, 2005).

28. Rush, *Account of the Bilious Remitting Yellow Fever,* 12.

29. J. Worth Estes, "Introduction: The Yellow Fever Syndrome and Its Treatment in Philadelphia, 1793," in Estes and Smith, *Melancholy Scene of Devastation,* 12–13.

30. Powell, *Bring Out Your Dead,* 13–15, 35–42.

31. Carey, *Short Account of the Malignant Fever,* 12–15.

32. For descriptions in this and the next paragraph, see ibid.; Powell, *Bring Out Your Dead,* 35–37.

33. John K. Alexander, *Render Them Submissive: Responses to Poverty in Philadelphia, 1760–1800* (Amherst: University of Massachusetts Press, 1980); Simon Newman and

Billy G. Smith, "Incarcerated Innocents: Inmates, Conditions, and Survival Strategies in Philadelphia's Almshouse and Workhouse," in *Buried Lives: Incarcerated in Early America,* ed. Michele Lise Tarter and Richard Bell (Athens: University of Georgia Press, 2012).

34. The next few paragraphs draw on Carey, *Short Account of the Malignant Fever,* 12–15; and Powell, *Bring Out Your Dead,* 57–63.

Chapter 9: Journal of the Plague Months

1. Edwin B. Bronner, ed., "Letter from a Yellow Fever Victim: Philadelphia, 1793," *Pennsylvania Magazine of History and Biography* 86 (1962): 205–7.

2. See, for example, Charles Brockden Brown's *Arthur Mervyn; or, Memoirs of the Year 1793, with Related Texts,* ed. Philip Barnard and Stephen Shapiro (Indianapolis: Hackett, 2008).

3. Daniel Defoe, *A Journal of the Plague Year* (New York: Oxford University Press, 1969), 75; Alexander Graydon, *Memoirs of His Own Time with Reminiscences of the Men and Events of the Revolution,* ed. John Stockton Little (Philadelphia: Lindsay and Blakiston, 1846), 365.

4. Mathew Carey, *A Desultory Account of the Yellow Fever, Prevalent in Philadelphia, and of the Present State of the City* (Philadelphia: Carey, October 16, 1793), 2, 5. The number of residents in individual streets, alleys, and lanes who fled were reported in Edmund Hogan, *The Prospect of Philadelphia and Check on the Next Directory* (Philadelphia: Bailey, 1795).

5. Martin S. Pernick, "Politics, Parties, and Pestilence: Epidemic Yellow Fever in Philadelphia and the Rise of the First Party System," in J. Worth Estes and Billy G. Smith, eds., *A Melancholy Scene of Devastation: The Public Response to the 1793 Philadelphia Yellow Fever Epidemic* (Philadelphia: Science History Publications, 1997), 119–46.

6. Ron Chernow, *Alexander Hamilton* (New York: Viking, 2005).

7. Pernick, "Politics, Parties, and Pestilence," 131–32.

8. Carey, *Short Account of the Malignant Fever,* 27.

9. Quoted in Powell, *Bring Out Your Dead,* 110. On Washington's death, see J. Worth Estes, "Introduction: The Yellow Fever Syndrome and Its Treatment in Philadelphia, 1793," in Estes and Smith, *Melancholy Scene of Devastation,* 14.

10. Quoted in Pernick, "Politics, Parties, and Pestilence," 132.

11. Carey, *Short Account of the Malignant Fever,* 27.

12. Ibid., 55–57; quoted in Powell, *Bring Out Your Dead,* 224–36.

13. *Independent Gazetteer and Agricultural Repository* (Philadelphia), September 21 and October 5, 1793; *Philadelphia Gazette,* September 25, 1793.

14. Susan E. Klepp, "'How Many Precious Souls Are Fled'?: The Magnitude of the 1793 Yellow Fever Epidemic," in Estes and Smith, *Melancholy Scene of Devastation,* 163–82.

15. Ibid.

16. Yellow fever deaths by streets are from Hogan, *Prospect of Philadelphia;* also see William Priest, *Travels in the United States of America; Commencing in the Year 1793, and*

Ending in 1797 (London: Johnson, 1802), 16; Carey, *Short Account of the Malignant Fever,* 27; English visitor, quoted in Richard Parkinson, *A Tour in America, in 1798, 1799, and 1800* (London, 1805), 486.

17. Carey, *Short Account of the Malignant Fever,* 27–28; Billy G. Smith, *The "Lower Sort": Philadelphia's Laboring People, 1750–1800* (Ithaca: Cornell University Press, 1990), 52–56.

18. Klepp, "How Many Precious Souls Are Fled."

19. Carey, *Short Account of the Malignant Fever,* 21–22; Priest, *Travels in the United States of America,* 9–20.

20. Carey, *Short Account of the Malignant Fever,* 17.

21. Estes and Smith, *Melancholy Scene of Devastation,* 24; British visitor, quoted in Parkinson, *A Tour in America,* 486; Carey, *Short Account of the Malignant Fever,* 59–60.

22. Carey, *Short Account of the Malignant Fever,* 27.

23. Bronner, "Letter from a Yellow Fever Victim," 205–6. Richard Wells, a bank cashier, welcomed the widow into his own home, where she later died of yellow fever. At the time he wrote the letter, Heston believed Wells had also fallen ill. Carey does not list Richard Wells as a victim of the epidemic in *Short Account of the Malignant Fever.*

24. Carey, *Short Account of the Malignant Fever,* 23. See also Sally F. Griffith, " 'A Total Dissolution of the Bonds of Society': Community Death and Regeneration in Mathew Carey's *Short Account of the Malignant Fever,* " in Estes and Smith, *Melancholy Scene of Devastation,* 45–60.

25. Jean Devèze, *An Enquiry into, and Observations upon the Causes and Effects of the Epidemic Disease, Which Raged in Philadelphia from the Month of August till Towards the Middle of December, 1793* (Philadelphia: Parent, 1794), 10.

26. Carey, *Short Account of the Malignant Fever,* 35–40.

27. Ibid., 7, 134, 235.

28. Ibid., 109.

29. Letter dated October 1, 1793, in L. H. Butterfield, ed., *Letters of Benjamin Rush* (Princeton: Princeton University Press, 1951), 809; "Memoirs of Charles Willson Peale from his original manuscript with notes by Horace Wells Sellers," Peale-Sellers Papers, American Philosophical Society, Philadelphia.

30. Anita DeClue and Billy G. Smith, "Wrestling the 'Pale Faced Messenger': The Diary of Edward Garrigues During the 1798 Philadelphia Yellow Fever Epidemic," *Pennsylvania History* 65 (1998): 243–68.

31. Jacquelyn C. Miller, "Passions and Politics: The Multiple Meanings of Benjamin Rush's Treatment for Yellow Fever," in Estes and Smith, *Melancholy Scene of Devastation,* 79–96; Lester S. King, *Transformations in American Medicine from Benjamin Rush to William Osler* (Baltimore: Johns Hopkins University Press, 1990), 52–54.

32. Powell, *Bring Out Your Dead,* 79.

33. Ibid., 118.

34. Rush, quoted in William Priest, *Travels in the United States of America,* 197–98; *Pennsylvania Gazette* (Philadelphia), September 20, 1797; Miller, "Passions and Politics"; Estes, "The Yellow Fever Syndrome."

35. Butterfield, *Letters of Benjamin Rush,* October 30, 1793.

36. Ibid.

37. Cobbett cited in Mary Alma Frances Mansfield, "Yellow Fever Epidemics of Philadelphia, 1699–1805" (master's thesis, University of Pittsburgh, 1949), 59. See also William Coleman, *Yellow Fever in the North: The Methods of Early Epidemiology* (Madison: University of Wisconsin Press, 1987).

38. Estes and Smith, *Melancholy Scene of Devastation,* 12–13; Devèze, *An Enquiry,* 54–56. For an argument that Benjamin Rush has received too harsh of a criticism from most scholars, see Bob Arnebeck, *Destroying Angel: Benjamin Rush, Yellow Fever and the Birth of Modern Medicine* (1999), online book available at http://bobarnebeck.com/fever1793.html.

39. Pernick, "Politics, Parties, and Pestilence."

40. Quoted in Powell, *Bring Out Your Dead,* 37–46; Isaac Cathrall, *Memoir on the Analysis of the Black Vomit, Ejected in the Last Stage of the Yellow Fever* (Philadelphia: Folwell, 1800); Benjamin Rush, *Medical Inquiries and Observations* (Philadelphia: Carey, 1809); Colin Chisholm, *An Essay on the Malignant Pestilential Fever Introduced into the West Indian Islands from Boullam, on the Coast of Guinea, as It Appeared in 1793 and 1794* (London: J. Mawman, 1795), 65.

41. Quoted in Powell, *Bring Out Your Dead,* xxvi.

42. Carey, *Short Account of the Malignant Fever,* 87. On Rush's death, see Eliza Cope Harrison, ed., *Philadelphia Merchant: The Diary of Thomas P. Cope, 1800–1851* (South Bend, Ind.: Gateway, 1978), 281.

43. Rush to Richard Allen, September 1793, Correspondence of Rush, unpublished manuscript, xxxviii, 32, Library Company of Philadelphia.

44. Quoted in *Philadelphia Gazette* and *Dunlap's American Daily Advertiser* (Philadelphia), September 11, 1793; Gary B. Nash, *Forging Freedom: The Formation of Philadelphia's Black Community, 1720–1840* (Cambridge: Harvard University Press, 1988), 121.

45. Nash, *Forging Freedom,* 122; Phillip Lapsansky, " 'Abigail, a Negress': The Role and the Legacy of African Americans in the Yellow Fever Epidemic," in Estes and Smith, *Melancholy Scene of Devastation,* 61–65.

46. Butterfield, *Letters of Benjamin Rush,* 2:654, 658.

47. Betty L. Plummer and James Durham, "Letters of James Durham to Benjamin Rush," *Journal of Negro History* 65 (Summer 1980): 261–69.

48. Devèze, *An Enquiry,* 54–56.

49. Absalom Jones and Richard Allen, *A Narrative of the Proceedings of the Black People, During the Late Awful Calamity in Philadelphia in the Year 1793* (Philadelphia: William W. Woodward, 1794), 18.

50. Ibid., 19–20.

51. Ibid., 16. Zachariah Poulson's Bills of Mortality show black burials for 1793 at 116 rather than the 305 claimed; see Billy G. Smith, ed., *Life in Early Philadelphia: Documents from the Revolutionary and Early National Periods* (University Park: Pennsylvania State University Press, 1995), 232–42; Klepp, "How Many Precious Souls Are Fled."

52. Bronner, "Letter from a Yellow Fever Victim," 206.

53. A subsequent account of the 1797 epidemic also condemned the conduct of blacks; see Richard Folwell, *Short History of the Yellow Fever, That Broke Out in the City of Philadelphia, in July, 1797* (Philadelphia: Folwell, 1797), 34.

54. An excellent account of the rhetorical strategies used by Allen and Jones is Jacqueline Bacon, "Rhetoric and Identity in Absalom Jones and Richard Allen's *Narrative of the Proceedings of the Black People, During the Late Awful Calamity in Philadelphia*," *Pennsylvania Magazine of History and Biography* 125 (2001): 61–90.

55. Jones and Allen, *Narrative of the Proceedings of the Black People*, 25.

56. Ibid., 25–27; Nash, *Forging Freedom*, 174–75; Gary B. Nash and Jean R. Soderlund, *Freedom by Degrees: Emancipation in Pennsylvania and Its Aftermath* (New York: Oxford University Press, 1991), 131–32, 180; Bacon, "Rhetoric and Identity," 75–77.

57. *Minutes of the Proceedings of the Committee . . . to Alleviate the Sufferings of the Afflicted with the Malignant Fever Prevalent in the City and Its Vicinity* (Philadelphia: Aiken and Son, 1794).

58. On higher mortality rate caused by fewer nurses in later epidemics, see DeClue and Smith, "Wrestling the 'Pale Faced Messenger.' "

59. Carey, *Short Account of the Malignant Fever*, 93.

60. Butterfield, *Letters of Benjamin Rush*, vol. 1, December 12, 1793.

61. Ibid., November 25, 1793.

62. Quoted in Estes and Smith, *Melancholy Scene of Devastation*, 99–100.

63. Quaker, quoted in Priest, *Travels in the United States of America*, 13; ministers, quoted in *Pennsylvania Gazette* (Philadelphia), December 4, 1793. See also the pamphlets by Thaddeus Brown, *Philadelphia Reformed or Else Destroyed* (Philadelphia, 1798); and William Marshall, *On the Propriety of Removing from the Seat of the Pestilence* (Philadelphia, 1799), both available at the American Philosophical Society.

64. A particularly impressive study of the political implications of the Philadelphia yellow fever epidemics is Simon Finger, *The Contagious City: The Politics of Public Health in Early Philadelphia* (Ithaca: Cornell University Press, 2012). Also see Michael McMahon, "Beyond Therapeutics: Technology and the Question of Public Health in Late-Eighteenth-Century Philadelphia," in Estes and Smith, *Melancholy Scene of Devastation*, 97–118.

65. John Ferling, *Adams vs. Jefferson: The Tumultuous Election of 1800* (New York: Oxford University Press, 2005); Margaret Humphrey, *Yellow Fever and the South* (Baltimore: John Hopkins University Press, 1992).

66. See the city's official report, *An Account of the Rise, Progress, and Termination of the Malignant Fever Lately Prevalent in Philadelphia* (Philadelphia, 1794); essay by Dr. William Currie, *Gazette of the United States* (Philadelphia), October 5, 1797; Carey, *Short Account of the Malignant Fever*; Chisholm, *Essay on the Malignant Pestilential Fever*.

67. K. David Patterson, "Yellow Fever Epidemics and Mortality in the United States, 1693–1905," *Social Science and Medicine* 34, no. 8 (April 1992): 855–65; J. Radcliffe, "A Note on the Recurrence of Yellow Fever Epidemics in Urban Populations," *Journal of Applied Probability* 11, no. 1 (March 1974): 170–73.

68. Gerald N. Grob, *The Deadly Truth: A History of Disease in America* (Cambridge: Harvard University Press, 2002); Douglas Carroll, "Yellow Fever Epidemics of the Late

Eighteenth Century in Baltimore," *Maryland State Medical Journal* 21, no. 9 (September 1972): 47–52; Patterson, "Yellow Fever Epidemics and Mortality"; William H. McNeill, *Plagues and People* (New York: Anchor, 1977).

69. William Marshall, *A Theological Dissertation on the Propriety of Removing from the Seat of the Pestilence: Presented to the Perusal of the Serious Inhabitants of Philadelphia and New-York* (Philadelphia: David Hogan, 1799), available at the American Philosophical Society.

70. Thomas Jefferson to Benjamin Rush, September 13, 1800, Butterfield, *Letters of Benjamin Rush,* vol. 2.

71. On the Louisiana Purchase, see Thomas Fleming, *The Louisiana Purchase* (Hoboken, N.J.: Wiley, 2003); Roger G. Kennedy, *Mr. Jefferson's Lost Cause: Land, Farmers, Slavery, and the Louisiana Purchase* (New York: Oxford University Press, 2003), 176–297; "Hamilton on the Louisiana Purchase: A Newly Identified Editorial from the New-York Evening Post," *William and Mary Quarterly,* 3rd ser., 12, no. 2 (April 1955): 268–81; Jed Handelsman Shugerman, "The Louisiana Purchase and South Carolina's Reopening of the Slave Trade in 1803," *Journal of the Early Republic* 22, no. 2 (Summer 2002): 263–90.

72. "Hamilton on the Louisiana Purchase."

73. Ibid., 269, 272.

74. Peter S. Onuf, *Jefferson's Empire: The Language of American Nationhood* (Charlottesville: University of Virginia Press, 2000); Dennis Brindell Fraiden, *The Louisiana Purchase* (Tarrytown, N.Y.: Marshall Cavendish, 2010); Fleming, *Louisiana Purchase.*

75. Livingston, quoted in Daniel Rasmussen, *American Uprising: The Untold Story of America's Largest Slave Revolt* (New York: Harper Collins, 2011), 52.

76. Anthony F. C. Wallace, *Jefferson and the Indians: The Tragic Fate of the First Americans* (Cambridge, Mass.: Belknap, 2001).

77. Ira Berlin, *Generations of Captivity: A History of African-American Slaves* (Cambridge, Mass.: Belknap Press, 2003).

Epilogue: The Living and the Dead

1. Colin Chisholm, *An Essay on the Malignant Pestilential Fever Introduced into the West Indian Islands from Boullam, on the Coast of Guinea, as It Appeared in 1793 and 1794* (London: J. Mawman, 1795); *Columbian Centinel,* June 6, 1799.

2. *Times* (London), November 9, 1793.

3. Reports appeared in *American Minerva* (New York), January 29, 1794; *Massachusetts Mercury* (Boston), February 7, 1794; and *Evening Post* (London), July 10, 1820.

4. *Times* (London), November 6, 7, and 9, 1793; *Evening Post* (London), July 10, 1820. Philip Beaver, *African Memoranda: Relative to an Attempt to Establish a British Settlement on the Island of Bulama, on the Western Coast of Africa, in the Year 1792 . . . and the Introduction of Letters and Religion to Its Inhabitants but More Particularly as the Means of Gradually Abolishing African Slavery* (London: Baldwin, 1805; repr. Westport, Conn.: Negro Universities Press, 1970), 192, 305–6.

5. *Times* (London), November 7 and 9, 1793.

6. Notices about the burning of the *Hankey* appeared in the *American Minerva* (New York), January 29, 1794; *Massachusetts Mercury* (Boston), February 7, 1794. The story was recounted later in the *Evening Post* (London), July 10, 1820.

7. Beaver, *African Memoranda,* 137, 145–47, 152–54, 157, 163, 279–81, 440–49.

8. *Times* (London), April 10, 1788; Beaver, *African Memoranda,* 9, 14, 39, 72–73, 112, 143–48, 157, 439–42. The will of the elder John Paiba can be found in PB 11/1249, page 365, Public Records Office, British National Archives, Kew, England.

9. *Proceedings of the Old Bailey, 1674–1913,* at www.oldbaileyonline.org (cited hereafter as *Old Bailey*), April 2, 1788, Thomas Blake t17880402-51; Beaver, *African Memoranda,* 163, 436, 438.

10. Glover, identified as a coach maker, appeared as a witness in the *Old Bailey,* December 4, 1805, t18051204-55.

11. Beaver, *African Memoranda,* 129, 144, 157, 173, 440–42, 448, 470.

12. *Times* (London), April 23, 1788; Beaver, *African Memoranda,* 118, 121, 140, 148, 159, 173, 176. After serving as the captain of the *Hankey,* Cox never again appeared as a captain either in *Lloyd's Register of Shipping* or any issue of the London *Times.*

13. C. B. Wadstrom, *Essay on Colonization, Particularly Applied to the Western Coast of Africa, with Some Free Thoughts on Cultivation and Commerce; Also Brief Descriptions of the Colonies Already Formed, or Attempted, in Africa, Including Those of Sierra Leona and Bulama* (London: Darton and Harvey, 1794; repr. New York: Kelley, 1968), 174; Beaver, *African Memoranda,* 49, 435–39.

14. This account of Beaver's life is from William Henry Smyth, *The Life and Services of Captain Philip Beaver* (London: John Murray, 1829); *London Gazette,* June 24, 1800, May 30, 1809, and January 21, 1812; J. K. Laughton and Andrew Lambert, "Beaver, Philip," *Oxford Dictionary of National Biography,* available at http://www.oxforddnb.com /public/index-content.html.

15. Beaver, *African Memoranda,* 305.

16. Beaver, quoted in Wadstrom, *Essay on Colonization,* 300. *Congressional Record,* vol. 428, session 3, February 28, 1843, U.S. National Archives.

17. *Times* (London), April 13, 1836, and July 20, 1850.

18. The literature on the ending of the slave trade is rich and vast. See, for example, David Eltis, "A Brief Overview of Slavery," Trans-Atlantic Slave Trade Database, http://www.slavevoyages.org/tast/assessment/essays-intro-08.faces; Linda Colley, *Britons: Forging the Nation, 1707–1837,* rev. ed. (New Haven: Yale University Press, 2009), 350–55; Adam Hochschild, *Bury the Chains: Prophets and Rebels in the Fight to Free an Empire's Slaves* (New York: Mariner, 2006).

19. Records of the Colonial Office, 879/2/16 L, British National Archives. Smyth O'Connor, "Notes on an Expedition down the Western Coast of Africa to the 'Bijuga Islands,' and the Recently Discovered River Kittafiny," *Proceedings of the Royal Geographical Society of London* 3, no. 6 (1858–59): 379–85; Edward Stallibrass, "The Bijouga or Bissagos Islands, West Africa," *Proceedings of the Royal Geographical Society and Monthly Record of Geography,* New Monthly Series 11, no. 10 (October 1889): 595–601.

20. "Arbitral Award Between Portugal and the United Kingdom, Regarding the Dispute About the Sovereignty over the Island of Bulama," April 21, 1870, *Reports of International Arbitral Awards* (New York: United Nations, 2007), 28:131–40.

21. Peter Mark, "The Evolution of 'Portuguese' Identity: Luso-Africans on the Upper Guinea Coast from the Sixteenth to the Early Nineteenth Century," *Journal of African History* 40 (1999): 173–91; Ed Vulliamy, "How a Tiny West African Country Became the World's First Narco State," *Guardian*, March 8, 2008; "Cocaine Capital: West Africa New Way Station for Drugs as Cocaine Use Soars," Associated Press, Guinea-Bissau, July 29, 2007; Brandon Lundy, "Bijagos of Guinea-Bissau: Resistance Is Fruitful," paper presented at the symposium *Prime Movers of the Atlantic World: Portugal and Africa*, State University of New York at Buffalo, April 22, 2006.

22. Lundy, "Bijagos of Guinea-Bissau."

23. Thomas Ruston, M.D., *Collection of Facts Interspersed with Observations on the Nature, Causes, and Cure of the Yellow Fever . . .* (Philadelphia: Bartholomew Graves, 1804), 26–27; J. Worth Estes and Billy G. Smith, eds., *A Melancholy Scene of Devastation: The Public Response to the 1793 Philadelphia Yellow Fever Epidemic* (Philadelphia: Science History Publications, 1997); James L. Dickerson, *Yellow Fever: A Deadly Disease Poised to Kill Again* (Amherst, Mass.: Prometheus, 2006); J. R. McNeill, *Mosquito Empires: Ecology and War in the Greater Caribbean, 1620–1914* (Cambridge: Cambridge University Press, 2010), 265–66.

24. William Pym, *Observations upon the Bulam Fever, Which Has of Late Years Prevailed in the West Indies, on the Coast of America, at Gibraltar, Cadiz, and Other Parts of Spain: With a Collection of Facts Proving It to Be a Highly Contagious Disease* (London: Callow, Medical Bookseller, 1815), 14–66; see also Robert Jackson, M.D., *Remarks on the Epidemic Yellow Fever, Which Has Appeared at Intervals on the South Coasts of Spain, Since the Year 1800* (London: Thomas and George Underwood, 1821), 1–25, 137.

25. McNeill, *Mosquito Empires,* 265–66.

26. Douglass C. North, *The Economic Growth of the United States, 1790–1860* (New York: Norton, 1966), chap. 1.

ↄ逨

Glossary of People and Places of West Africa

Algerians: A term used in the seventeenth and eighteenth centuries for people living in North African states, often designated by the English as the Barbary powers (Morocco, Algiers, Tripoli, and Tunisia). English polemicists of the time condemned Algerians as barbarians.

Barbary pirates: Muslim corsairs or privateers who preyed on nonmilitary shipping in the Mediterranean, seizing both crew and passengers and holding them to ransom, enslaving any who could not pay. Both Britain and the United States paid tribute to protect their ships from raids, although there were no guarantees of safe passage. European shipping continued to be disrupted by Barbary pirate captures and demands for crew ransoms well into the nineteenth century.

Biafada (Bafatá, Beafada, Biafar, Bidyola, Bedfola, Dfola, Fada): An ethnic group in central and south Guinea-Bissau, and the language spoken by this group. There are approximately 41,000 Biafada who speak this language in Guinea-Bissau today (2002 estimate).

Bidyago (Bijago, Bijogo, Bijougot, Budjago, Bugago, Bijuga): A language with several dialects spoken in the Bijagos Archipelago. By estimates in 2002, approximately 28,000 Bijago speak these dialects in Guinea-Bissau.

Bijago (Bijagó, Bissago, Bisago, Bijuga, Bidjugo, Bidyago, Bidyogo, Bidyugo, Bidjougo, Bojago, Bujago): An ethnic group that has lived on the Bijagos Archipelago since at least the thirteenth century. Because the Bijago were separated from mainland Africa, they were isolated and protected enough to form and preserve a unique identity, maintained today in part through matrilineal social arrangements, the Bidyago language, and specific cosmological beliefs. It was estimated that there were 30,000 Bijago in 2006.

Bijagos Archipelago (Bissagos Islands): More than thirty islands extending thirty miles from the West African coast of Guinea-Bissau. The archipelago is now a UNESCO World Biosphere Reserve.

Bissau (Bissao): A city located on the Upper Guinea coast at the mouth of the Rio Geba. The Portuguese founded Bissau as a fortified trading post in the seventeenth century, using it primarily for the slave trade. It was contested territory among European colonizers throughout the eighteenth century. Portugal designated Bissau as a "captaincy" at the beginning of the nineteenth century to shore up its tenuous colonial hold against potential claims by France and Great Britain. After 1836, a district governor of Portuguese Guinea resided in Bissau, reporting to the governor-general of Cape Verde. Bissau became capital of Portuguese Guinea in 1941. It has been the capital city of the Republic of Guinea-Bissau since the country's independence in 1974.

Bolama (Bulama, Bulam, Bullam, Boullam): An island in the Bijagos Archipelago that is now part of Guinea-Bissau. The term also refers to the contemporary name of the island's major town and to the encompassing administrative region of Guinea-Bissau.

Canabac Island (Bubaque, Kanabak, Canhabaque): An island in the Bijagos Archipelago. Bubaque (Canabac) is also the name of the island's main city, the largest contemporary town in the archipelago. A World Gazetteer 2008 population survey estimated that the island had 9,000 inhabitants.

Canabacs: Bolama colonists used this name to refer to Bijago who lived on the neighboring island, which the colonists called "Canabac" but today is usually anglicized as "Bubaque."

Canary Islands: An archipelago belonging to Spain near the northwest coast of mainland Africa. These islands, especially Tenerife, were important as way stations for eighteenth-century European shipping to and from Africa as well as for voyages across the Atlantic.

Cape Verde: A nation made up of ten islands located 280–450 miles west of the coast of Senegal. The Portuguese discovered these uninhabited islands in the mid-fifteenth century, and Portuguese farmers, exiles, and criminals began colonizing them in the 1460s. Portuguese plantation owners used slave labor from the Upper Guinea coast to grow sugar, cotton, and indigo on two of the rain-fed, larger islands, Santiago (São Tiago) and Fogo. The slaves also tended livestock, labored in the salt flats on the island of Sal, and produced cloth. The World Bank estimated the 2011 population to be 501,000.

Creole (Crioulo, Kriolo, Kriulo, Kiryol, Portuguese Creole): A Guinea-Bissau Creole language with several dialects. It was spoken by grumettas working for the Bolama colony and is spoken today in the Bijagos Archipelago, the Gambia, Senegal, and the United States; nearly 200,000 inhabitants of Guinea-Bissau claim it as their first language. *Crioulo* is also used to designate a Luso-African or mixed-race person.

Gabu: *See* Kaabu.

Gambia: Both a major river and a contemporary nation (Republic of the Gambia) in West Africa. British presence along the river dated back to the sixteenth century. In the eighteenth century, the area was part of Senegambia. The Gambia won its independence from the United Kingdom in 1965. In 2011 the World Bank estimated the national population as 1.8 million. The official language is English, while Mandinka, Wolof, and Fula are the major ethnic groups and languages.

Gorée Island: A French possession that was used as a trading post from 1817 to 1960 located south of the Cape Verde Islands near the coast of Senegal; today it is administratively part of Senegal's capital city, Dakar. The town of Gorée occupies most of the island. Historians estimated that millions of slaves were shipped from this tiny island to the Americas from 1536, when the Portuguese launched the Atlantic slave trade, until slavery was made illegal in Senegal in 1848. Recent research has brought the size of the number into question, although the island was a major embarkation point. Gorée Island became a UNESCO World Heritage site in 1978.

grumetta: Anglicized form of the Creole/Portuguese term *grumete* (canoe-hand), designating an African or mixed-race person who worked primarily for coastal traders.

Guanche: The name Europeans gave to the people they found living on Tenerife and the other Canary Islands. *See* Vincheai.

Guinala (Ghinala): A town on the Rio Grande (Rio Grande de Buba) in what is now Guinea-Bissau that served as an entrepôt for African coastal people and long-distance African traders. Biafada merchants brought kola, fish, mollusks, salt, and other products to Guinala, while Mandinka merchants brought meat, hides, cotton, cloth, gold, iron, and many other trade goods found or produced in the interior. Guinala also served as an important center for the export of slaves.

Guinea (Guiné, Guinée): Fifteenth-century Portuguese mariners called the West African coast south of the Sénégal River "Guiné," and the name entered English and other European languages from the Portuguese. The Portuguese established their first colonial footholds on the Guinea coast in the sixteenth century; French, British, and Dutch trading posts followed in the seventeenth. In the eighteenth century, European geographers did not agree on the specific area of the western coast to be so designated; they divided "Guinea" into two regions— Upper and Lower Guinea. The Bolama colony was situated in Upper Guinea. Colonial rivalries over Guinea territory were not settled until the nineteenth century; the entire area won its independence in the twentieth, although indigenous people were not represented when the boundary lines for the three new nations of Guinea, Guinea-Bissau, and Equatorial Guinea were drawn. The country today called Guinea, often referred to as Guinea-Conakry—using the name of its largest city to distinguish it from similarly named nations—was formerly a subdivision of French West Africa called French Guinea. It won its independence in 1958. It is located southeast of Senegal and is also bordered by Guinea-Bissau, Liberia, Sierra Leone, and the Ivory Coast. The World Bank estimated its 2011 national population to be 10 million, comprising Fulu, Mandinka, Susu, and several other ethnic groups. Its official language remains French.

guinea: A British gold coin minted between 1663 and 1813 (eventually valued at one pound plus one shilling). The general geographical area known as Guinea was the main source of gold for Europe and the Mediterranean region in the seventeenth century.

Guinea-Bissau: A small West African country that today comprises about 14,000 square miles (roughly half the size of South Carolina). Senegal borders the nation to the north, Guinea to the south and east, and the Atlantic Ocean to the west. The country is a mainland strip of the African coast composed of rain forests, swamps, and mangrove-covered wetlands, in addition to about thirty nearby coastal islands. The area was part of Portuguese Guinea until it won its independence in 1974. Indigenous peoples of Guinea-Bissau include Biafada, Bijago, Mandinka, Manjaco, Nalu, and Papel, as well as several others. The World Bank 2011 national population estimate for Guinea-Bissau was 1.6 million, including all ethnic groups.

Kaabu (Gabu): A Mandinka-dominated confederation that broke away from the Mali Empire in the fifteenth century. Founded in the eleventh century and stretching from the Niger River area to the Atlantic, the Mali Empire was based on inter-African trade. Kaabu had been one of the Mali Empire's most distant provinces. It claimed land along the West African coast, which Portugal seized in the sixteenth century, though it was primarily an inland confederation. Kaabu threatened the security of Upper Guinean coastal people, but they were largely able to remain free of political control from both the confederation and other colonizers until the nineteenth century.

Mandinka (Mandinga, Mandingue, Mandingo, Mandinque, Manding): An ethnic group and a language spoken by peoples of north-central, central, and northeastern Guinea-Bissau and other West African countries. Many became Muslims after the fourteenth century.

Manjaco (Mandjak, Mandjaque, Manjaca, Manjiak, Mandyak, Manjaku, Manjack, Ndyak, Mendyako, Kanyop): An ethnic group and a language spoken by an estimated 170,000 people living west and northwest of the city of Bissau in Guinea-Bissau. Today the language is also spoken in France, the Gambia, and Senegal.

Nalu (Nalou, Baga): An ethnic group and a language. A 2002 estimate counted 8,000 Nalu in southwest Guinea-Bissau near the coast. Larger numbers of Nalu live in contemporary Guinea, the Gambia, and Senegal.

Papel (Pepel, Papei, Moium, Oium): An ethnic group and a language in Guinea-Bissau. Papel have historically played an important part in African trade, negotiating commerce between coastal peoples and the African interior. In 2002, there were an estimated 125,000 people speaking the Papel language in Guinea-Bissau.

Portuguese: An ethnic group and a language spoken by peoples living in Portugal and its former colonies, many in West Africa. Portuguese has historically been an important language in Guinea-Bissau and the Cape Verde Islands, where dialects were distinguished as either Guinean Portuguese or Cape Verdean Portuguese. Today there are approximately 240 million Portuguese speakers in the world, making it the sixth most-spoken language.

Rio Geba: A West African river that runs through Guinea, Senegal, and Guinea-Bissau. It has been an important trade and transportation link from the Atlantic Ocean to the African interior.

Rio Grande (Rio Grande de Buba): A West African river that flows through Guinea-Bissau. The island of Bolama is located at the mouth of the river.

Rio Nuñez: A West African river south of Guinea-Bissau that empties into the Atlantic along the Guinea coast. Like the Rio Geba, the Rio Grande de Buba, the Sénégal, and the Gambia, the Rio Nuñez was a major conduit for trade between the West African coast and interior peoples. At the end of the eighteenth century (when some Bolama colonists sailed to one of the river's trading posts), it was the end point for caravans bringing slaves to the coast and remained so until 1840. Nalu live in the area around the river.

Santiago (São Tiago; Portuguese for "Saint James"): The largest of the Cape Verde Islands. At the time of the *Hankey*'s voyage, as well as of Charles Darwin's later visit, it was called Saint Jago. The Portuguese constructed settlements on the uninhabited island in the fifteenth century; it has always had the largest population of the Cape Verde Islands, with a 2011 World Bank estimate of 210,000.

Sénégal/Senegal: A major West African river (Sénégal) and a West African nation (Senegal) of 75,955 square miles, divided into a hot, dry north and a moist, tropical south. In the seventeenth century, the French first established trading posts at the mouth of the river and then seized Gorée Island from the Dutch. The French established the town of Dakar on the coast across from Gorée in 1857. They pushed inland along the Sénégal River to the Niger River, claimed the newly explored territory as part of French West Africa in 1895, and made Dakar its capital in 1902. Senegal won its independence from France in 1960. According to the 2011 World Bank estimate, the major languages spoken by its approximately 13 million citizens are French (the official language) and Wolof.

Senegambia: The term Europeans used to refer to the area between the Gambia and Sénégal Rivers. Before the fifteenth century, several Mandinka and other African polities were located near these rivers. British presence along the Gambia River dated back to the sixteenth century and in the eighteenth century led to the establishment of a colony called Senegambia around the river. In 1783 the largest part of British Senegambia was turned over to France, but Britain held on to the land closest to the Gambia River, making it a British protectorate in 1820 and a British crown colony in 1886. Britain and France drew boundaries between the Gambia and Senegal (then a French colony) in 1887. Senegambia was also the name of a short-lived (1982–89) confederation between the contemporary nations of Senegal and the Gambia.

Sierra Leone: A West African nation named by a Portuguese explorer in the fifteenth century. Like most of western Africa, its interior was dominated by African states, while the coast was dotted with Portuguese, Dutch, French, and other European slave forts until the end of the eighteenth century. The first settlement in 1787 of former slaves and free blacks from North America and Britain did not prosper, but Freetown, the capital, founded in 1792, endured and became a British crown colony in 1808. Sierra Leone's interior became a British protectorate in 1896, but local peoples won their independence in 1961. Political disagreements within the Republic of Sierra Leone led in 1992 to a brutal civil war between the Revolutionary United Front (RUF), with support from the special forces of Charles Taylor's National Patriotic Front of Liberia (NPFL), and the Sierra Leone army that lasted until 2002. Today Sierra Leone is a constitutional democracy, and English is the official language, although it is spoken only by a small minority. The ethnic groups and African languages in Sierra Leone differ almost completely from those of Guinea-Bissau. The World Bank 2011 population estimate for the nation was approximately 6 million inhabitants.

Upper Guinea: As a geographic unit, Guinea or Guinée was named by Europeans. By the early seventeenth century, "Upper Guinea" had become the English term for the coastal area between the Sénégal River and Cape Palmas, the headland of the extreme southeast end of the coast of contemporary Liberia. "Upper Guinea" is no longer used to refer to this coastal area, but is still currently used to describe a region within the independent nation of Guinea. *See* Guinea.

Vincheai: The indigenous people living on Tenerife and the other Canary Islands at the beginning of European conquest; Europeans called them Guanches. Their ancestors probably floated to the archipelago from southern France, the Iberian Peninsula, and northwestern Africa about three thousand years ago. Approximately 80,000 Vincheai lived in the seven inhabited Canary Islands (out of thirteen) when the Genoese and Portuguese began invading the area both for land and for slaves in the fourteenth century. By the sixteenth century, the Vincheai had virtually been destroyed as a people.

ↄ০ↄ

Index

Page numbers in **boldface** indicate illustrations.